NURSING HOME ADMINISTRATION

Fifth Edition

James E. Allen, MSPH, PhD, CNHA, is Associate Professor of Health Policy and Administration Emeritus at the University of North Carolina at Chapel Hill and President of Long-Term Care Education.com, a national resource Web site for information on the long-term care field. He has 30+ years experience teaching and conducting research in the field of health care administration. He taught courses at the University of North Carolina at Chapel Hill in long-term care administration, medical ethics, and the organization and financing of health care delivery in the United States.

The Web site www.longtermcareedu.com (or easier, www.ltce.com) provides 500 pages of state-by-state, up-to-date information on such subjects as:

- becoming a nursing home administrator
- becoming an assisted-living administrator
- exploring a career in long-term care
- contacting the state licensing authority in each state
- enrolling in college programs in each state
- obtaining key publications in the long-term care field
- getting continuing education units

Additional resources available to persons preparing to become long-term care administrators are:

Nursing Home Federal Requirements: Guidelines to Surveyors and Survey Protocols, 6th ed., Springer Publishing Company, 212–431–4370, 877-687-7476; a user-friendly rendering of the Centers for Medicare and Medicaid Services nursing home inspection requirements.

The Licensing Exam Review Guide in Nursing Home Administration (current edition) Springer Publishing Company, 212–431–4370, 877-687-7476; 800+ practice questions for national examination preparation.

Instructor's Guide—20 case studies plus several hundred questions for college instructors' classroom use. Instructors: go to www.ltce.com to order a copy.

Springer also publishes similar text and exam review guides for assisted-living administrators.

Continuing education units for both nursing home and assisted-living administrators are available through the Web site www.LongTermCareEducation.com.

For further information visit the Web site www.ltce.com. Dr. Allen can be reached via email on the Web site, directly at jeallen@mindspring.com, or 1-919-815-0387; FAX 919-933-6825.

Nursing Home Administration

Fifth Edition

James E. Allen, MSPH, PhD, CNHA

SPRINGER / PUBLISHING COMPANY

NEW YORK

Springer Publishing Company, LLC
11 West 42nd Street
New York, NY 10036
www.springerpub.com

Acquisitions Editor: Sheri W. Sussman
Project Manager: Carol Cain
Cover design: Joanne E. Honigman
Composition: Apex Publishing, LLC

08 09 10 / 5 4 3 2

Library of Congress Cataloging-in-Publication Data

Allen, James E. (James Elmore), 1935–
   Nursing home administration / James E. Allen. — 5th ed.
      p. ; cm.
   Includes bibliographical references and index.
   ISBN-13: 978-0-8261-5394-4 (alk. paper)
   ISBN-10: 0-8261-5394-1 (alk. paper)
   1. Nursing homes—Administration.   I. Title.
      [DNLM: 1. Nursing Homes—organization & administration.   WX150
A427n   2008]
RA999.A35A45   2008
362.1'6068—dc22   2007022457

Printed in the United States of America by Maple-Vail Book Manufacturing Group.

The ideas that shape this work grow out of the concept of nursing home administrator as hero.

To these individuals this book is dedicated.

Contents

Part I. Management, Governance, Leadership

Part III. Finance/Business

Part IV. Environment: The Industry: Its Laws and Regulations

Part V. Patient / Resident Care

Foreword

Knowledge requirements for nursing home administrators continue to be impacted by the increase in government regulations and the changing demands of residents and their families. The new administrator is required to have a working familiarity with these changing regulations as a means of understanding the government's rationale "that no harm come to the public" and that the tax dollars are spent appropriately.

At the same time, the administrator must develop and test his or her philosophy of care within this environment. Toward this end, the entry-level person begins preparation for licensure in their state to become a licensed nursing home administrator. A major component of the licensure is successfully passing the national examination administered by the National Association of Boards of Long Term Care Administrators (NAB). This national exam tests the candidate's ability to integrate this knowledge within their decision-making process as a means of providing quality care. The administrator has to cope with an increasing circle of stakeholders whose demands require the ability to keep demands in balance, while delivering quality care.

This 5th edition of *Nursing Home Administration,* by James E. Allen, continues to be one of the best texts in the field of nursing home administration. It incorporates a scholarly treatment of the five Domains of Practice developed by the National Association of Boards of Examiners for Long Term Care Administrators. This text is a good review of the core of knowledge of gerontology. Insights gained from mentors active in the field of nursing home administrators are incorporated in this text.

The value of this text is five fold:

- It is an excellent text for the candidate in their preparation to take the national NAB examination (this exam is required in all 50 states).
- It has bibliographical references to help the reader explore in-depth any area of nursing home administration.
- It is a current guide to the best practices in nursing home administration.
- It is an up-to-date resource on regulations and *Life Safety Code*® standards.

In addition to being valuable to persons preparing to become licensed nursing home administrators, this 5th edition is a practical reference resource for the practicing administrator.

This 5th edition has the following new insights into the field of nursing home administration.

Part One: Management

- A major emphasis on the current state of federal regulations and these regulations' impacts on the nursing home industry;
- 2006 industry data from the Centers for Medicare and Medicaid Services (CMS);
- A series of trends analyses for the years 1993, 1999, and 2006;
- Updates on quality measures used by the Centers for Medicare and Medicaid Services;
- Inclusion of numerous Web sites important to long-term care providers that facilitate the reader exploring various topics in more depth;
- A section on acronyms currently in use in the long-term care industry; and
- Inclusion of the Scope and Severity grid used by surveyors.

Part Two: Human Resources

- Trend data for 1993, 1999, and 2006 in each of the facility's departmental functions; and
- New diet data.

Part Three: Finance

- New risk management data;
- New section on corporate compliance; and
- New section on the Sarbanes-Oxley Act of 2002.

Part Four: Environment

- More in-depth analysis of the possible impacts of the Baby Boomer generation on the nursing facility;
- Updated section on the major organizations in the long-term care field;
- New Medicare Plan D section;
- Updated information on the various government acts and unionization data; and

- New *Life Safety Code®* section: 2000 *Life Safety Code®* specified by Congress as the code year to be used in governmental surveys of nursing facilities.

Part Five: Resident Care

- Updated drug lists;
- Updated information on prevalence and incidence of diseases among the aging;
- Updated information on levels of disability;
- New sections on distinguishing delirium from dementia and distinguishing psychosis and agitation;
- New sections on Gastroesophageal reflux disease (GERD), glycemic control, and hand washing data; and
- Expanded sections on decubitus ulcers/pressure sores, urinary tract infections, and data on depression.

I have been working in the field of long-term care since 1965 as an administrator, teacher, and as a board member of a state licensing agency, and I am active in and have served as an elected officer of the National Association of Boards of Examiners for Long Term Care Administrators (NAB).

I find the Allen text meets the learning needs of the entry-level administrator. The reader will find the scope of the text to be challenging to their knowledge base, in addition to being an enhancer of personal philosophy of care and operation of the nursing facility. Studying this text will strengthen the administrator's ability to meet the demands of the regulations and residents. Open this text, and begin your journey to richer understandings of the important field of nursing home administration!

Philip S. Brown, ThM, MA, NHA
Retired director of Penick Village,
North Carolina;
past officer of NAB; and
retired Methodist minister

Acknowledgments

For more than two decades, I have interacted with countless long-term care personnel, from nursing assistants to corporate leaders, in an effort to absorb as much as possible about the industry in all its complexity.

For several years I was privileged to participate in the daily life of a local nursing facility where my name tag reads "James Allen, PIT" (Professor in Training). It is impossible for one person to know all that is required to successfully operate a nursing facility. This PIT will remain in training for the rest of his professional career, seeking to understand how to achieve excellence in the administration of the nursing home.

Introduction

Along with the other components of the American health care system, the nursing home has entered an extended period of change. Already second in size only to hospitals, it has rapidly moved beyond being over a $100 billion-a-year industry.

Administrators of a nursing home have one of the most demanding as well as exciting positions in the health care field, with the quality of life of over one million Americans depending on their leadership skills.

This text provides an introduction to the practice of nursing home administration. The book is divided into five segments: management, human resources, finance, the industry's environment, and patient/resident care. Each section offers a working vocabulary and detailed description of activities associated with it. Each term is defined as it is introduced. A set of learning objectives follows.

The sections are self-contained and may be studied in any sequence.

The book contains the knowledge essential toward preparation for licensure or employment as a nursing home administrator.

Successfully administering a nursing home is one of the most complex and challenging tasks that can be undertaken and one of the most rewarding professional commitments available in the health care field. The nursing home administrator, together with the director of nursing, is uniquely responsible for the quality of care and quality of life of residents/patients and staff in their facility.

This text, together with additional publications by the author, covers the current domains of practice on which the national nursing home administrator examination is based.

The Nursing Home Administrator's Challenge

Leadership By Vision

For many centuries, a village was known far and wide for its porcelain. Especially sought after were its urns: tall as a person, graceful in form, they were admired for their delicate beauty. But what was the potter to do when, on occasion, a carefully made piece would break? A master potter solved the problem by pouring gold between the shards and thus restoring the urn.

What seemed a broken vessel, useless for any purpose, became with the gold filigree, a unique work of art.

—from ancient Chinese legend

The nursing home administrator's task is that of the creative master potter of legend, restoring as if with gold filigree the joy of living to what appeared to be the shattered life of a patient/resident.

Leadership By Walking Around

Typically, it depends on who the administrator and director of nursing are. If they're doing their job, and forceful enough, then you have a good, well-managed facility. But if they're weak individuals, or not paying attention, then care doesn't get up to the rate one would expect.

—Carol Scott, a contemporary experienced observer of the nursing home industry

List of Figures

List of Tables

PART I

Management, Governance, Leadership

1.1 Management Functions

The skilled administrator of a nursing facility is a person capable of organizing the resources and finances available to best meet the needs of the residents. In successfully accomplishing this, the administrator makes innumerable decisions.

Management is decision making (Dale, 1969, p. 5; Hitt, Ireland, & Hoskisson, 2001, p. 3; Robbins & Coulter, 2007, pp. 156–161). What the administrator does for the nursing facility is make decisions about what ought to happen in the facility (Johns & Saks, 2001, p. 363; Robbins & Coulter, 2007, pp. 161, 176).

Although there is by now an extensive literature describing the field of management theory, authors have returned again and again to a basic set of activities as the best explanation of what managers do (Hitt et al., 2001, p. 3; Robbins & Coulter, 2007, p. 174).

Luther Gulick, an early 20th-century author, defined the manager's tasks as:

Planning
Organizing
Staffing
Directing
Coordinating
Reporting
Budgeting

Several decades later Earnest Dale, in his textbook *Management Theory and Practice,* differed only slightly in his description. He agreed on the importance of the tasks, but consolidated the last four under three rubrics: controlling, innovating, and representing (Dale, 1969, pp. 5–7).

Very briefly, at the core, this is what an administrator does:

Forecasts—Projects trends and needs that the facility management must meet in the future.
Plans—Decides what needs to be done and makes a set of plans to accomplish it.

Budgets—Projects costs and establishes categories with dollar amounts for each.

Organizes—Once a plan has been made, the administrator decides how to structure a suitable organization to implement the plan and put it into action. This will include the number of people needed for the staff and the materials with which to build or to work.

Staffs—Attempts to find the right person for each defined job.

Directs—Provides direction (preliminary training and ongoing supervision) through communication to each employee who thereby learns what is expected.

Evaluates—Judges the extent to which the organization is accomplishing its goals (usually set by corporate).

Controls Quality—Takes steps to assure that the goals are accomplished and that each job is done as planned (Robbins & Coulter, 2007, p. 543).

Innovates—Leads the staff to develop new ideas that enable the facility to enhance its attractiveness to the community served.

Markets—Assures that the facility successfully attracts and admits to the extent feasible the persons it seeks to serve.

The nursing facility administrator is responsible for assuring that all of these activities are accomplished by the facility. Assuring that forecasting, planning, organizing, staffing, directing, evaluating, controlling, innovating, and marketing are successfully accomplished is providing leadership to the facility (Argenti, 1994, p. 251).

An approach to leadership of particular value in the nursing facility setting is leading by walking around (LBWA). LBWA allows the administrator to assure himself that facility resources and finances are successfully being used to best meet the needs of the residents. This is a part of the quality assurance process set by the facility, corporate, and payers such as Centers for Medicare and Medicaid Services.

Another explanation of the manager's function is that "management is getting things done through other people" (Hitt et al., 2001, pp. 23–33; Robbins & Coulter, 2007, p. 9). A staff member who becomes a manager may or may not continue to give direct care, but does assume new duties that are entirely managerial in character. The new manager is no longer directly responsible for doing specific work, such as patient care, but ensures that such care is accomplished. For example, when a nurse who has been giving direct care to patients becomes the director of nurses, this new job entails supervision of other employees to provide the nursing care needed by the residents. This distinction is especially important when, typically, the director of nurses becomes the licensed administrator.

According to another group of management theorists (Hitt et al., 2001, pp. 37–38), the general manager (such as a nursing home administrator) performs five functions:

- planning for future operations
- designing and administering decision-making structures (organizing)
- developing human resources and capabilities (staffing, directing)
- supervising current operations (controlling)
- representing and holding an organization responsible to its various constituencies (p. xvi) among whom the most important are the residents, corporate, and Centers for Medicare and Medicaid Services.

The administrator's job is to ensure that the appropriate employees do the tasks of the organization at an acceptable quality level (Hitt et al., 2001, pp. 210–213; Robbins & Coulter, 2007, p. 48). Many volumes have been written about managing, because it is one of the more complex tasks in modern society. Three professors at the Harvard Graduate School of Business Administration state that administrators ask three questions:

- Where are we now?
- Where do we want to go?
- How do we get there? (Christensen, Berg, & Salter, 1980, p. 12).

A Detailed Look at What Managers/Administrators Do

We have described in very general terms what administrators do. What is actually involved in forecasting, planning, organizing, staffing, directing, evaluating, controlling, innovating, and marketing? Consider the following basic functions of the manager:

Forecasting (projecting trends into the future): The administrator forecasts the economic, social, and political environment expected for the facility and the resources that will be available to it.

Planning (deciding what is to be done): The administrator decides what is to be accomplished, sets short-and long-term objectives, then decides on the means to be used for achieving them.

Budgeting (deciding acceptable costs): All facilities must operate on plans that have been translated into budgets that are realistic, yet functional.

Organizing (deciding the scheme of the organization and the staffing it will require): The administrator decides on the structure the organization will take, the skills that will be needed, and the staff positions and their particular duties and responsibilities. This includes coordinating the work assignments, i.e., the interrelationships among the departments and their workers (Johns & Saks, 2001, p. 454).

Staffing (the human resources function): The administrator attempts to find the right person for each defined job.

Directing (providing daily supervision and employing good communication, people, and skills): The administrator provides day-to-day supervision of subordinates, makes sure that subordinates know what results are expected, and helps the staff to improve their skills. In short, the administrator explains what is to be done, and the employees do it (in the ideal world) to the best of their abilities. Daily reality in the nursing facility is much more complex, of course.

Evaluating (comparing actual to expected results): The administrator determines how well the jobs have been done and what progress is being made to achieve the organization's goals as stated in its policies and plans of action.

Controlling Quality (taking necessary corrective actions): The administrator revises policies, procedures, and plans of action and takes necessary personnel actions to better achieve the facility goals. Over time, the administrator writes many "plans of correction" for corporate and the many agencies that survey the facility.

Innovating (the effective administrator is always an innovator): The administrator develops new ideas, combines old ideas to form new ones, searches for useful ideas from other fields and adapts them, and acts as a catalyst to stimulate others to be as creative.

Marketing (identifying and attracting the persons to be served): The administrator assures that the facility identifies the group(s) of persons to be served and successfully attracts (to the extent market place realities will allow) and serves the residents it seeks.

These are the basic functions of administrators/managers. The reader may wish to use other words and concepts to describe these functions, or even improve on the model. Certainly administrators do much more than has been described above (Hitt et al., 2001, pp. 492–495).

However, if forecasting, planning, organizing, staffing, directing, evaluating, controlling, innovating, and marketing are not successfully accomplished, the minimum leadership responsibilities of a nursing home administrator have not been fulfilled.

The skilled long-term care administrator is capable of providing leadership that accomplishes each of these tasks in a manner that meets facility financial, resident care, corporate, and surveyors' needs and requirements.

In his book *A Passion for Excellence,* Tom Peters, advocates a simple four-part scheme of management's role: care of customers, constant innovation, turned-on people, and leadership. He observes that in both the for-profit and not-for-profit sectors, superior performance, over the long haul, depends on two things: (1) taking exceptional care of residents in the facility via superior service and superior quality of care; and (2) and constant innovation.

He observes that financial control is vital, but that one does not sell financial control but rather a quality service or product (excellently cared for residents). A facility seldom sustains superior performance merely by having all the beds full; the superior facility sustains itself through innovation in ways to serve residents and promote market development. Efficient management of the budget is vital in an organization such as a university (a nursing facility), he observes, yet a great university (nursing facility) is never characterized by the remark, "It has a good budget" (Peters, 1985, p. 4). Just as the superb university is superb only by virtue of its success in serving its ultimate customer—the student—the superb nursing home is superb only by virtue of its success in serving *its* ultimate customers—the residents and their families/significant others.

Peters (1985) advocates a management model based on what he calls "a blinding flash of the obvious" (p. 3). Giving every employee the space to innovate, at least a little. Answering the phones and resident call buttons with common courtesy and timeliness. Doing things that work (giving quality care). Listening to residents and families and asking them for their ideas, then acting on them. Soliciting staff input, then, as appropriate, implementing it. Wandering around: with residents, staff, suppliers, visitors, inspectors. Common sense, obvious? Yes. But the obvious must not be so obvious or more would practice it. All of these are "people skills" based on an ability to facilitate communication among staff and residents. All too often, common sense is very scarce.

To achieve Peters' "blinding flash of the obvious" in the nursing facility environment, the administrator normally must cultivate good people skills (communicate successfully with both residents and staff) to achieve excellence in service to the facility residents and their significant others.

1.1.1 LEVELS OF MANAGEMENT

Two additional concepts are worth noting at this point: upper–middle–lower levels of management and line–staff relationships. The administrator of a large nursing home might assign some of these responsibilities to others. The administrator need not personally perform each of the management tasks, but rather must assure that these tasks are successfully carried out. To accomplish this, management is often divided into three layers: upper, middle, and lower (Hitt et al., 2001, pp. 492–495; Robbins & Coulter, 2007, p. 8).

Upper-Level Management

The upper-level manager is responsible for the overall functioning of the facility, normally interacting directly with the board of directors or owners and multiple inspectors. This person is responsible for formulating policies that will be applied to the entire facility. The nursing home administrator is an excellent example of upper-level management (Hitt et al., 2001, pp. 492–495).

Middle-Level Management

Middle-level managers report to upper-level managers and at the same time interact significantly with lower-level managers. A good example in the nursing home is the director of nursing who reports to the facility administrator and in turn has managers—for example, nurse supervisors and charge nurses—reporting to them (Hitt et al., 2001, pp. 493–495).

As the name implies, this staff member interfaces with upper-level and lower-level managers. The middle-level manager normally does not make policies affecting the entire facility, as does the facility administrator. However, the middle-level manager does make decisions on policies for managers responsible to them. The middle-level manager must have good communication skills to deal successfully with both the administrator of the facility and the lower-level workers.

Some nursing home chains allow local facility administrators wide latitude in decision making, in which case the local administrator functions primarily as an upper-level manager. In other chains, decision making is more centralized in the corporate offices, in which case some dimensions of the local administrator's role more nearly resemble that of the middle-level manager.

Lower-Level Management

As a rule, lower-level managers have direct supervisory responsibilities for the staff who do the actual work, for example, the nurse's aide who physically takes care of the resident in the room. The nurse supervisor or charge nurse is a good example of lower-level management in a nursing home facility. At this level managers deal directly with those at the middle level, but not with administrators at the upper level. That is, they are expected to conduct their business through the channel of their middle-level managers.

If the charge nurse wants a change in a policy, they will discuss the matter with the nursing supervisor, who in turn will bring it to the attention of upper-level managers, should this be desirable. The middle-level manager might also make a policy decision without consulting upper-level management, for example, to change the bathing schedule to accommodate an additional workload due to increased occupancy.

Management decisions in nursing home facilities are, of course, noticeably more complicated than the simple establishment of lower, middle, and upper levels of management. The presence of several professions, for example, physicians, nurses, physical therapists, dietitians, and others, causes decision making in nursing home facilities to be a complex and often delicate task.

1.1.2 LINE–STAFF RELATIONSHIPS

Line–staff relationships constitute a second important concept in understanding management functions (Hitt et al., 2001, pp. 492–495; Robbins & Coulter, 2007, p. 278). A person who is empowered by the administrator to make decisions for the organization is said to have line authority. A person is said to have a staff role if they are advisory to the manager and do not have authority to make decisions for the organization.

A Line Position

The administrator must assign to other employees some of the decision-making authority to accomplish the work of the organization. Such employees are line managers. They are empowered to make decisions on behalf of the administrator. The director of nurses is a line position. Therefore, decisions by the director of nursing have the same force as if the administrator made them. The administrator still remains responsible for all decisions made on their behalf by persons to whom decision-making authority has been delegated.

A Staff Position

A staff position, on the other hand, is an advisory role. None of the administrator's authority to make decisions on behalf of the facility is delegated to persons in a staff position. An accountant in the business office is an example of a staff position. Persons who are paid consultants, such as a local pharmacist or a registered dietitian, hold staff positions. These persons are expected to advise the administrator or appropriate others in the facility on what to do, but they have been given no authority by the administrator to make decisions on behalf of the facility.

Smaller nursing home facilities typically do not employ as their food services director a person eligible for registration by the American Dietetic Association. Consequently, to meet federal regulations, they hire such a person as a consultant on a periodic basis. Although the consulting dietitian may be the better trained person, if the nursing home administrator allows this consultant to give direct orders to the food service director, lines of authority in the facility may become confused, and staff morale will suffer. Matters, however, are slightly more complicated. Only a person eligible for registration by the American Dietetic Association may designate diets as prescribed by physicians, and in this case the consultant is making decisions for the facility that an unqualified food service director is not permitted to make.

Or, again, in a very large facility the administrator might hire a specially trained geriatric nurse practitioner to advise the administrator or the director of nursing on nursing functions in the facility. This nurse would normally have no authority to ask or order anyone to do anything in the facility.

It is the director of nursing to whom power and authority to make nursing decisions has been delegated and who therefore makes decisions on behalf of the administrator in the nursing area. The director of nurses can hire and fire, assign work, and give whatever orders are needed to make the facility nursing activities function, because line authority to do so has been delegated to that employee.

If, for example, the administrator permitted the geriatric nurse practitioner, to whom a staff role had been assigned, to tell the director of nurses what to do or to give orders to nurses on the halls, the authority of the director of nurses would be undermined. The director of nurses and nursing staff would be understandably confused about the role of the director of nurses: Does the director of nurses represent the authority of the administrator or is the staff advisory nurse practitioner actually the manager of the director of nurses?

Again, life in the nursing facility is seldom this seemingly uncomplicated. A large number of nursing facilities in the United States are operated by chains with corporate staff who often visit or are assigned to assist a facility for a short period of time. Technically, these corporate representatives may be there only to advise, but facility staff are hardly free to ignore such "advice." Some chains expect their corporate staff to function more nearly as consultants to local facilities they visit; other chains want them to function as if they exercised line authority in their area of expertise while in one of that chain's facilities. Or, again, when the facility is functioning smoothly the corporate representative might be comfortable with a "take it or leave it" approach to advice given, but in times of crisis that same representative might come in and exercise direct line authority in the day-to-day operation of that facility.

We turn now to a more detailed discussion of some of the activities and skills involved in the management functions. We will begin to further explore some of the complexities of these functions.

1.2 Forecasting

Managerial success belongs to those who successfully prepare for the future. In the nursing home industry, the future belongs to administrators who can anticipate and successfully prepare for rapid change.

Trend Analysis

After nearly two decades of more gradual evolvement, the pace of change in the long-term care field increased visibly with reforms to Medicare and Medicaid contained in the 1987 Omnibus Budget Reconciliation Act and subsequent amendments. The long-term care industry has entered a period in which rapid and far reaching changes can be expected.

Forecasting involves trend identification and analysis. Clues to the future are present in trends, which the alert administrator can observe. The skill needed in forecasting is the ability to accurately predict the future implications for the nursing facility of new trends to which the current environment may offer clues. For example, several states have moved to reimbursement for public paying patients based on acuity level of their illness(es). The federal government is actively employing this reimbursement method after the Balanced Budget Act of 1997. Alert administrators in states using other reimbursement approaches can estimate the likelihood that this method may be adopted in their state and make contingency plans to adapt if this occurs.

One apparent certainty is that conventional perceptions of the nursing facility's roles will be challenged in the American health care system. In the past, developments occurred more incrementally, at a slower pace. During the 1970s and 1980s, administrators had the luxury of making long-range projections during a period of relative stability in the health care industry under less limited Medicare and Medicaid reimbursements from the federal and state governments. In today's world, the rate of transformation in the health care field is exponential, shifting so rapidly that it is ever more difficult to predict the shape of the nursing home industry, even from year to year, as Congress, states, and the Centers for Medicare and Medicaid Services modify, sometimes radically, the reimbursement rules.

The Changing Core

Consider the following. Every 10 years, one-fourth of all current knowledge and accepted practices in the health care and other industries will be obsolete. The life span of new technologies is down to 18 months and decreasing (Kriegel, 1991, p. xvi). Estimates are that people under 25 can expect to change careers every decade and jobs every 4 years, either by choice or because the industry in which they work will disappear and be replaced by others yet unimagined. The "core" business of the nursing home of the 21st century may be entirely different from that in the second decade of the 21st century (Kriegel, 1991, p. xvi; Robbins & Coulter, 2007, p. 212).

As Kriegel has observed, nursing home administration is in a new and unpredictable world, an arena in which we have not played before. The rules will be different. The game itself is changing—the nursing home we went to work for 5 years earlier may have changed entirely. Everything is moving faster in the health field. New technologies are replacing current technologies ever faster. What the nursing home administrator needs to know to act effectively is changing. The Centers for Medicare and Medicaid are rapidly moving to a totally electronic system both for monitoring resident care and reimbursing the facility for care given. The shape of the final system is unknown. Relying on the "tried and true," observes Kriegel, is dangerous because what was tried yesterday is no longer true today (1991, p. xvi). Nursing homes that continue to rely on conventional formulas for success will both miss opportunities for new markets and find themselves in the backwash of the health care industry as it metamorphoses into constantly new permutations.

The truth is that for the first time in human history, the capacity exists to provide more expensive and effective health care than any nation, including the United States, may be able to afford. The roles possible for hospitals, nursing homes, the myriad forms of multiunit senior housing, assisted-living facilities, home health agencies, managed care organizations, and other providers are endless and will remain up for the taking for the next few decades as society struggles to absorb health care costs and technologies.

Change Itself

Change at a laser-fast pace will continue. As one chief executive officer observed, mankind's cumulative knowledge doubled in the decade 1985–1995—and may double as rapidly as every 5 years (Kriegel, 1991, p. 1). In the health sciences field this may occur even more rapidly. The U.S. Congress's Office of Technology has warned that the rate of development is too fast for proper monitoring of the effects and will threaten the foundations of even the most secure American businesses. The staff in nursing facilities are experiencing culture shock: In the 1980s their nurses were considered to be working at a lower technological level than hospital nurses. Today nursing home nurses are busy learning high-tech skills just to be able to treat the subacute care residents being admitted to nursing facilities. Almost as soon as rules are established, they become obsolete. By the time we notice that a nursing home could be started with as little as $12,000 cash from the owner (when combined with now no-longer-available federal government incentive loans), a new facility costs $6 million or more dollars.

Survival in the nursing home industry will depend on the ability to forecast the future and to learn entirely new ways of thinking, behaving, motivating, and communicating in the nursing facility. Survival will depend on ability and willingness to change . . . something both owners and staff do with great reluctance.

1.3 Planning

1.3.1 WHY PLAN?

An Integrated Decision System

The purpose of planning is to provide an integrated decision system that, based on the changes forecast by the administrator, establishes the framework for all facility activities. Plans, in essence, are statements of the organizational goals of the facility.

A Means of Coping With Uncertainty

Plans are a means of coping with the uncertainty of the future (Hitt et al., 2001, pp. 377–378; Robbins & Coulter, 2007, p. 169). All organizations must deal with the outside world in order to survive. Inevitably, events beyond the control of the nursing home will shape the range of options available to the facility and set the context within which it will be obliged to function.

A plan is a prediction of what the facility's decision makers believe they must do to cope with the future. A carefully developed plan makes it possible to compare what actually happens to what was expected to happen. The plan may then be altered to achieve the set goals when external conditions change.

Strategic Planning

To survive and prosper, the nursing facility must engage in strategic planning (Noe Hollenbeck, Gerhart, & Wright, 2000, p. 42; Robbins & Coulter, 2007, p. 189). Strategy comes from the Greek word *strategos,* referring to a general (the administrator's) grand design behind a campaign or battle. Strategic management is conceiving and implementing the pattern or plan that integrates the facilities' major goals, policies, and action sequences into a cohesive whole (Noe et al., 2000, p. 42). It is the process of analyzing the facility's competitive position, developing the strategic goals, devising a plan of action and allocating the resources that will best achieve those goals (Noe et al., 2000, p. 43).

Break-It Thinking

It is important to have a plan. Sometimes it is even more important to abandon it! As Kriegel (1991) has observed, today change is coming at such a fast pace that today's innovations are tomorrow's outworn models. He observes that, if it ain't broke today, it will be tomorrow! He cites an architect who finds the pace of change so fast that he feels like a gunfighter dodging bullets, and an electronics manager who does little besides come up for air and catch his breath in the momentary lull before the next storm (p. 3). The nursing facility administrator in this new millennium is faced with so many new regulations from the federal and state governments and the financial pressures merely to survive, that it seems difficult to do more than just dodge these bullets.

1.3.2 STEPS IN PLANNING

Phase One: Decide What Ought To Be Done

Few people have the opportunity to plan for an organization from the very outset. Typically, in the nursing home field, an individual is hired as administrator of an ongoing facility. For the purposes of illustration, however, let us follow the planning process that might occur in the creation of a new nursing home.

Suppose that one is asked by the regional vice-president of a mid-sized publicly traded for-profit chain of nursing homes to evaluate a medium-sized community (about 50,000 residents) for the purpose of recommending or advising against the building of a nursing facility there. Assume that sufficient funds are available if the decision is favorable. The assumption is further made that, if a home is built, the person doing this assessment would serve as its initial administrator.

This individual must appraise the present competitive, economic, and political environment in that community. We will not attempt to provide a complete checklist for arriving at an assessment of a community, but among the major planning considerations might be the following factors.

Governmental Permissions

Numerous governmental bodies must grant permission to build a facility. Zoning requirements, building codes, and local fire codes must be met. If Certificate of Need, or similar governmental permission to build a new nursing facility legislation exists, the likelihood of obtaining this is an early consideration. Will approval of all required federal, state, and local government permits be forthcoming (Hitt et al., 2001, p. 72)? What is the political climate in the town? Is the proposed nursing facility likely to be welcomed, or if not, would permits probably be delayed, disapproved, or interpreted so strictly that costs rise unacceptably?

Competition

What is the level of unmet need for nursing facility beds in the community and its environs? How many competitors are there? What are their present and projected bed capacities? Is there enough unmet bed need to expect that a new nursing home would fill up sufficiently quickly and maintain the desired level of occupancy over an extended period of at least 5, preferably 10, years? What expansion plans do present facilities have? Are other competing nursing homes apt to be built over the next 3 to 5 years? In many communities assisted-living facilities are being built beyond capacity to absorb. Are licensed and unlicensed multiunit senior living facilities whose residents will want to "age in place" (thus avoiding admission to a nursing facility) being built? What is known about local hospitals? Are they likely to enlarge, shrink, or stay the same? Are hospitals themselves in the process of opening long-term care beds or expecting to do so? What is known about local home health care agencies? Is it probable that they will aggressively siphon off patients who might currently be candidates for nursing home placement? Is there an active hospice agency? Will they be competition or is a cooperative effort possible, placing selected hospice patients in the proposed nursing facility?

Economic Considerations

Are the expected residents apt to have the present and future income to keep the occupancy level high and with the desired mix of residents? Based on the company's projected daily charges for care, would the facility, if built, be competitive with charges by its competitors? Will the community and its surrounding area maintain or improve its economic condition over the next several years? What are the public and third-party reimbursement trends in this community and state? Can your company build a facility and charge competitive prices based on present and anticipated trends in reimbursement for nursing home care?

What are the trends among third-party payers in this community? Are health maintenance organizations, preferred provider organizations, and similar third-party reimbursement groups such as health insurance companies hiring case managers to place persons in nursing facilities and controlling their length of stay and type of care? Are these case managers placing patients at favorable negotiated rates based on acuity levels of care needs in this community? Is it possible to negotiate bed-hold contracts with other providers such as hospitals or health maintenance organizations that would guarantee payment for a specified number of the facility's beds whether occupied or not? To what extent are veterans' administration patient contracts available in this community?

Market Considerations

The evaluator must visualize the desired roles of the proposed nursing facility in this environment. The considerations mentioned amount to conducting a *needs assessment* for the proposed nursing home. The perceived unmet needs will influence the role planned for the proposed facility. Unmet need, however, is not the sole criterion. The company may seek to create new markets for nursing facility care not currently existing in that community. Increasingly, the nursing facility census is made up of a profile of several types of residents. The long-termed resident is increasingly only one of several types of residents for which a facility might be planned. Nursing facility care is now more frequently characterized by niche marketing in which facilities offer Medicare funded rehabilitative care and other identifiable increasingly specialized types of care for subacute conditions, ventilator care, Alzheimer's disease, wound care, and numerous others.

Phase Two: Set Short- and Long-Range Objectives

Let us assume that a decision to build a new 100-bed facility has been made. A next step is to develop broad goals, objectives, and plans that will direct the efforts. A broad goal might be to build, keeping with the architecture of the community in a location convenient to the local hospital.

From a set of broad goal statements such as these, more specific objectives and plans can be developed. A short-range objective (Hitt et al., 2001, pp. 366–367; Robbins & Coulter, 2007, p. 527) might be set to have a 100-bed facility in operation within 18 months, and, as a long-range objective, a new wing of 60 additional beds within 10 years.

Phase Three: Decide on the Means to Achieve the Objective

The next logical step is to translate broad planning goals into functional efforts on a more detailed basis. It is at this stage that allowable cost levels are determined, detailed plans for the building drawn, and the building site purchased.

The planning process has moved from the general to the specific: from broad goals to architectural plans that are detailed enough to direct every person connected with the project. In this way, broad goals are translated into specific and detailed behaviors for everyone who takes part in realizing these goals.

Planning for Next Year

We have used planning for a new facility as the example, because this demonstrates the entire planning process. Most planning is of shorter range (done for the next year). As a practical matter, this planning is usually accomplished when the budget for the next fiscal year (next 12 months) must be developed.

Once plans have been crystallized, the next step is to put them into effect, to make them operational. This is the process of giving plans an organizational form. The form depends on the administrators' perceptions of that structure in particular and behavior of organizations in general.

Plan to Change Your Plans

No matter how carefully we plan, at any moment circumstances can change. The three main sources of residents today may be entirely different tomorrow. Perhaps this is why administering a nursing facility will remain a challenging job: Nothing remains stagnant in the health care field.

Consider Kriegel's (1991) experiences in teaching people how to prepare mentally for difficult rock climbing. Looking up the mountain from the bottom one mentally constructs a plan to reach the top. Once the climb begins, however, the view becomes different. Other, more promising routes to the top begin to appear. So one would change the route. Mountain climbers come to expect that no matter how well they plan from the bottom of the mountain, they can count on running into the unexpected on the ascent. To those who enjoy finding new ways and improving current modes of doing things in the nursing facility, this is an exciting prospect, an opportunity for creativity. Nursing home administrators who learn to deal with the unexpected, even to thrive on it, will endure in the profession. As the management guru Peter Drucker has observed, "No other area offers richer opportunities for successful innovation than (the) unexpected" (Kriegel, 1991, p. 211).

Successful nursing home administrators can assume that once they begin to implement any plan they will meet new people, receive new information, learn of new developments and see possibilities about which they could not have known at the outset. The unexpected cannot be controlled. In the nursing home industry of today, uncertainty and surprise, from both the public and private sectors, are normal. What can be controlled is one's attitude toward the unanticipated. If one accepts that change is integral to living, one can look forward to it and be ready to take advantage of the new opportunities it offers. Accepting the inevitability of change is an attitude that will serve the administrator well.

1.4 Organizing

Organizing is a method of ensuring that the work necessary to achieve a goal is broken down into segments, each of which can be handled by one person (Hitt et al., 2001, pp. 33–34; Robbins & Coulter, 2007, pp. 17, 371). There must be no duplication of work. Efforts are then directed toward accomplishing the goal by dividing the work up so that each job can be done by one person and providing a means for coordinating the jobs done by different people—the task of the managers.

Descriptions are written for each job. A job list for each position usually includes the following:

- the objectives (result to be accomplished)
- the duties and authorities of the position
- its relationship to other positions in the organization

As a rule, an organizational manual containing all job descriptions and several charts is prepared.

It is argued in William Gulick's text that job analysis consists of answering the following questions:

- What does the worker do? (worker functions)
- How does the worker do it? (methods and techniques)
- What aids are necessary? (machines, tools, equipment)
- What is accomplished? (products, services produced)
- What knowledge, skills, and abilities are involved? (qualifications)

Organizing is the first step in implementation of a plan. It is the process of translating plans into combinations of money, materials, and people.

All administrators organize their facilities according to some theory of organization. Their understanding of organization is reflected in their day-to-day and year-to-year direction. For some administrators this is a very thoughtful process; for others it is quite superficial. Nevertheless, all of them apply their concept of organization through their behavior in daily decision making.

Systems

Organizations are systems of interactions among the three available inputs: people, materials, and money (Hitt et al., 2001, pp. 259, 292; Johns & Saks, 2001, p. 495; Robbins & Coulter, 2007, p. 38).

A great deal has been written in recent decades about systems theory. This literature appeared after World War II and has paralleled the development of computer applications to management tasks. The systems concept is primarily a way of thinking about the task of managing any organization. It offers the manager a framework for visualizing the internal and external environment of the organization.

A *system* has been defined as an organized or complex whole, an assembling or combining of things or parts forming a complex or single whole (Johns & Saks, 2001, p. 487; Robbins & Coulter, 2007, p. 39). Stated more simply, the idea of systems helps us to figure out how things are put together. How, for example, do all of the departments in the nursing home relate to each other, to the community, and to the rest of the world that affects them (Johns & Saks, 2001, p. 454; Robbins & Coulter, 2007, p. 38)?

Systems theory is a tool for making sense out of our world by helping to make clearer the interrelationships within and outside of the organization. The administrator uses systems theory to determine what is going on inside the facility and between the facility and the larger outside community.

1.4.1 DESCRIPTION OF THE ORGANIZATION AS A SYSTEM

Systems descriptions vary from completely nonmathematical to highly sophisticated mathematical models demanding specially trained personnel and computers (Hitt et al., 2001, p. 175; Robbins & Coulter, 2007, p. 38). The model we present does not require quantification, although numerical weights could be given each of its elements (Hitt et al., 2001, p. 175; Johns & Saks, 2001, pp. 509–515).

Overview

In Figure 1.1, we illustrate a systems model that may be useful to the nursing home administrator in daily management of the facility. This model consists of the following elements: inputs, processor, outputs, control, plans of action, feedback, and environment.

Organizations such as nursing homes use inputs to get work done, which results in outputs, which can be the desired outputs or undesired/unintended

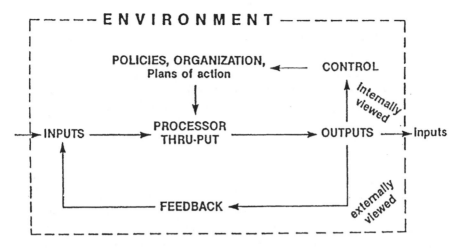

FIGURE 1.1 Simplified systems model.

outputs. The quality and acceptability of outputs are evaluated by the residents, their significant others, and the public, which then reacts, and the facility receives feedback. The outputs are also evaluated by the administrators and compared to what was sought. If the results, or outputs, do not conform to organizational policy and action plans, the administrator takes control (plans of correction) actions to bring the outputs into line with those planned. All of these activities occur within the constraints placed on the organization by the external environment.

Inputs

The inputs to any organization can be described as three elements: money, people, and materials. Inputs are elements the facility administrators can change and use to advantage.

How Can Inputs Be Increased?

A primary concern of the system's administrator is how inputs can be renewed and increased. To accomplish this, organizations take in resources (Hitt et al., 2001, pp. 21–23; Robbins & Coulter, 2007, pp. 244–252). Just as the human body must have oxygen from the air and food from the environment, the nursing facility must constantly draw renewed supplies of energy from other institutions, people, and the material environment.

As residents are rehabilitated and return home, or die, more residents must be admitted into the facility if it is to continue to function. As food is consumed in the dining rooms, more food supplies must be brought in, so that the work of the facility (caring for residents) may continue. As employees leave for other jobs, new staff must be recruited. As the month's cash income is spent paying the facility bills, more revenue from residents must be brought in.

Processor

The *processor* is the work the organization accomplishes. Organizations transform the energy (inputs) available to them, just as the human body converts starch and sugar into heat and action. The nursing facility cares for residents. Work is accomplished. Inputs are reorganized (e.g., food supplies are blended into recipes for the next meal). This is sometimes called the throughput. It is the actual work that the organization performs (Hitt et al., 2001, pp. 21–23; Robbins & Coulter, 2007, p. 244).

The nursing facility takes its inputs (staff, money, and materials) and reorganizes them into active caring for residents. In essence, what nursing facilities do is take money resources from residents and other sources and use those funds to hire staff and provide materials needed (buildings, beds, food, syringes, tissues) to give resident care.

Output

The results of the work (caring for residents) that nursing facilities do is the *output,* the product of the work accomplished by the organization. The organization exports some product (service) to the environment. The output can be good care or "bad" care. The surveyors' come primarily to identify bad care and plans of correction as to how the good care the facility failed to provide can become the good care the facility was seeking to, but failed to give.

Nursing homes produce services to residents. This service may take many forms, as we have noted elsewhere, such as day care as the output for an adult day program, mobility as the output of a physical therapy program, self-feeding as the output of a restorative feeding program, meals served to senior citizens in the community, and so forth. Nursing facilities can and do provide an increasing variety of outputs.

Control of Quality

Control will be discussed at greater length in a later section. For the purposes of exploring the systems diagram in Figure 1.1, it will be described only briefly here. Control is a most important tool available to administrators in the process of keeping the organization on course. *Control* is the corrective action taken after evaluation of outputs by the organizational decision makers. The intended output may not be achieved.

In the nursing home the administrator exercises control of quality by comparing the care given residents actual output with the care called for in the organizational policies and plans of action. This, in our view, is at the very heart of what administrators do. Just as important, every nursing home administrator has the responsibility of comparing the ultimate financial results with the expected financial results.

Put simply, control of quality is the process of asking if the work accomplished (actual output) by the facility is up to expected standards and, if not, taking corrective actions to remedy the problem (Hitt et al., 2001, pp. 210–213; Robbins & Coulter, 2007, p. 48). Here we are discussing the actual standards the organization has established for itself through its policies and plans of action.

There are several "standards of care" that exist for nursing homes. Among them are the federal requirements for care and the standards imposed by each state for a license to operate.

Policies and Plans of Action

For the purpose of illustrating the system configuration we use, let us simply refer to *policies* and plans of action as the guidelines the administrator uses to compare the output (e.g., actual patient care or financial results achieved) with the expected (i.e., the policies and plans of action developed and put into operation by the facility). As the arrows in Figure 1.1 indicate, the administrator uses the organization's *policies* (broad statements of goals and procedures) and *plans of action,* which are the more specific procedures designed to govern the implementation of the policies (Robbins & Coulter, 2007, p. 165).

There are numerous organizations geared to set policies and impose plans of action for nursing homes in the United States. This has been a response, in part, to the financing of nursing home care by the Centers for Medicare and Medicaid Services.

Congress imposed detailed operating regulations, called requirements, on facilities prepared to accept Medicare patients. Individual states, at the request of Congress, have also issued very specific sets of policies and detailed requirements for facilities that wish to serve Medicaid patients. A number of states surveyors leave little room for the exercise of discretion, while others have dealt with a more permissive hand.

Nevertheless, there are many areas in which nursing facilities must develop and implement their own policies and plans for action. One such area is food services. Every facility develops policies by which it hopes to control the quality of food served its residents.

To summarize: Administrators compare the results obtained with the results expected and then take steps to reorganize the inputs and reorganize the processor (the work itself) to better achieve the desired standards.

Feedback

Feedback is a form of control, but feedback is used here to refer to the external responses to the output ("good" or "bad" resident care provided, etc.) by the nursing facility.

Nursing facility outputs have many dimensions, such as roles played in long-term care in the community and in providing short-term, and increasingly, subacute and rehabilitative care to patients who have been hospitalized before they return home.

Resident Council Feedback

Feedback from residents and their families represents a key source of evaluative help to the administrator and staff. Federal survey data indicate that at least 92% of U.S. nursing facilities have resident councils, and 45% have family groups as an additional form of feedback (Harrington, Carrillo, Thollaug, Summers, & Wellin, 2000, p. 30).

Regulatory Feedback

Inevitably and systematically members of the community and other individuals, such as state inspectors, complaint investigators, and ombudspersons, evaluate the results of nursing home efforts to provide quality care to residents. In the 1960s Congressional feedback to the nursing home industry resulted in considerable reshaping of the inputs in the industry when these lawmakers established the requirements then called the Conditions of Participation.

The 1987 Omnibus Budget Reconciliation Act, which contained Medicare and Medicaid reforms, imposed even more stringent requirements. Laws passed by Congress and subsequent regulations prescribe how nursing homes must configure inputs (e.g., sufficient staff hours per patient day, square feet or floor space per patient, and similar issues). As a consequence, the potential freedom to determine operating policies is reduced. It is frequently asserted that the nursing home industry is the second most heavily regulated industry, nuclear power plants being the first.

External Feedback

Typically, external feedback to an industry is not manifested in such powerful and influential terms as stringent federal and state regulations. Hospitals, for example, are lightly regulated by comparison to nursing facilities. The feedback is normally expressed through reactions in the community about quality of work (outputs) being produced. This appears as

- word of mouth evaluations
- newspaper articles and radio and TV commentary
- the reputation enjoyed by the facility's staff, which leads potential employees to consider it as a desirable or undesirable place to work
- the number of potential residents applying for admission to the facility
- willingness of hospital discharge workers to refer patients to a facility

The reader can add to the list. All of these elements constitute what is referred to in Figure 1.1 as the environment.

Environment

The *environment* consists of all relevant external forces that affect the nursing home facility.

Defining the Environment

Defining the relevant environment of one's organization is perhaps the most complex and least obvious aspect of viewing organizations as systems. The environment consists of opportunities and constraints. One way to conceptualize this is to ask two questions:

1. Does it relate meaningfully to my objectives? If so, it is an opportunity.
2. Can I do anything about it? If not, it is a constraint.

If the answer to the first question is yes and the second question is no, it is a constraint in the relevant environment. If the answer to both questions is yes, it is an opportunity for the facility.

From the systems perspective the entire world is interconnected in one large network. The challenge is to identify the aspects of the external world that now affect or may eventually affect the facility in its attempt to achieve objectives, such as serving patients and making a profit. This is the first step in the management process: forecasting.

The environment, then, is both a set of constraints within which the facility must operate and a set of opportunities that the facility administration may seize (Hitt et al., 2001, pp. 187–190; Robbins & Coulter, 2007, p. 73).

Some easily recognizable constraints in a nursing facility's environment might be

- federal, state, and local regulations
- the number of other facilities operating in the area
- the availability of qualified applicants for positions to be filled in the home
- the availability of foods at affordable prices
- state and federal Medicare and Medicaid practices and reimbursement policies
- availability and costs of money
- inflation or deflation rates

Some recognizable opportunities might be

- increasing availability of managed care contracts for individual patients at negotiated rates
- the opportunity to offer "higher-tech" services
- the opportunity to identify and serve niches in care needs
- the unprecedented increasing number of frail elderly who will need nursing care
- pressures for increased number of beds due to the aging of the "baby-boom" population explosion that followed World War II (1945–1963)

1.4.2 IDENTIFYING SYSTEMS

The outputs of one system normally become the inputs for the next system (Hitt et al., 2001, pp. 23–26; Robbins & Coulter, 2007, p. 38), for example, the set of relationships that normally exists among hospitals, nursing homes, home health agencies, and hospice providers.

Hospital patients who no longer need acute care and who need facility-based nursing care (the outputs of the hospital) can become the inputs of the nursing facility—new patient admissions. The rehabilitated nursing home resident who no longer needs facility-based nursing care, but requires follow-up home care (the nursing home output) becomes the input of the home health agency, or perhaps the hospice agency.

We have been using the nursing home as an entity to illustrate the systems concept. We could have selected another level of function within the facility, for instance, the department of nursing.

Who Defines the System?

The selection of what is to be viewed as the system is left entirely to the discretion of the person who describes or analyzes it. This may be one of the more subtle concepts in systems theory. The fact is that the user decides what to designate as a system for their own purposes. The Center for Medicare and Medicaid, because they pay 80 to 90% of all nursing home bills in the United States, define "the system" as the Minimum Data Set (MDS) and the Resident Assessment Protocols (RAPs). The chief executive officer of a large nursing home chain is accustomed to thinking of the several hundred homes as the system. The individual nursing home administrator may conceive of the departments operating in the facility as the system. The maintenance department manager may consider their department as the system.

One of the virtues of the systems concept is that it is almost infinitely adaptable to the needs of the individual user. Anybody can define any set of interrelationships as the system for purposes of description or analysis. All of us use systems analysis in our everyday thinking about the interrelationships of things around us. The systems theory and model described here is an analytic tool that the administrator can use to solve organizational problems as they arise.

In 2006, the Centers for Medicare and Medicaid Services (CMS) found the following 10 systems in 15,021 nursing facilities to be functioning the worst.

- F371 store/prepare/distribute food sanitarily (5,124 facilities; 34% were deficient in practice)
- F281 services provided meet professional standards (4,005 facilities; 27% were deficient in practice)
- F426 acceptable pharmaceutical services (1,587 facilities; 11% were deficient in practice)
- F498 proficiency of nurse aides (728 facilities; 5% were deficient in practice)
- F309 achieve highest feasible resident functioning (4,155 facilities; 28% were deficient in practice)

- F324 preventing resident accidents (3,144 facilities; 21% were deficient in practice)
- F253 acceptable housekeeping and maintenance services (3,078 facilities; 20% were deficient in practice)
- F141 resident dignity (2,417 facilities; 16% were deficient in practice)
- F323 facility is free of accident hazards (3,025 facilities; 21% were deficient in practice)
- F312 providing additional care for dependent residents (1,728 facilities; 12% were deficient in practice) (Department of Health and Human Services [DHHS], 2006b)

1.4.3 ADDITIONAL CHARACTERISTICS OF SYSTEMS

Social science researchers have identified several characteristics of systems that the reader may find useful as analytical tools.

The output of each system furnishes the stimulus for repeating the cycle (Katz & Kahn, 1967, p. 20; Robbins & Coulter, 2007, pp. 534–537). In the case of nursing care facilities, the successfully cared for resident (the desired outcome of the nursing home's efforts) furnishes the source of more inputs: Other persons apply for admission to the facility to replace the resident who has left (Argenti, 1994, p. 225). The new resident brings renewed energy in the form of a renewed source of continuing income to the facility and thereby furnishes a renewal of the capacity of the facility to continue to pay employees and provide services.

The administrator can view the nursing facility as a dynamic system whose essence is the cycle of activities (providing care to residents, making sufficient income) for which they are responsible.

Organizational Growth

A nursing home and similar social organizations can grow indefinitely.

Scientists speak of the *entropic process,* a universal law of nature that all organisms move toward death (Hitt et al., 2001, p. 219). All of us, for example, realize that one day we will die because one or more of our vital systems comes to a halt.

In sharp contrast, a nursing facility or chain not only does not have to die, but can keep on growing, with no time constraints, as long as it receives more energy from the environment than it consumes. In this way, organizations can be said to acquire negative entropy.

Organizations tend to try to grow, not in every case, of course, but in general. Organizational theorists have called this the tendency of organizations to maximize the ratio of imported to expended energy. One social scientist (Miller, 1982, pp. 513–531) has observed that the rate of growth of an organization, within certain ranges, is dramatic if it exists in a medium that makes available unrestricted amounts of additional inputs. The significance for administrators is that organizations, unlike people, are not subject to disintegration as long as they can keep adding to their resources, and like people, they tend to try to grow. Between 1965 and 1983, American hospitals added vastly to their expensive equipment and procedures, because Congress had made virtually unlimited resources available through reimbursement for whatever they chose to charge under Medicare. Since 1984 Congress has been progressively limiting what it will reimburse hospitals. Growth may be qualitative (better care) or quantitative (a larger patient census or more facilities being added to the chain).

Maximizing Basic Character

Another important aspect of organizations is that organizations, as they grow, attempt to accommodate the world around them to meet their own needs (Hitt et al., 2001, pp. 505–508; Robbins & Coulter, 2007, p. 217). For example, in planning for an extended care system, the nursing home associations place themselves at the heart of the system. The American Hospital Association, on the other hand, envisions the American health care system with hospitals at its core. The insurance companies are similarly convinced of their own strategic importance at the very center of such a system.

Maintenance Functions: "Atherosclerosis," "Congestive Heart Failure"

Once in place, organizations become creatures of habit and develop a tendency to resist change. There can be a strong effort to keep the current pattern of relationships with others from changing at all. Sometimes this is called organizational hardening of the arteries (atherosclerosis). Organizations that have become set in their ways will try to maintain the status quo through several devices:

1. Any internal or external situation that threatens to force a change in the organization is countered by employees seeking to retain their old patterns and modes of operation (Johns & Saks, 2001, p. 523; Robbins & Coulter, 2007, p. 64). For example, the nursing home faced with a

"disruptive employee" agitating for change will dismiss that employee and resist change (Hitt et al., 2001, pp. 505–508).

2. Administrators, when confronted with external changes that might affect the organization, will try to ignore them. For example, if their patient census declines while it increases in nearby homes, the tendency will be to find excuses rather than to examine if the others are offering better services.

3. Resisting change, many organizations will attempt to cope with external forces that might force them to change by acquiring control over them. For example, if a nursing home chain is losing patients to a competing freestanding group of facilities, the chain might attempt to acquire those other facilities rather than remedy its own situation (Hitt et al., 2001, pp. 505–508; Robbins & Coulter, 2007, p. 60).

Rapid and unanticipated changes are a permanent fixture of the managerial landscape of today.

We've Always Done It That Way

Once firmly in place, systems, policies, procedures, plans, organizational approaches, and assumptions become the standard operations of the facility—its sacred cows. They are sacrosanct because it has *always* been done this way. They are created by the training received in nursing, medical, or physical therapy school. In this way creativity is stifled and competitive strength weakened. Today, anything that remains unchallenged or untouched for very long can become the sacred cow of tomorrow.

Sacred cows are difficult to round up for a variety of reasons. For too many adult children putting mother or daddy in physical restraints so they won't fall is one such sacred cow.

Sacred cows may be untouchable, because the state inspectors want operations done the federal and state way, or are the administrator's special concerns, or relate to one department's closely guarded turf.

You cannot move fast if you are following a herd of sacred cows. Paper trails represent people trying to keep tabs on other people. All this when the real purpose of systems, as we have described them previously, is to empower, not control people, to liberate staff to experiment with new ways to meet resident needs, not to tie them down. The nursing home industry is full of sacred cows; federal, state, and local officials, physicians, registered dietitians, the daughters, and a host of other well meaning individuals see to that. Finally, two other characteristics of organizations should be briefly mentioned.

Organizations Grow Increasingly Complex

New organizations tend to be simple at their start, then become more and more complex as they grow. The human personality is similar. As infants we have few perceptions. As we grow, we begin to build ever more complex and complicated perceptions of the world around us. The personality we develop is a system with no physical boundaries. A social organization such as a nursing home is also a system with no physical boundaries (Hitt et al., 2001, pp. 240–242; Johns & Saks, 2001, p. 38; Robbins & Coulter, 2007, pp. 266, 278, 283).

Just as the human personality becomes progressively more sophisticated, social organizations move toward the multiplication and elaboration of roles with greater specialization of functions. For example, the mom-and-pop nursing homes of a few decades ago are giving way to increasingly larger and more sophisticated facilities offering medically complex, highly computerized services.

The organization of American medicine provides another illustration. In 1870, 80% of all American physicians were general practitioners. Only a few were specialists. Today, with the explosion of medical technology, the reverse is true: 80% of American physicians are specialists, and only 20% are general practitioners. As was bound to happen, today one must become a 3-year trained specialist to become a general practitioner who today is called a family practice specialist!

The process of nursing homes grouping into increasingly larger and competing chains (i.e., multiplication and elaboration of roles) has led to multiplying the number of possible management jobs available to persons interested in such a career. Middle-level and upper-level positions are now available in corporate nursing home management offices.

Organizations Are Difficult to Predict

There need not be a single strategy for an organization to achieve an objective. We have argued that organizations are dynamic systems of social interactions. Because the situation is volatile, there is low predictability (Hitt et al., 2001, pp. 7–9; Robbins & Coulter, 2007, p. 283).

An organization can reach its goals from different starting points and by a variety of routes. If, for example, a small, financially weak nursing home chain management staff wanted to take over a financially stronger and larger chain, there are many possible alternatives. They could try to compete more successfully, thus weakening the larger chain, making it more susceptible to takeover. They could attempt to raise enough venture capital to buy out the larger group (Hitt et al., 2001, pp. 541–542). They could arrange to be taken over by an unrelated corporation with considerable liquid assets, thereby enabling them to buy out the currently stronger and larger chain.

The listing of the 10 largest nursing home chains has changed rapidly over the past several years. Predictability is equally low in a number of fields, for example hospitals, the assisted-living industry, multiunit senior housing, the home health care industry, and health maintenance organizations, to mention a few.

Summary

In the process of looking at the function called organizing we have suggested that thinking of organizations as systems is a useful approach to the task of understanding how a nursing facility operates. The systems model is a useful way to visualize the inputs (money, materials, and people) that are available to administrators. The way in which administrators configure and use money, materials, and people will depend on their beliefs about how organizations function.

1.5 Staffing

Staffing is hiring the right persons for the jobs in the organization. It is one of the most difficult tasks the administrator and their department managers face, because it is seldom possible to predict from an interview and recommendations how a person will work out on the job. The number of variables is almost infinite, and many of them are difficult to recognize beforehand: Many poorly qualified candidates are skillful at presenting themselves well in initial interviews.

Staffing patterns of nursing homes are more prescribed than for most other health care institutions. This is the result of the federal requirements and state regulation, which carefully delineate qualifications for each type of staff position and require minimum staffing (or, in the judgment of the surveyors, sufficient staffing) in nearly every area of the facility.

One thing is quite clear: The success of the nursing home depends directly on adequate staffing. Nursing care is looking after people. The interactions between residents and staff determine the quality of life in the nursing home. Physical facilities are important, but once they are in place at a minimally adequate level, the patient's satisfaction with the facility varies directly with their satisfaction with the staff performance.

The administrator may choose to delegate coordination of the hiring process to a personnel director or assign it to the individual department managers (normally) with the advice and consent of the administrator.

1.6 Directing

Directing is the process of communicating to employees what is to be done by each of them and helping them to accomplish it. An earlier step, organizing, included breaking down the work necessary to achieve the organizational goals into work assignments that can be handled by one person. Directing is an aspect of the organizational activity in which the actual work is done.

Several important management concepts will be included under this heading:

- policy making
- decision making
- leadership
- power and authority
- communication skills
- organizational norms and values
- additional related concepts

Directing involves reference to each of these key concepts to arrive at the goal of a successful program.

1.6.1 POLICY MAKING

The ultimate goal of the administrator is to design a program in which every member of the organization makes the same decisions given the same set of circumstances. To this end, the administrator attempts to persuade the entire staff to carry out their responsibilities exactly as the administrator would like them to.

Purpose and Function

It is impossible for the administrator to be everywhere at once, 24 hours a day throughout the facility. It is possible, however, for the administrator to make policies that direct the activities of the employees everywhere in the facility 24 hours a day. The purpose and function of these policies is to communicate to each employee as exactly as possible what the management expects in any situation on the job.

It is, of course, neither possible nor desirable to establish policies for every conceivable situation. However, a person can provide guidelines or policies that become the framework within which the employee decides what to do in each situation requiring action on behalf of the nursing home facility. G. R. Terry, in his book *Principles of Management* (1969), has defined policy as a verbal, written, or implied overall guide that sets up boundaries supplying the general limits and direction in which managerial action will take place.

Policies are used to help keep decisions within the areas intended by the planners, because they provide for some consistency in what employees decide in particular situations usually under repetitive conditions. Policies reveal the facility administrator's intentions with respect to the behavior of employees, residents, and the public in the future. Policies are decided before the need for employee knowledge arises. A simple illustration might be useful.

It is not possible for management to know when, where, or even whether a fire will break out in the facility. By developing a complete set of procedures for personnel to follow in case of fire, the administrator is able to communicate before the occasion arises precisely what each employee in the facility must do if a fire should occur.

Defining Policies and Procedures

The reader may have noticed the use of the word procedures previously, rather than policies. Writers in the field of management use policies, procedures, and plans of action as terms to indicate movement from generalized statements of intention (*policies*) to a specific spelling out of the method, step by step (*procedures*), for carrying out those policies or plans of action.

It may be useful to think of the following set of concepts, which moves from the general to the specific behaviors the manager wishes the employees to exercise.

Example of Policies and Procedures

Fire Preparedness

General goals or objectives may be stated for the facility. In the area of fire preparedness it might be: "to have our facility employees completely prepared to take appropriate action in case of fire." The administrator might then draw up a general policy statement indicating that the head of the housekeeping department would develop a step-by-step plan of action based on Life Safety Code requirements for every department to follow in case of fire. This plan is a *set of procedures*, a highly detailed plan of specific actions that each employee would be expected to follow in case of fire.

Notice that at each level the degrees of freedom within which decisions can be made are reduced. The head of housekeeping could develop a variety of configurations for employee responsibilities, but by the time the individual employee becomes involved, the degrees of freedom have nearly vanished. The responsibility in case of fire moves from the general goal or policy of fire preparedness to a detailed set of instructions or procedures to be followed to the letter. "The moment you hear the fire alarm, proceed immediately to station J on the Blue wing and report to the nurse in charge" is an example of a procedure.

Food Preparation

The board of directors might set a policy goal of offering an outstanding selection of first-quality food to the residents of the facility. It becomes the responsibility of each progressively lower level of management to actually implement this policy. The food service director must take this communicated policy or goal and develop a series of policies for decision making by the kitchen staff that result in the actual service of an outstanding selection of first-quality food to the residents.

General policies are developed at each level of management. Normally, the amount of specificity increases at each lower level. The food service manager may, for example, announce a policy to the food service supervisor responsible for salads that there be a sufficient variety with specified proportions of crisp fresh lettuce every evening. The supervisor may then write out a step-by-step set of procedures for the kitchen worker who prepares salads.

The set of steps the salad worker is to follow is an example of a *set of procedures,* for instance, at 4:00 P.M. each afternoon, the salad worker should begin by removing the lettuce from the refrigerator. The broad policy of excellence in food service promulgated by the administrator has now been translated into a set of procedures or individual steps for the salad worker in the kitchen to follow at 4:00 P.M. each afternoon to assure the crispness of the lettuce to be served each evening. Sounds simple, but ask the residents. Too few nursing facilities succeed in serving a sufficient variety of salads with crisp lettuce. Interesting salads 365 days a year is but one of hundreds of complex tasks that must be successfully accomplished each 24 hours.

Insertion of a Peripheral Device

A policy statement regarding peripheral devices might read as follows: "It is the policy of this facility to permit nurses to insert peripheral devices only after 20 hours of specialized training and certification by the director of nursing that the nurse has qualified."

A procedure statement regarding insertion of a peripheral device and administration of continuous solution might read as follows:

1. Verify physician's orders. Check for allergies.
2. Compare label on solution with order.
3. Wash hands.
4. Assemble equipment and supplies.
5. Inspect solution and container.
6. Close flow clamp on tubing.
7. Attach administration set to fluid container. Hang on IV pole.
8. Prime intravenous therapy tubing by squeezing drip chamber to fill 1/2 full; open flow clamp until tubing is primed; close flow clamp.
9. Explain procedure to patient, position resident.
10. Apply tourniquet to extremity (optional).
11. Select catheter insertion site, cleanse site with antimicrobial swab; start at center of the site, use a circular motion moving outward.
12. Repeat with antimicrobial swab. Allow to completely dry on skin at least 30 seconds.
13. Don gloves.
14. Place thumb below intended venipuncture site; gently draw skin toward you.
15. For wing-tipped needle, hold needle by the wings, with bevel up, at 45 degree angle to skin surface, penetrate the skin surface, lower the angle of the needle almost parallel with the skin, pierce the vein. Observe for blood return; release the tourniquet if one has been applied. Secure wings with tape.
16. Attach IV tubing or extension set, if used for intermittent infusion. Start solution at a slow rate.
17. Observe for signs of infiltration at venipuncture site. Anchor wings of needle with tape.
18. Cover venipuncture site with transparent dressing. Make a small loop with infusion tubing and secure with tape.
19. Check and regulate flow rate according to physician's orders.
20. Place label on dressing, indicating the following: date and time, type, length and gauge, initials of nurse.
21. Discard used equipment appropriately.

Documentation

Record procedure in the resident's medical record. Include the following:

- type, length, and gauge of device
- date and time of insertion
- site of insertion
- resident's response
- number of attempts
- type of dressing applied
- solution and rate of administration
- nurse's initials/signature.

Summary

Policies serve as general statements or understanding that guide or channel subordinates' thinking as they make decision. Policies limit the area within which a decision is to be made and seek to assure that it will be consistent with the overall objectives. Policies tend to decide issues beforehand by establishing the framework and scope of the actions.

The decisions made at each level of management establish the framework for decision making at each successively lower level of management, generally with progressively less and less discretion to do so. However, each level of management does participate in the policymaking process, and policies are made at every level of management. Policy is made by persons at upper, middle, and lower levels of management within the nursing home facility. Defining policy making is complicated by this fact.

When do policies become procedures? Sometimes these are separated by a fine line that is hard to distinguish. Generally, a policy is a statement that contains some degree of freedom and some further need for interpretation. Procedures are step-by-step instructions on how a specific task is to be carried out.

A Cautionary Note

Most health care facilities write their own policies and procedures. Well enough. It is important for every facility to individualize its mission and how to achieve it by developing appropriate policies and procedures to achieve their goals.

It is important to note, however, that if a facility policy or procedure sets a higher standard than the state or federal requirements, the facility will be held to that higher standard both on federal and state surveys and in courts of law. Our view is that the federal government has done a remarkably detailed and excellent job setting the appropriate policies for nursing homes in the United States over the past 30 years. Facility policies should conform as closely as possible to federal and state policies. Even so, most corporations and facilities write their own policies and procedures.

1.6.2 DECISION MAKING

Although decision making can be synonymous with managing, it is difficult to define. Shackle (1957, p. 105) defines *deciding* as the focal creative psychic event in which knowledge, thought, feeling, and imagination are fused into action (see also Hitt et al., 2001, pp. 26–27, 36–37; Robbins & Coulter, 2007, p. 163). Both Dale (1969) and Shackle point out the impossibility of a useful formula for decision making. Inevitably, we are left with an imprecise definition of the process. Even so, administrators do make numerous decisions every day.

To make the *right* decision in a given situation is often difficult. It is the nursing facility administrator's job to assure that all employees make the right decisions for the organization as often as possible (Kotter, 1982, p. 9; Robbins & Coulter, 2007, p. 170).

We define a successful manager as a person who is able, on balance, to make enough right decisions for the organization and *no* disastrously wrong ones.

Successful Decision Making: Enough Right Decisions

In the day-to-day world of the nursing facility, decision making translates into successfully implementing corporate, federal, and state policies and procedures. The successful nursing home administrator will achieve successful inspections from the many entities whose policies and procedures the nursing home must implement. An inspection by the Centers for Medicare and Medicaid Services (the federal and state surveyors) resulting in few or no deficiency citations, for example, Level A deficiencies, which are defined as isolated (involving few residents) and no actual harm with potential for minimal harm, is deemed a successful administrator—making enough right decisions.

Unsuccessful Decision Making: Disastrously Wrong Decisions

An example of disastrously wrong decision making would be for an inspection by Centers for Medicare and Medicaid Services to result in deficiency citations revealing patterned bad decisions (Level K) or widespread bad decision making (Level L) resulting in immediate jeopardy to resident health or safety. Citations for deficiencies at Levels K and L can be disastrous inasmuch as the facility is typically given notice that Medicare / Medicaid certification will be terminated within 30 days if deficiencies are not satisfactorily corrected.

1.6.3 LEADERSHIP

Organizations that thrive over an extended period of time (years) depend on *effective leaders*—persons who have foresight combined with an ability to guide the organization to successfully take advantage of the opportunities the future offers.

The Great Leadership Theory of History

Just as a satisfactory description of *deciding* is elusive, so is a satisfactory description of leading. There are, however, those who propose the "great leadership theory of history," suggesting that history is *made* or measurably influenced by individuals who become leaders. Whatever one might think of their accomplishments, persons such as Alexander the Great, Genghis Kahn, Confucius, Joan of Arc, George Washington, Abraham Lincoln, Margaret Sanger, and Winston Churchill seem to have assumed leadership roles that affected the course of history.

Leadership in the business world seems to be no less crucial to the success of organizations. Between the years 1915 and 1973, Thomas Watson, Sr. and Thomas Watson, Jr. provided leadership to an organization, International Business Machines Corporation (IBM), that came to dominate the computer world only during their tenure, because this father and son had foresight (successfully predicted the future) combined with an ability to guide the organization to successfully take advantage of the opportunities offered by the future. It was not until being discharged from a job he had held for 14 years that Tom Watson, Sr. joined a company that manufactured scales, meat slicers, time clocks, and punch cards for data sorting. He envisioned that these punch cards could revolutionize the future. He borrowed money and renamed the company. At the time, 1924, his son, Tom Watson, Jr. commented "What a big name for a pip-squeak company that makes meat grinders" (Kriegel, 1991, p. 39). International Business Machines Corporation had just been born.

As another example, William McWhorter was given responsibility for 103 hospitals that Hospital Corporation of America believed to be irreversibly unprofitable in 1987. Through his personal leadership these hospitals became both profitable and major leaders in the hospital industry.

The leadership provided to the nursing facility by the administrator, director of nurses, and other department managers is no less critical to the success or failure to thrive of each nursing facility.

The Administrator and the Director of Nursing Theory

There is scant research literature to prove the assertion that leadership by the administrator, director of nurses, and the department heads is key to the success of any nursing facility. There apparently exists, even in the absence of such data, a broad consensus among observers of the industry, especially the federal and state inspectors, that quality care in a nursing facility does depend on its administrators being able to exercise good leadership skills. Federal inspectors normally try to inspect a nursing facility within 6 months after a change in the administrator or director of nurses, believing that leadership (or lack of it) from these administrators does directly affect the quality of care in a facility. When IBM's leadership changed after 60 years under the Watsons the giant lost its leadership position. IBM had ridden the wave of change for 60 years with them at the helm.

When the Watsons led IBM, it usually was ranked #1 in *Fortune Magazine's* annual survey of America's Most Admired Corporations. Lou Gertsner, IBM president in the mid-1990s, stated several times that he did not have to have a vision to lead the corporation. By 1995, out of the 500 ranked companies, IBM had dropped from #1 most admired corporation to the 281st most admired corporation! Leadership counts. The Watsons inspired IBM to six decades of greatness with a vision. Vision, it seems, also counts (America's Most Admired Corporations, 1995, p. 66; Hamel & Prahalad, 1994). Gertsner later developed and implemented a vision of IBM becoming the service leader in the computer industry, and to some extent IBM has regained its place as one of several moderately successful industry leaders, but not as *the* industry leader.

Through forecasting, planning, organizing, staffing, directing, evaluating, controlling quality, innovating, and marketing decisions the administrator is providing leadership to the nursing facility. There are various styles of leadership (e.g., democratic, authoritarian, or laissez-faire), and these will be discussed in the following paragraphs (Robbins & Coulter, 2007, p. 490).

Leadership By Walking/Wandering Around

One effective style is leading by walking around (LBWA). When walking around and observing such things as staff interaction with residents and with families, volunteers and other employees, one can personally evaluate the quality of care being rendered. This is also an opportunity to see if the residents are having any problems and to physically inspect the building and equipment (observations by Karen Weddle, RN, Middletown, MD).

Leadership by wandering or walking around provides opportunity to the staff to speak with the administrator informally. It allows time to observe what is going on and to let the staff know the administrator is interested in them, the residents, and the facility. Leading by walking around is not new to the nursing facility setting. In many nursing facilities, each shift is expected to make rounds reporting on each resident's condition over the preceding 8 hours. This is how nursing keeps informed of and anticipates care needs for the coming shift.

Through LBWA, the administrator receives a daily update on the real world of the facility—in the rooms, hallways, departments, loading dock, and restrooms. This positions the administrator to uncover problems before they become major problems, for example, the NO SMOKING sign has fallen down and staff are smoking next to the oxygen cylinders. Administrators who do not take the initiative to keep informed about facility affairs on a daily basis often become involved in a style of management known as fire fighting. Once small issues become hot issues a lot of time must be spent extinguishing flames.

In making daily rounds, the administrator can do naive listening, gaining raw impressions of what is happening in the facility and sensing how things are going. Not enough time is available to get the paperwork done, meet all the other administrator requirements, and still make time to walk daily around the facility sensing its pulse? Sam Walton, the originator of The Wal-Mart Corporation visited every one of his stores at least once a year when he had 18 stores. By the early nineties he owned over 800 stores, and he was still visiting each one at least once a year, riding cross country with Wal-Mart truck drivers having donuts at 3:00 A.M. He thought the check-out clerk (read nursing assistant, CNA) to be the most important employee. Until his death in the early 1990s, every check-out clerk knew that sometime each year Mr. Sam might be the next customer waiting in the checkout line, observing how the customer ahead of him was being treated!

The future doesn't just happen: Leaders like Tom Watson, Sam Walton, and the local nursing home administrator dream it, shape it, and sculpt it!

Walking, Yet Maintaining the Chain of Command

Wandering around the facility talking with residents, visitors, and staff appears to violate the traditional concept of chain of command. The administrator is there to hear it firsthand and to communicate firsthand. Ed Carson, a former airlines chairman, who used LBWA, took lots of notes on scraps of paper, but he never told people down the line what to do or change. He never corrected on the spot what he disliked. But he did promise to get back to the "resident, visitor, or employee" in a few days. He then discussed each situation with his department head and charted with them a course of action to resolve any problem. And after a few days he would check with the "resident, visitor, or employee" to see if appropriate action had been taken. He was practicing what he called "visible management" (Johns & Saks, 2001, p. 310; Peters, 1987, p. 386; Robbins & Coulter, 2007, p. 270).

The basic benefits of LBWA are listening (finding out what's happening on the firing line), teaching (communicating the facility's values), and facilitating. Through LBWA the administrator can facilitate the work of employees by asking naive questions, finding out what is frustrating the staff, then running interference and knocking down small hurdles for them. Only the facility that pays excessive attention to details can achieve excellence in resident care. Quality of care is staff paying attention to the details that lead to excellent care as they emulate their administrator.

Choosing to Lead

Deciding on one's approach to leading is one of the more important decisions managers ever make. Kriegel compares leading an organization to riding the waves of change (1991, pp. 5–9). The time to change is when you don't have to, he asserts, when you are on the crest of a wave, not when you are in the trough. In the world of health care delivery administration the surf is up! Waves of change are coming from government, third-party payers, and the residents and their families.

The best surfers (nursing home administrators) are not necessarily the best swimmers (best management theoreticians). The best surfers are persons with the following mind-set.

Riding the Wave of Change

Passion rules. Catching and riding a wave is fairly simple, but there are many who give lip service to the art. They have the correct equipment and stylish outfits, the right jargon, but spend most of their time on the beach talking about surfing. The best surfers spend their time out in the water, rough or calm, looking for the next wave. They are totally committed to surfing, body, mind, and spirit.

No dare / no flair. Good surfers constantly push their limits, continuously trying new moves, going for bigger and bigger waves. They know that no two waves are ever the same, so that each one is ridden a little differently. Keeping ahead of the wave involves risk taking and constantly challenging oneself and those around you.

Expect to wipe out. For every successful ride there will likely be two or three wipe-outs. Sand is part of every surfer's diet. A changing ocean with its dynamic wave patterns and shapes is a source not of fear but of challenge that provides the thrill of surfing. Successful surfers know that if they do not wipe-out several times each day they are playing it too safe to keep improving.

Don't turn your back on the ocean. Surfers know that they are dealing with an environment beyond their control. They understand that uncertainty and unpredictability are part of the game. They respect the ocean and its power, never taking it for granted. They never turn their backs on the ocean.

Keep looking "outside." The outside waves are those on the horizon. It is important to pay attention to the wave closest to you, and also to what is coming. First, there may be a bigger and better wave coming in on the horizon. Second, the wave on the horizon may crash over you as you come up for air after riding the wave closest to you.

Move before it moves you. Surfing is forecasting and planning for the future. You have to begin moving yourself while that big wave is still on the horizon or it will surge by you leaving you in its trough.

Never surf alone. It is not smart to tackle the complexities of life alone. One needs back-up help when emergencies arise. By pooling one's knowledge and insights surfers can learn about and get more exotic spots, trade tips, and techniques that work. It is also a lot more fun to have a friend along to "talk story" with as you navigate the complexities of the nursing facility operations. Having someone to share your hopes, dreams, and frustrations leads to more creativity, joy, and effectiveness.

As Kriegel (1991) has suggested, the future is coming at us like enormous waves of change in set after set, and they are getting bigger. The surf is up in the hospital industry, the assisted-living industry, the life care communities, the multiunit senior housing industry, the home health care industry and the managed care industry. The future belongs to those who decide to ride, to those who welcome the unexpected.

John F. Welch, as president of General Electric, became widely regarded as the leading master of corporate change through shedding 200,000 employees while tripling GE's market value over a 12-year period. He believed that every business must be fast and adaptable to survive. People ask, he observed, if the change is over (at GE), can we stop now? He responded that change has just begun, that it is never ending. Change, he asserted, is a continuing process, not an event. He sees the administrator's job as listening to, searching for, and spreading ideas—the process of exposing people to good ideas and role models (Welch, 1993, p. 83).

As observed by Dennis Kodner in the *Journal of Long Term Care Administration,* the days of "business as usual" in the long-term care industry are over. He foresees that success in today's world depends on understanding where the industry is heading, having a vision of the future and developing the capacity to implement change as an ongoing aspect of managing a facility (1993, p. 82). Connie J. Evashwick thinks that facilities that resist change and continue to function in isolation may survive, but will not thrive in this 21st century (1993, p. 13).

Fire in the Heart

To be a successful nursing home administrator over a sustained period of years requires that one be excited and passionate about the profession. Top performers in all fields have one quality in common: passion. Their drive and enthusiasm is what distinguishes them. As numerous executive recruiters have observed, "The thing that makes the difference between a good manager and an inspiring, dynamic leader goes beyond competence. It's passion. That is the single quality that is going to lift a person head and shoulders above the rest" (Kriegel, 1991, p. 13).

Passion brings complete commitment to one's work: physical, emotional, and mental. It sustains the successful administrator through the outrages of regulations and an abusive public image of the field. Passion is contagious. An administrator who is enthusiastic about the work can inspire excitement in the nurses and nursing assistants. Knowledge of the field, competence, and experience make a good manager, but a greater commitment gives one the necessary edge to provide the leadership necessary in today's nursing facility.

Of course, passion is not a scientifically measurable component of nursing home administration, but then, management is not yet exactly a science. What the nursing home administrator needs is a fire in the heart for continuously improving the quality of the daily life of each resident.

A Continuum of Leadership Styles

In *Leadership and Organization,* Tannenbaum, Wechsler, and Massarik (1961) discuss a continuum of leadership styles. This allows us to characterize seven possible positions along the continuum, from manager-centered to employee-centered leadership. Several dimensions are portrayed in Figure 1.2. Under manager-centered leadership, the manager retains a high degree of control and uses authority extensively.

Manager-Centered Leadership

Position 1. The manager simply makes the decision, then announces it (autocratic style; Robbins & Coulter, 2007, p. 490).

Position 2. The manager attempts to convince the employees of the value of the decision made.

Position 3. The manager presents ideas and invites questions, in effect engaging the employees actively in the decision-making process.

Employee-Centered Leadership

Position 4. The manager presents a tentative decision, subject to change. Here the employees are further involved in the decision-making process itself.

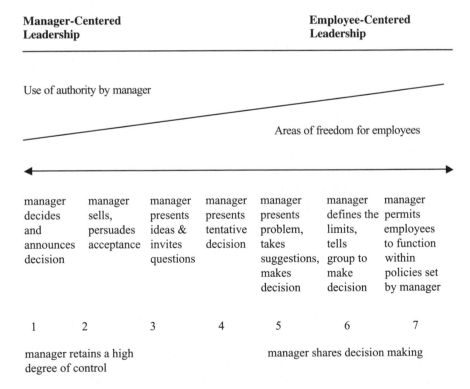

Manager-Centered Leadership

Employee-Centered Leadership

Use of authority by manager

Areas of freedom for employees

manager decides and announces decision	manager sells, persuades acceptance	manager presents ideas & invites questions	manager presents tentative decision	manager presents problem, takes suggestions, makes decision	manager defines the limits, tells group to make decision	manager permits employees to function within policies set by manager
1	2	3	4	5	6	7

manager retains a high degree of control

manager shares decision making

FIGURE 1.2 Range of decision-making strategies open to the manager.

Position 5. The manager presents the problem requiring a solution, invites suggestions, then makes the decision.

Position 6. The manager permits the subordinates to make the decision and function within the limits defined by the manager (laissez-faire leadership style; Johns & Saks, 2001, p. 183; Robbins & Coulter, 2007, p. 512).

Deciding How to Lead

At least the following three levels of considerations should be taken into account by the administrator who is selecting the leadership style for a particular situation.

First level forces in the administrator:

- the administrator's own values
- the administrator's confidence in the department heads
- the administrator's own feelings of security or insecurity

Second level forces in the employees:

The facility administrator can permit greater freedom to department managers who:

- have a need for independence (e.g., the director of nurses)
- are ready to assume responsibility for decision making (are professionally licensed)
- are interested in the problem and consider it is important (take resident care seriously)
- understand and agree with the mission statement / goals of the facility
- have the necessary knowledge and experience (e.g., the RN who comes with 2 years' intensive care experience)
- are prepared and expect to make decisions (e.g., a trained, licensed physical therapist)

Third level forces in the organization

- expectations of the organization's management (position taken by corporation or the board)
- ability of subordinates to function as a group (eight competent department heads who have worked together for 3 years versus five new and three continuing department heads)

- the problem itself (excessive medication errors or excessive in-house acquired decubitus ulcers rates cannot be permitted)
- time constraints (e.g., plans of correction for deficiencies all have correction dates)

Three Levels of Leadership Skill Requirements

We have already discussed three levels of management—upper, middle, and lower level—each with its own particular skill requirements. Figure 1.3, adapted from Katz and Kahn (1967), shows three different levels of leadership skills.

The Upper-Level Manager. The nursing facility's upper-level administrator is primarily responsible for creating and changing the organization's structure.

The Middle-Level Manager. The head of dietary, head of housekeeping, or other department head is responsible for development of more specific policies that interpret administration policy implications for their departments.

The Lower-Level Manager. The charge nurse who supervises a specific group of nurses or nursing assistants, for example, has the responsibility of applying the policies provided by the director of nursing to the hour-by-hour care given.

As Figure 1.3 suggests, different skills are needed at the three distinct levels of management.

Upper-Level Management's Job. The chief administrator must understand not only how the organization accommodates to the external environment, but also how all of the subsystems function within the nursing facility itself.

Middle-Level Management's Job. The middle-level manager is responsible for implementing the policies of the administration by devising ways to put them into action within the facility. This level of management translates the broader institutional policies by developing more specific ones to control employee behavior. The administrator, for example, may set a goal of preventing acquired decubitus ulcers. The middle-level manager must understand how the subsystems of the organization fit together to achieve such overall goals. They have the difficult task of representing to upper-level management the needs of those supervised.

FIGURE 1.3 Three levels of skill requirements for managers.

To function effectively, middle-level managers must realize that they are the conduit through which action travels in both directions.

Lower-Level Management's Job. Lower-level managers guide employees according to established policies of the facility. To accomplish this, the rules must be thoroughly understood and applied evenhandedly to all employees under their direction. One particularly important key to effective leadership at the lower level is the sense the employees have of their manager's advocacy for the employees they supervise. It is not enough to be their advocate, however; the manager must be their effective spokesperson.

Procedures can be written by any level of management; in most cases, procedures are written by both middle-level and lower-level managers.

Characteristics of the Effective Leader

Katz and Kahn (1967, pp. 325–327; Robbins & Coulter, 2007, p. 502) have characterized an effective leader as a person who

- mediates and tempers the organizational requirements to the needs of persons in a manner that is organizationally enhancing (the facility assists employees having family crises through unplanned time off and other support not just because the Family and Medical Leave Act provides for such action)
- promotes group loyalty and personal ties (working for the facility becomes a personally satisfying experience)
- demonstrates care for individuals (knows each employee by name and something about that employee's interests)
- relies on referent power (respect from employees and residents) rather than the power of legitimacy and sanctions alone (discussed later; Robbins & Coulter, 2007, p. 504).

Tannenbaum et al. (1961, ch. 5) conclude that a successful leader is a person who is keenly aware of relevant forces in the situation, understands themself and the individuals with whom they are dealing, but also is able to behave appropriately vis-à-vis the situation, making decisions where needed and sharing the decision making where appropriate.

Tannenbaum et al. consider the successful leader as being neither strong nor permissive, but rather as endowed with a strong "instinct" (gut level feeling) for determining appropriate personal behavior and capable of acting accordingly.

Day-to-Day Leadership Requirements

In the daily administration of the typical long-term care facility the administrator will face a variety of situations with differing leadership needs. Recognition of appropriate leadership behavior for any specific situation is a valuable insight; the capacity to behave in differing leadership styles is an accomplishment of a high order indeed. Much of the flexibility the administrator can exercise in distinctive leadership styles depends on how comfortable they are in wielding power and authority in the management of the facility.

Charismatic Leadership

Although charismatic leadership cannot be consciously chosen by the administrator, it is worth mentioning here (Johns & Saks, 2001, p. 288; Robbins & Coulter, 2007, p. 512). This quality has been described by Max Weber as a magical aura with which people sometimes endow their leaders. It appears when a group has an emotional need for a person who, they feel, will make the right decision for them. The acts of charismatic leaders are typically unexamined. Their followers do not scrutinize their acts as they would those of their immediate supervisors. Charisma is not an objective assessment by the followers and normally requires a psychological distance between the followers and the leader. When charisma is assigned to a leader, the power and authority of the organization is enhanced.

1.6.4 POWER AND AUTHORITY

Power is the ability to control the behavior of others. A person has power when they are able to make other people do what they want them to. Several writers say this is the ability to motivate someone to do something that they would otherwise not do (Argenti, 1994, p. 310; Robbins & Coulter, 2007, p. 510). The administrator of a nursing facility has the power to order employees to act to implement the goals of the facility as expressed in the policies and plans.

Webster's *New World Dictionary* (1968) (1968) gives 14 definitions for the word *power*. An additional half-dozen synonyms indicate that power denotes the inherent ability or the admitted right to rule, govern, determine, control, regulate, restrain, and curb. Power is a complex concept in our culture.

The administrator has the power (from the board or the ownership) to tell employees what to do and to expect them to do it. It is well known that although an organization theoretically provides equal legitimating power to all administrators at the same level, the administrators do not in fact remain equal.

For example, a board of directors controlling five nursing facilities, in theory, delegates equal authority to the administrators to act on its behalf in the five facilities. Some of these five administrators might have firm control over employee behavior, while others might be having difficulty convincing employees to do what they request. Why?

Reciprocity

Power is a reciprocal relationship. The board of directors or the owners can confer power on the administrator, but the employees and residents must accept that power as permissible if it is to be meaningful. This does not imply disrespect or chaos. The concept of authority or power is more complicated than the mere announcement that power has been given to the administrator by the board or the owners.

French and Raven (1960, pp. 607–623), Robey (1982, p. 147), and other writers have identified at least five types of power: legitimate, reward, punishment (coercive; Robbins & Coulter, 2007, p. 504), referent, and expert. In light of this, it is important for administrators to be familiar with these types of power and their applications.

Legitimate Power. This describes authority given to a particular position and is associated with the person's position in the organization (Argenti, 1994, p. 310; Johns & Saks, 2001, p. 378; Robbins & Coulter, 2007, p. 495). Organizations expect each person to yield to the appropriate authority. The administrator has more legitimate power than the director of nurses and so on. When employees or residents respond to legitimate power their actions are motivated by the level or position of the manager, not to any personality, knowledge, or other characteristics of that person.

Reward Power. The fact that reward is a second type of power is testimony to the mundane reality that employees do not always respond correctly. Administrators are given reward power to induce or persuade employees or residents to do what the administrator asks. If not, certain desired approval(s) may be withheld (Robbins & Coulter, 2007, p. 404; Robey, 1982, pp. 382–383). For example, if the administrator has authority to give a 15% year-end cash bonus to the three supervisors who have best achieved the facility's goals (translation: Those who most often responded acceptably to the administrator's instructions), then they have reward power.

Punishment Power. Sometimes known as coercive power, this exists when the employee believes that a manager has the ability (and inclination) to punish unacceptable behaviors. The ultimate punishment power is firing the employee or requiring the resident to leave the facility, but there are many intermediate, less drastic means. The employees who do not observe the manager's rules for functioning in the facility may receive a written warning, a copy of which is placed in the human resources file. Use of punishment power is normally a last resort—used after other types of uses of power have failed. Extensive use of punishment power leads to distrust and fear (Argenti, 1994, p. 310; Johns & Saks, 2001, p. 379; Robbins & Coulter, 2007, p. 412)—circumstances clearly not conducive to quality resident care.

Referent Power. Power to influence is often based on liking or identifying with another person. When the employees like the administrator and identify with them, they are more apt to do what the administrator wishes. Referent power exists to the degree employees and residents identify with the administrator. This is both simple and powerful. Employees who do not admire an administrator or do not identify with the administrator are more difficult to control, that is, it is harder to make them do their work as the organization wishes (Johns & Saks, 2001, p. 379).

Expert Power. Power can derive from recognition by the employees and residents that the administrator is very skillful, has had considerable training, and is quite knowledgeable in the field of nursing home administration. For the nurse, this acknowledgment comes from the registered nurse (RN) license, for the physician, the license to practice medicine (Johns & Saks, 2001, p. 379).

Power From Outside the Organization

It is important to note that expert and referent power, to the extent they are present in the facility, are additions to the power of organizationally given rewards and punishments because expert and referent power cannot be conferred by the organization (Katz & Kahn, 1967, pp. 302–303). There is literally an increase in the amount of power or control that can be exerted over the personnel and residents, and it is a persistent factor in increased organizational performance.

Expert and referent power can be substituted for power based on punishment. This can mean fewer negative, or undesired, or unintended organizational consequences. It is desirable to promote referent power in addition to, or instead of, power based on rewards and punishment or organizational dictates. Remember, the task of the administrator is to motivate the members of the organization to achieve the organization's goals.

Expert and referent power are available to all members of the staff. Referent power, in particular, depends on personal and group characteristics and is available to *peers* (persons at the same level) in the organization. Peer influence is often more readily accepted than influence from superiors. If, for example, one of the nurses is particularly skillful in creating a cheerful atmosphere in the facility, their leadership through referent power gives the nursing facility greater control over the quality of life achieved.

The Administrator's Power Is Real

Administrators do have power over other people's lives. Christensen et al. (1980) have characterized the power of the chief administrator as potentially "irresponsible" (p. 49), not necessarily because of the use of power in any particular decision or even because of the motives of the administrators but because those affected by the decisions (the employees, residents and their significant others, and even the board or owners) very often have little or no real immediate voice in the making of some decisions (e.g., when to finally tell employees that the cumulative effect of their behaviors renders them unfit to work at that facility). This can be especially true when most of the power is centralized in the office of the administrator. There are limitations, however, to the administrator's power.

The Administrator's Power Is Constrained

As we discuss elsewhere, nursing facilities have quite complex lines of authority because of the presence of several professional groups within the facility: physicians, nurses, dietitians, physical therapists, and others. All these groups have professional organizations and loyalties that influence their behavior in the nursing facility. They have "authority" within their own professional spheres.

The facility administrator's authority is constantly constrained or limited by the influence of the medical, nursing, and other professions, respectively, over the behavior of its physicians, nurses, nutritionists, and other professionals within the facility. Membership in these professional groups means that, in the last analysis, the doctors' behavior may be governed more by professional standards enforced by the medical profession than by policies or goals of the nursing facility (Williams & Torrens, 1980, pp. 277–279). Similarly, nurses are governed by the state nurse practice act and enforcement board, rather than by the policies or goals of the nursing facility when there is a conflict between the two. The same, of course, is true of the other professionals. This does not mean that the administrator has little or insufficient control, but rather that the authority or power to act is always circumscribed or constrained by the presence of the controls over behavior exerted by the professional groups (Gordon & Stryker, 1983, pp. 136–137).

The task of achieving control over the behavior of the professional employees is a complicated one, requiring tact and ingenuity on the part of the administrator.

1.6.5 COMMUNICATION SKILLS

Directing is the process of communicating the organizational objectives to the staff, residents, and their significant others. *Communication* is the exchange of information and the transmission of meaning.

Communication is essential for the survival of any social system. The skills of the administrator in communicating what is to be accomplished and the manner in which it is to be carried out have much to do with the success of the administration in achieving the plan for the facility. Unless the plans of action are successfully communicated to the staff, the plans will, at worst, not be implemented at all, or, at best, be only partially carried out.

Steps in the communication process are that: (a) someone initiates it, (b) it is transmitted from its source to its destination, and (c) it has an impact on the recipient. Unless, or until, a communication has made its intended impact on the recipient, it has, for all intents and purposes, not taken place.

Communication = Information = Power

Communication is the transmission of information, and information is power, because it provides sounder bases for judgments. The informed person is on sounder ground and therefore more powerful. The withholding of information is also a form of power, inasmuch as the person with the information is in a superior position to make decisions. Good communication is sometimes described as active listening, that is, listening with (1) intensity, (2) acceptance, (3) empathy, and (4) a willingness to assume responsibility for understanding the speaker's complete message (Argenti, 1994, p. 25; Robbins & Coulter, 2007, p. 293).

Systems of Communication

Organizations are described as having at least two systems of communication existing side by side: the formal and the informal communication processes.

The *formal communication* process closely resembles the formal organizational structure of the nursing facility. The administrator may send memoranda to the department managers, or the department managers may send them to their staff.

The *informal communication* process exists in nearly every organization. The social groups within the facility define the informal communication process. Nurses chatting in their lounge communicate informally and exchange much important information in the course of their casual conversation.

Communication is the flow of information in the organization, which social scientists describe as flowing upward, downward, and horizontally. As the words themselves suggest, *upward communication* flows from subordinates upward to the next level(s) or administration. *Downward communication* flows from upper-level management to lower-level members of the staff (Robbins & Coulter, 2007, p. 303). *Horizontal communication* is information flowing between peers or persons of equal rank or status.

The closer a person gets to the organizational center of control, the more pronounced the emphasis on the exchange of information. Administrators process information and use it in their decision making. Communicating is at the heart of the management process.

Communicating is an art that managers must master. Communications between administrators and personnel are full of subtleties and shades of meaning. Most communication also has numerous levels of meaning and function and is essential to building a relationship. Any act of communication may answer a question at the moment, but it has different meanings for the persons involved. Managers need to be aware that there are many barriers to full, clear communication. Seldom does any single communication have only one level of meaning (Johns & Saks, 2001, p. 313; Robbins & Coulter, 2007, p. 293).

Barriers to Communication

Agenda Carrying. Each person carries their own agenda(s) into every communication situation, preoccupied with their own concerns and life experiences. Each individual filters what is communicated through their own perceptions.

Selective Hearing. Persons hear selectively; that is, they tend to hear what they want to hear, thereby filtering out the unpleasant. A nursing supervisor may wish to communicate to an aide dissatisfaction with one aspect of the aide's performance. To soften the effect, the supervisor may first praise the employee for some other work. The employee may hear the praise and effectively screen out the criticism.

Differences in Knowledge Levels. Persons who have only sketchy knowledge about a topic may process information quite differently from persons who may be more knowledgeable. That is, degrees of sophistication vary among listeners and the "information" they process from a single communication may differ significantly.

The Filter Effect. The manager may be told what the employees believe they want to hear. It is not easy to give bad news to a superior when one already knows such news is not welcome. Ancient Greek literature recounts how frequently the messenger bringing bad news to the king was killed. The implications of this reaction have not been lost on most organizational members.

It seems that no matter how much middle-and upper-level administrators insist they want to hear bad as well as good news, the employees filter the information toward the known bias of the next level(s) of management. When there are several layers of management through which unwelcome news must filter, the upper management may receive less accurate information. (Another good reason for the administrator to manage by walking around doing naive listening in the hallways!)

Subgroup Allegiance. Each one of the subgroups in the organization (nurses, housekeepers, residents on a hall) demands allegiance from its members. Tangible and intangible rewards are given in each group, so when a communication arrives, it is interpreted in light of the goals and needs of each subgroup and usually not from the viewpoint of the organization as a whole (Johns & Saks, 2001, p. 328; Robbins & Coulter, 2007, p. 425).

Jay Jackson, in "The Organization and Its Communication Problems" (1960, pp. 443–456), concluded that:

- people communicate far more with members of their own sub-group than with any other persons (e.g. the nurses have difficulty in learning what the nurses' aides are thinking and feeling)
- people prefer to communicate with someone of higher status than themselves (the aides prefer to talk to the nurses)
- people try to avoid having communication with those lower in status than themselves (the nurses prefer to talk to the doctors, not to the aides except when giving instructions to them)
- people will communicate with those who will help them achieve their goals—higher status persons have power to create either gratifying or depriving experiences
- people communicate with those who can make them feel more secure and avoid those who make them anxious

Status Distance. The nursing home staff is comprised of a broad range of professional and nonprofessional groups (Johns & Saks, 2001, p. 326; Robbins & Coulter, 2007, pp. 293, 431). At the top of the status ladder is the physician on whose orders the majority of nursing facility activities depend. Numerous health professionals at the mid-level are present in the facility: nurses, Geriatric Nurse Practitioners,

RNs, LPNs, therapists of several types (e.g., physical, occupational, and recreational), dietitians, pharmacists, physician assistants, and others. Toward the lower end of the status ladder are the nurses' aides and housekeepers, few of whom have any formal training. It is difficult for lower-level employees to communicate upward. The administrator must be aware of the status sensitivities of these many groups and be capable of successfully fostering the needed communication among all of them.

Language Barrier. Doctors and nurses speak "medicalese." The pharmacists speak yet another language; the physical therapists have their jargon (Johns & Saks, 2001, p. 323; Robbins & Coulter, 2007, p. 66). In short, given the great variety of professional specialists who must by regulation be employed or retained as consultants, the nursing home administrator and the staff who deal with them have an especially difficult task in assuring that resident care is not compromised through miscommunication among these occupations .

Self-Protection. Persons often fail to communicate information that might reflect badly on them, their friends, or the organization (translation: The administrator should be certain that the accident report portrays what actually occurred.).

Information Overload. The abundance of information flowing in the facility (as many as 50 to 100 separate forms) may produce an information overload that results in the staff's compromised ability to distinguish among communications requiring prioritizing and attention. Bad news travels fast. Good news hardly travels at all.

Others. The administrator must bear in mind that all communication is multidimensional, needing appropriate interpretation to be of use.

In sending out a memorandum to employees or engaging in any communication, the administrator must take into account that its effect depends at least on the following:

- feelings and attitudes of the parties toward each other
- expectations
- how well the subordinate's needs are being met by the organization—if the nursing facility is supportive, the employee receiving administrative communications may be less defensive and more problem-oriented, that is, readier to absorb the communication and comply with the organization's request.

1.6.6 ORGANIZATIONAL NORMS AND VALUES

Developing Loyalty to Facility Goals

Administering an organization such as a nursing home facility is a complicated process. We have discussed some of the problems encountered by administrators as they attempt to lead employees to do the tasks required. One of the impediments to accomplishing this is that the organization can never count on the individual employee's undivided attention. This is known as the concept of partial inclusion, or the segmental involvement of people in the job role.

Limitations on Employee Participation

The nursing home defines behaviors that require only a portion of a person's 24-hour day. The facility asks only that during each shift employees perform the tasks or roles prescribed for them and that they have agreed to do. Unavoidably, however, the whole person must be brought into the work situation (Katz & Kahn, 1967, p. 50; Robbins & Coulter, 2007, p. 429). To deal with this, the employee is asked to set aside the nonjob aspects of life while at work. This is literally a depersonalizing demand that most employees find difficult to accomplish, so informal "organizations within the organization" develop in defense of personal identity.

The result is that people behave less as members of the nursing facility and more in terms of some compromise of their many commitments. For example, when asked about the sources of satisfaction from their jobs, employees often rate their interpersonal relationships with their fellow employees as the most important aspect of their work. Association with the residents follows, with the goals and values of the nursing home facility itself tending to be somewhat low on the list of employee motivations. Administrators and supervisors engage in a constant struggle to gain loyalty from employees to the goals of the facility.

There is yet another important limitation to employees' full participation. People tend to interpret the facility as a whole from the viewpoint of their particular section of the organization. This is another reason why upper-level administrators who collect information only from their immediate subordinates may never know what is actually transpiring or taking place.

People tend to exaggerate their importance to the organization as a whole. Loyalties develop to the work area rather than to the whole facility. This is a major source of conflict among departments. The nursing department views the organization from its unique perspective, as do the maintenance, food service, and other groups.

To enable staff to accomplish necessary work, organizations develop and specify roles (job descriptions) that are carefully prescribed forms of behavior associated with the tasks the organization wants performed. *Roles* are standardized patterns of required behavior (Katz & Kahn, 1967, p. 49; Robbins & Coulter, 2007, p. 429). The nurse's aide is told very clearly what their role is during the 8 hours on the job.

Connecting Roles to Norms

To build loyalty, organizations try to identify roles and persons filling them with the *norms* or values of the organization, general expectations for all employees.

Professional standards for nurses and nurse's aides are examples of such norms. They are behavior patterns to which all members of the group are expected to adhere. Respecting the personal privacy of patients would be an example of such a norm. Sam Walton, by standing in a checkout line in all his Wal-Mart stores each year, was constantly teaching and reinforcing an important norm: Assure that check-out is a pleasant experience thus stimulating the customer to feel favorable toward Wal-Mart.

Norms are justified by *values,* which are more generalized statements about the behavior expected from staff members. Values furnish the rationale for the normative requirements. Treating all patients with respect for their rights as persons is an example of a broad value statement, justifying the more specific norm that nursing personnel ought to respect each resident's personal privacy. For Sam Walton, building customer loyalty and repeat business might be the general value under which he established a pleasant check-out experience as a norm to be enforced.

System norms and values are attempts to connect employees with the system so that they remain within system values while carrying out their role assignments. It could be said that norms and values furnish "cognitive road maps" (ways to think about the organization and its goals). Norms help personnel adjust to the system.

Nursing facilities' norms and goals revolve around providing the highest quality of life achievable for residents. Under Tag F241 the federal government defines resident dignity as care for residents in a manner and in an environment that maintains or enhances dignity and respect in full recognition of their individuality. This involves assisting residents to be well groomed, dress appropriately, promote independence in dining, allowing private space and property, speaking and listening respectfully, and focusing on the individual's communication. In 1993, 19.1% of facilities received deficiencies for this, declining to 13.2% in 1996 and rising to 16% in 2006.

The reader may want to study Table 1.1. Dignity, like many of the federal standards, is a complex concept interpreted differently state to state and differently over time. Using the same federal definition, some states recorded dramatic decreases in dignity deficiencies while other states recorded dramatic increases over the same period of time using the same criteria.

Justification of the Facility: "Soft" and "Hard"

Another contribution of organizational norms and values is the moral or social justification for the activities of the nursing facility. This is often put in the form of a mission statement for the facility, defining the purposes and values held by the facility. The mission statement often appears at the front entrance and often in the front of the human resources handbook—it becomes the first impression the visitors and prospective employees have of the purposes of the facility.

When nursing homes are attacked in the newspapers or subjected to public criticism, staff members look to their administrators for reaffirmation of the facility's worth, enabling them to feel good about themselves and their work there.

The administrator demonstrates what is important, the values that actually guide the day-to-day behavior of staff, by the way they behave to what they give attention. If the administrator constantly moves around the facility assuring that each resident is getting quality care and enjoying a high quality of life, the employees will probably follow suit. Likewise, if the administrator concentrates instead on getting the paperwork done, meeting regulations, and saving money, that is what the staff will give their attention. To develop pride in the facility and enthusiasm for its works is the goal of *people management*.

When it comes to achieving long-term success with personnel, soft is hard. Quality care and a high quality of life are soft, but the administrator must be uncompromising and implacable in implementing them. Administrators care deeply about and respect their staff and residents. Yet they must enforce a "no excuses" environment when it comes to patient care. The successful

TABLE 1.1.   Percent of Nursing Facilities in the U.S. Deficiency Group = Quality of Life: F241, 1993, 1999, Percent and Number of Facilities 2006

	Percent of Facilities with Deficiencies = Quality of Life
1993	19.1%
1999	13.2%
2006	15.96%; 2,542 facilities

Source: DHHS, 2006b.

administrator is at once tough on values, yet tender in support of staff who try to implement those values.

Dreams, Vision, Goals

Another way to conceptualize values, norms, and roles is to equate them to dreams/vision, goals, and behaviors respectively. Employees are more motivated by and able to accept a vision or dream held by the facility. A dream or vision is a motivating abstract or belief. Dr. Martin Luther King, Jr., could not have so highly motivated the unprecedented number of demonstrators on the Washington, DC mall by telling the marchers that he had this or that goal, or this or that well devised plan of action. Rather, he moved them by telling them that he had a dream of equality for all Americans. A dream or vision of constantly improving the daily life experiences of residents and staff in the facility can motivate. Specific goals, such as having a full activities program, are secondary to the dream. Goals give employees specific targets to shoot for and provide feedback, but goals must be guided by something larger—a dream or vision that inspires. Dreams, then, can become goals with wings. Each goal is a step toward a dream.

Most nursing home corporations publish mission statements that resemble a list of goals more than a vision or dream (e.g., "We seek to be the provider of choice for each community in which we have a facility"). Fine for the corporate level, but not very motivating to the nursing assistants in their day-to-day struggles to provide care. Deming has observed that goal statements from the corporate level seldom motivate. Many local facilities have corporate goal statements in large print on well-designed posters on the walls, but these may not be their own goals. Corporate generated goal statements are subject to the NIH phenomenon (not invented here). Each facility must generate its own vision of what it is seeking.

One major nursing home chain does have a corporate vision that can motivate all employees as long as the highest level of management stands behind it: "whatever it takes." By that the corporation promises to assist every employee to give the best quality of care possible to their residents by the corporate commitment to assist each employee, no matter what it takes at the corporate level. As long as each employee believes they will be supported in their own individual effort to improve the daily lives of residents and staff, each employee can participate in the dream.

Why Organizations Need Administrative Leadership

Once all the plans have been developed and staff hired and trained, why doesn't the organization just run smoothly? Although there are a number of dimensions to any answer of this question, we will discuss only a few that seem especially relevant.

All organizational designs are imperfect (Demski, 1980, p. 58; Hitt et al., 2001, pp. 499–500; Robbins & Coulter, 2007, pp. 266, 278). Differences between the organizational chart, the written policies, and the organization's actual functioning are easily seen. It is commonly recognized that the new worker, after being instructed by the supervisor, turns to the group's members to learn what the job requirements really are.

Actual behavior, the actual functioning of the organization, is infinitely more complex, inconclusive, and variable than the plan. An illustration of this is organizational sabotage. Any worker who wants to sabotage the facility can do so by merely following organizational law to the letter—doing what is formally stipulated, no more and no less.

Nursing facilities, like all organizations, need administrative leadership to cope with the constantly changing external environment that requires internal adjustments. When, for example, three new assisted-living facilities open in an area and one's own occupancy rate drops from 92% to 72%, organizational leadership is in order.

Organizations also need leadership to accommodate to the changes constantly occurring within them. Employees retire or find work elsewhere, the needs of staff and residents change, conflicts develop, physical systems break down, and decisions to repair or replace are called for.

As Kriegel (1991) has pointed out, change is here to stay. To meet current challenges it is necessary to constantly adapt. Whether one feels one has reached the top, or is still climbing, you cannot stay still. The old saying "if it ain't broke, don't fix it" needs to be changed to "if you don't fix it all the time, it will break."

1.6.7 ADDITIONAL RELATED CONCEPTS

We turn now to several additional concepts worth reviewing in any consideration of attempts by administrators to direct the efforts of the organization.

Corporate Culture

Corporate culture is the overall style or atmosphere of a facility. The corporate culture governs how people relate to each other in the organization, for example, "this is how we do things in this facility." Corporate culture is important to the organization's survival. The corporate culture at IBM, for example, changed dramatically away from Tom Watson, Sr. and Tom Watson, Jr.'s commitment to "respect to the individual" once they retired (Argenti, 1994, p. 116; Robbins

& Coulter, 2007, pp. 63, 91, 99, 103). For the nursing facility to have the best chance of succeeding it needs a stable staff (low turnover) with all staff members participating in the facility culture and taking personal responsibility to make the corporate culture a daily reality. In a sense, the CNAs (the nursing assistants who deliver the majority of hands on care in the facility) may be the most key staff member in implementing the corporate culture (DePorter, 2006).

Delegation

The concept of *delegation* is permitting decisions to be made at the lowest possible level. Such authority is given to middle-level and lower-level managers, allowing them to make decisions for the organization, as appropriate. The essential issue is the determination of the nature of the decisions to be made at whatever level (Johns & Saks, 2001, p. 353; Meal, 1984, pp. 102–111; Mintzberg, 1979, pp. 212–213; Robbins & Coulter, 2007, p. 270).

Delegating can be both beneficial and disadvantageous. At optimum operation, delegation channels decision making to staff members who are best informed and most skilled to make a particular decision or set of decisions. The negative aspect of this practice is that because the managers have only a partial view of the organization, they consciously or unconsciously may make decisions in a manner that maximizes their area of the organization, to the possible detriment of the facility as a whole.

Ultimate responsibility cannot be delegated. The chief administrator is held accountable for the acts of all persons working under facility auspices.

Unity of Command

The concept of unity of command emphasizes the importance of each person being accountable to only one supervisor (Hitt et al., 2001, p. 489; Simon, 1960, pp. 23–26). Because it is functionally difficult for any employee to answer to two managers, the facility must be organized to assure this relationship.

Span of Control

How many immediate subordinates with interrelated work should a manager supervise? This has been a point of contention for decades. The British World War I general Sir Ian Hamilton insisted that six was the maximum span of control (Argenti, 1994, p. 361; Hitt et al., 2001, pp. 405–410). Others have proposed different numbers. Decisions by a number of state governments illustrate this issue. Several states had expanded operations to the point that perhaps 100 persons were reporting directly to the governor. It was realized that in this circumstance no one, in actual practice, was supervising these 100 persons. To regain control, several states reconstituted their organizational pattern to include a department of human resources to whose supervisor most of the former 100 reported, leaving perhaps a dozen persons reporting directly to the governor. In the last analysis, the administrator must be certain that each employee is effectively supervised.

Short Chain of Command

This principle asserts that there should be as few levels of management as possible between the chief administrator and the rank and file (Hitt et al., 2001, p. 493). Certainly, for the communication purposes of upper-level management, this seems a good principle to follow. It minimizes the number of interpreters through whom information for upper-level managers must be sifted (Johns & Saks, 2001, p. 310).

Balance

Advocates of the principle of balance assert that there is a need for continual surveillance to maintain balance among the following:

- size of the various departments
- standardization of procedures and flexibility
- centralization and decentralization
- span of control and short chain of command

Management by Objectives (MBO)

This approach emphasizes setting specific, jointly developed goals with a time period for goal achievement and performance feedback (Argenti, 1994, p. 264). The theory is to create a process of participation beginning with the lowest levels of workers whose recommendations are constantly moved upward until final selection of the goals to be put into place is made by upper management.

Management by objectives was first put into practice (under this rubric) by Lyndon Johnson. As President of the United States he wished to gain meaningful control of the largest bureaucracy under his management, now known as the Department of Health and Human Services (DHHS; Johns & Saks, 2001, pp. 186–191).

While MBO, in theory, meaningfully involves lowest level employees/ managers in recommending organizational goals, the real effect is to shift power upward (Swiss, 1983, p. 238). This occurs because it is the upper level managers who actually make the final choice among (and modify if necessary) recommendations from the lower levels.

Management Information Systems (MIS)

The phrase *management information systems* (MIS) originally came into the literature as a description of computer-based information processing for managers in making their decisions (Argenti, 1994, pp. 266–267). Withington (1966, p. 3) defined MIS as the study of how the organization communicates and processes information to maximize the effectiveness of management and to further the objectives of the organization.

The point recognized in MIS is that the manager needs a constant rationalized and organized flow of information in order to make appropriate decisions. In Levey and Loomba's view (1984, pp. 386–387), developing an MIS is as simple as

1. determining one's need for information
2. identifying the sources of information
3. deciding on the amount, form, and frequency of information needed
4. choosing the means of information processing
5. implementing the system

Management by Exception

Every day the manager receives numerous verbal and written reports, which usually contain routine information about the functioning of the facility. One way managers can effectively use their time is by giving attention to exceptions to the plan. If the census, the number of meals served or their costs are within plan, there may be no need for action. There are multitudes of detailed tasks being accomplished in acceptable fashion by the staff every day. What merits the administrator's attention are the exceptions to the policies and plans of action originally established for the organization.

The budget is one of the more useful tools for spotting exceptions (Gordon & Stryker, 1983, pp. 100–113). Getting information about the amount of money that has been spent in the last time period is a reasonably exact control measurement. As long as any department is spending within the agreed-on budget there may be no need for the administrator's attention. Whenever a departmental budget falls short or exceeds the amounts allocated to it, the administrator should give attention to the exception and take whatever steps may be necessary to bring expenditures back within the budgeted limits. Nursing having to hire unexpected numbers of "pool" nurses for weekends (nurses hired by the day from an agency that supplies temporary nursing help), for example, is a frequent cause of budget overage. However, too little expenditure by nursing or by, for example, the food service, might be as much a cause for alarm as too great an expenditure. In the first case the facility might be short on the required number of nursing personnel hours per day, in the second case the quality of food being purchased and prepared might be unsatisfactory.

Management by exception does not mean that the routine and within-specification behaviors of the facility remain unexamined. It is the routine behaviors of the organization that are being examined for deviations from the norm.

PERT / CPM

Program Evaluation and Review Technique (PERT) and Critical Path Method (CPM) are control tools showing the relationship among the activities that make up a project. The renovation of a wing of a facility, for example, may be mapped out with time estimates for completion of each necessary step, the critical path. This aids in allocating resources (Argenti, 1994, p. 322).

Concepts of Efficiency and Effectiveness

Efficiency is the ability to produce the desired effect with a minimum of effort, expense, or waste (Webster's *New World Dictionary,* 1968). Efficiency can be measured by the ratio of effective work to the energy expended in producing it. In systems terms this simply means getting the maximum outputs with the minimum inputs (Hitt et al., 2001, pp. 6, 131, 145).

Effectiveness is the power or ability to bring about the desired results. A nursing home that sets a goal of achieving excellence in resident care and then does so is said to be effective. The effective home may not, however, be efficiently achieving excellence of patient care. The home may, for example, be employing a large number of nurses and aides to accomplish excellence in resident care. Yet, studies in human resources reveal that when more people are placed on a work shift than are needed, the quality of care is not necessarily improved. The staff may simply divide the work up to lighten the load for everyone, or take more frequent breaks and not actually give additional attention to the residents. In this case, the too heavy staff/resident ratio may lead to both inefficiency and ineffectiveness.

The solution is to assign the optimum number of staff known to be needed to provide excellent care to a specified number of residents, and then, to manage their time so that the amount of work and quality are optimized. In this way, the manager achieves both efficiency (the desired effect with a minimum of effort, expense, or waste) and effectiveness (the desired results). Given enough resources and appropriate consultation, almost any nursing home administrator can achieve effectiveness. What is essential today is to be both effective and efficient.

1.6.8 HISTORY OF THE CONCEPT OF MANAGEMENT

Administrators have been managing organizations, large and small, for thousands of years.

It is believed that some 5,000 years ago the Sumerian civilization (Iran and Iraq of today) developed a script to control business accounts (George, 1972, p. 143). Clay tablets recording business transactions of that ancient time have been found by archaeologists. We have records of Cheops, the Egyptian king who built the Great Pyramid about 2900 B.C. We know that this monument covered 13 acres and employed 100,000 laborers for 20 years and that 8,368 lower-, middle-, and upper-level managers administered the project (George, 1972, p. 5; Robbins & Coulter, 2007, p. 28). In ancient Greece music was used to govern motions in the production lines.

In the fifth century B.C., Plato reports in *The Republic* a dialogue between Socrates and a Greek general about the extent to which management is a transferable skill. The general, it seems, was incensed that the Athenian Assembly had just appointed the manager of the Athenian chorus as the commander-in-chief of the army, because he had shown himself to be an excellent fundraiser and chorus director. Socrates argued that if the man could run the chorus well and raise the necessary revenue, then he could also be a good general (George, 1972, p. 16). Fifteen upper-level executives of General Motors more recently expressed the same view of their own ability to manage almost anything during a 15-month study of their skills conducted by a Harvard Business School professor (Kotter, 1982, p. 8). Managers' opinions of their capabilities have not changed much over the last 5,000 years.

Scientific Management

By the 1800s the early scientific management movement was underway in England as an outgrowth of the industrial revolution. The managers at Soho Foundry of Boulton, Watt, and Co. were concerned with market research and forecasting, planned site location, machine layout study, production standards and planning, standard components, cost controls, cost accounting, employee training, work study and incentives, and employee welfare (Argenti, 1994, p. 348; George, 1972, p. 59; Robbins & Coulter, 2007, p. 30).

During that epoch a management literature began to appear, but there was little recognition of the principles of management we have discussed. Current management philosophy in the West seems to have evolved from four schools of thought, although various writers refine them even further (Levey & Loomba, 1984, p. 495).

Human Relations Management

At the end of the 19th century a group of writers who believed management could be an exact science emerged. They focused on the physical activities involved in production. Frederic Taylor (Robbins & Coulter, 2007, p. 39) conducted research in a Philadelphia machine shop, demonstrating with time and motion studies that work then done by as many as 450 shovelers at Bethlehem Steel could be accomplished by as few as 150 persons, provided they received instructions to improve their effort. Frank Gilbreth's time and motion studies are well known. Henry Gantt developed his now widely used Gantt Chart with its task and bonus plan and standard hour concept (Robbins & Coulter, 2007, p. 246).

Early in the 20th century, Henri Fayol identified management "universals" as: to plan, to organize, to command (tell others), and to coordinate (control; Robbins & Coulter, 2007, p. 14). Fayol thus developed one of the earliest formulations of a general theory of management. The Process School members, such as Fayol and James Mooney, focused on departmentalization, coordination, and organizational form—the issues we have discussed under "organizing" (Johns & Saks, 2001, p. 455).

During the 1920s and 1930s, a group of theorists led by Elton Mayo described management as consisting primarily of human relations skills. According to them, successful organizations fulfill not only the employees' economic needs but also their social and psychological needs.

Sponsored by the National Research Council, Mayo conducted several experiments at the Hawthorne manufacturing plant to determine the effect of illumination on output (Johns & Saks, 2001, p. 568; Robbins & Coulter, 2007, pp. 36, 39). He found that production rose for the experimental group when illumination was increased. But the control group also produced more, although it had no increase in illumination. Illumination was then reduced to the barest minimum in both groups, yet their production continued to rise, the apparent reason being the increased attention they were given by the managers (George, 1972, pp. 136–137; Robbins & Coulter, 2007, p. 36). His experiments convinced Mayo that human factors exercise the most powerful influence on employee behavior, because the workers need to participate in social groups. Work arrangements, he concluded, besides meeting production requirements, must meet the employee's need for social satisfaction on the job. Unfortunately, the Behavioral School experienced a low predictability rate (Johns & Saks, 2001, p. 568).

Computers and Management

Various names are applied to management theory emerging after World War II (Johns & Saks, 2001, p. 487). Its major thrust has been systems theory—our approach here. Mathematical quantification is the hallmark of these theories. This is made possible by the development of computers capable of processing enormous quantities of intricate data (Johns & Saks, 2001, p. 512). Some members of the management science schools believe that almost everything can be quantified. This may be so. However, the problem remains that people assign the mathematical weights to each factor quantified, and then others must interpret for themselves the meaning they attach to the quantified results (Demski, 1980, p. 29; Robbins & Coulter, 2007, p. 100).

Whatever one's personal views about quantification, it is clear that computers are affording managers access to much information previously too laborious, too expensive, or too slow to obtain on a timely basis. Computers are a major management tool at regional and national offices of nursing home chains. Computerization of the local nursing facility is now nearly mandatory to process the Minimum Data Set, patient care planning, and other types of necessary reporting. Computers are the only means to keep up with the regulatory process. Others view the computer as a way to expand communication capabilities and perform data analyses that enhance decision making (Hegland, 1995, p. 4; Johns & Saks, 2001, pp. 346–350).

Managing is an exceptionally complex, multidimensional task not yet fully understood by the social sciences. Much has been learned, however that can be useful to the nursing home administrator in their efforts to assure a caring environment while running the nursing facility as a good business operation.

Nursing facilities will, of necessity, enter the e-commerce business in seeking admissions and developing marketing strategies (Hitt et al., 2001, pp. 3–5, 18). The Internet is increasingly driving mergers and acquisitions in industry, and nursing homes are not exempt (Hitt et al., 2001, p. 273).

Computer systems are now virtually mandatory at both the corporate and local facility level. Worker skill in the use of new technologies such as computer-aided med passes, government required computer-to-computer reporting not only for billing, but for resident care through the Minimum Data

Set (MDS) patient record, must be anticipated and supported by the administrator (Maddox & Sussman, 2001, p. 689; Noe et al., 2000, p. viii).

In addition, facilities are increasingly expected to have not only their own (or corporate) Web site, but also their own Blog, or online journal (Robbins & Coulter, 2007, pp. 100, 308).

The nursing facility front office will need to utilize advanced office technology to keep up with Medicare, Medicaid, and other third-party billing. In 2007, for example, Medicare changed to a new billing form UB-04 in tandem with the National Provider Identifier Number (NPI) with which the administrator must cope. Computerization of most aspects of resident care is being mandated by Congress.

Summary

In this section, we have examined a number of concepts: policy making, decision making (Argenti, 1994, p. 251), styles, power, authority, and the need for communication skills, norms and values. We have touched lightly on a number of concepts guiding the administrator in attempts to direct the efforts of the nursing facility and have indicated that the administrator, in providing day-to-day guidance for the staff, assures that they know what is expected of them.

Having done this, administrators may be tempted to rest on their oars. This could be a fatal error in judgment. We have demonstrated that organizations are volatile systems that may or may not respond to the administrator's direction. The only way an administrator can be certain that the nursing facility is in fact making appropriate progress toward implementing its policies and plans of action is by comparing the outputs (results of organizational work) with the intended results. This is the process of evaluating and controlling for quality.

1.7 Comparing and Controlling Quality

Because all organizational designs are incomplete, the quest for quality is frustratingly elusive, both in industry and in the health care setting. The quest for quality in the nursing facility is especially challenging because of the facility's organizational complexity and, more often than not, too limited resources.

Even so, or perhaps because of this circumstance, perhaps the most valuable functions managers perform for the facility are comparing (evaluating) and controlling the quality of facility outputs. *Comparing* is judging the extent to which actual results of the facility's efforts achieve the outcomes proposed in the plans. Controlling quality follows comparing. *Controlling* is successfully taking the steps necessary to adjust the policies and plans of action to more satisfactorily achieve stated goals.

One problem in controlling quality is that it obliges the manager to take sometimes unpleasant corrective actions to keep the facility on target. This may involve advising staff members that the work result is not suitable, or informing department managers that the actual outputs (level of performance) are unsatisfactory. This is invariably an awkward business and avoided by managers who hope the situation will correct itself or that the problem will simply disappear. But matters usually get worse and require attention for solution.

1.7.1 SOME REQUIREMENTS FOR EFFECTIVE CONTROL OF QUALITY

We will discuss several of the current methods used for controlling quality such as the Deming method, benchmarking, reengineering, and continuous quality improve (CQI) / total quality management (TQM; Johns & Saks, 2001, pp. 190–195, 540–541; Robbins & Coulter, 2007, p. 566).

There are at least nine conditions that any method for effective control of quality should observe.

1. Goals must be translated into policies and plans of action that are clearly stated, known, and measurable.

2. The appropriate measurements must be identified. If the wrong measurements to compare actual to expected outputs are used, no quality control system, however sophisticated, can truly inform and manage quality.

3. Limits to deviations from the goal/policy/plan of action have to be set. The manager must have predetermined and known outside limits for each output (quality goal) being controlled.

4. Information in useful form must go to staff at appropriate levels. It needs to be timely, easily understood, and unambiguous, so that the employee cannot use lack of clarity as a pretext for nonconformity.

5. Policies of actions to be taken when limits are exceeded (quality not achieved) must be known to the managers responsible for controlling outputs. Clear statements of policies are crucial for influencing staff members to take corrective actions when needed.

6. Corrective actions must be taken. To maximize the probability that managers will take needed corrective actions, an effective system of rewards and punishments is needed to encourage them to do so. When middle- and lower-level managers sense any softening in the administrator's determination to enforce the quality control policies, there will be a simultaneous softening of the quality control effort.

7. A system must be set up for constant renewal of control measures to account for any changing organizational goals (as expressed in new or modified plans of action) that are responses to changes in the external or internal environments of the organization. Middle- and lower-level managers may interpret portions of the quality control system being discarded as evidence that all of the quality control system is no longer in force. Eternal vigilance is the price of a quality control system that remains effective over an extended period of time.

8. The quality control mechanisms themselves must be functional and valued at each level of management to remain effective. If the staff responsible for enforcing quality controls do not feel the measures are acceptable and productive, excuses will be found not to rely on them.

9. Limitations of the scope and capabilities of the quality control system itself must be kept constantly in mind. They are never perfect. It is not possible to devise an organizational quality control system that does not need the good judgment of concerned employees to arrive at an interpretation of what the organization "really wants" in any situation (Hitt et al., 2001, p. 213; Robbins & Coulter, 2007, p. 48).

1.7.2 DIAGNOSING / ORGANIZATIONAL QUALITY

In caring for their patients, physicians base their treatment protocols on their medical diagnoses, which they interpret from the patient's presenting symptoms. In the same way administrators are organizational diagnosticians who manage the nursing home facility by using judgments based on their interpretation of presenting organizational symptoms. Physicians diagnose and treat patient illnesses; administrators diagnose and treat organizational illnesses. In the literature, organizational illnesses are often referred to as organizational pathologies. Organizational pathology is the study and diagnosis of what is believed to be a problem adversely affecting the nursing facility (Johns & Saks, 2001, pp. 264–265; Robbins & Coulter, 2007, p. 283).

In this section we will compare organizational care concepts to diagnoses. Three diagnoses that affect us all also affect organizations:

- atherosclerosis (narrowing and hardening of the arteries, allowing less blood to flow),
- aortic stenosis (a stiffening of the main blood vessel supplying the body, reducing the amount of blood reaching the limbs), and
- congestive heart failure (CHF; a progressive reduction of the heart's ability to pump enough blood), which often leads to peripheral vascular diseases (reduced blood flow to the limbs).

Organizations suffer from similar pathologies (disease processes), reducing their effectiveness and ability to function.

Managers have always sought to achieve quality control in their organizations, but this remains one of the more elusive aspects of successful managing. A number of studies have been conducted to discover quality indicators for nursing facilities.

For more than three decades the Centers for Medicare and Medicaid Services (CMS) have sought to measure and improve quality measures through data collection and assessment using forms developed by CMS using information collected pertaining to the residents' physical, clinical conditions and abilities. The quality measures change from time to time. In 2006 CMS focused on the following as quality measures

- Percent of residents whose need for help with daily activities has increased (national average in 2006 was 17%)
- Percent of residents who have moderate to severe pain (national average in 2006 was 5%)

- Percent of high-risk residents who have pressure sores (national average in 2006 was 13%)
- Percent of low-risk residents who have pressure sores (national average in 2006 was 2%)
- Percent of residents who are physically restrained (national average in 2006 was 6%)
- Percent of residents who are more depressed or anxious (national average in 2006 was 15%)
- Percent of low-risk residents who lose control of their bowels or bladder (national average in 2006 was 48%)
- Percent of residents who have/had a catheter inserted and left in their bladder (national average in 2006 was 6%)
- Percent of residents who spend most of their time in bed or in a chair (national average in 2006 was 4%)
- Percent of residents whose ability to move about in and around their room worsened (national average in 2006 was 14%)
- Percent of residents with a urinary tract infection (national average in 2006 was 9%)
- Percent of residents who lose too much weight (national average in 2006 was 9%)
- Percent of long-term stay residents with delirium (national average in 2006 was 3%)
- Percent of short-stay residents who had moderate to severe pain (national average in 2006 was 22%)
- Percent of short-stay residents with pressure sores (national average in 2006 was 18%)

Beginning in 2007 CMS also made hospital quality indicators available to the public at www.hospitalcompare.hhs.gov, which might be a valuable tool for the administrator to use in deciding to which hospitals to send residents.

The W. Edwards Deming Approach to Assuring Quality in Organizations

Born in 1900, the late Dr. W. Edwards Deming helped the U.S. Census Bureau prepare for the 1940 census with statistical techniques that used sampling rather than 100% surveys. After World War II he was invited to Japan by the Supreme Command for the Allied Powers to assist preparations for the 1951 Japanese census. In brief, Dr. Deming became a major force in the quality control movement in Japan that, it is believed by many, helped vault Japan into its position as a world leader in the production of quality products.

Dr. Deming was not "discovered" in the United States until his appearance on June 24, 1980, on a television documentary titled "If Japan Can … Why Can't We?" (Molloy, 1994, pp. 36–37). This led to his immediate broad popularity in the United States. Dr. Deming lectured on his 14 points and 7 deadly organizational diseases to enthusiastic American corporate executives even while wheelchair bound until a few weeks before his death at 93. His 14 points and 7 deadly organizational diseases, along with their potential application to the nursing home industry, are explored in the following paragraphs (Robbins & Coulter, 2007, p. 566). At first blush, Deming's points may seem too focused on the manufacturing plant. The thrust of his observations have application to nursing facility operation.

Deming's 14 Points

1. *Create and publish to all employees a statement of the aims and purposes of the … organization. The management must demonstrate constantly their commitment to this statement.* The role of the corporation, he argued, rather than making money, is to stay in business and provide jobs through innovation (Argenti, 1994, p. 224), research, constant improvement, and maintenance. The nursing home chain goal, then, is to stay in business and to provide jobs. This is to be accomplished through innovation (discovering current health care needs and foreseeing future health care needs), research (finding out how effective current care is, finding new ways to give better care), constant improvement (of the experience of being a resident in their facilities), and maintenance (keeping everything in working order).

2. *Learn the new philosophy, top management, and everybody.* Don't tolerate poor caregiving and sullen service to residents. Mistakes and negativism in approaching residents and other staff are not acceptable.

3. *Understand the purpose of inspection, for improvement of processes and reduction of cost.* Focus on the resident's daily experience, not on nursing summaries and plans of care. Mass inspections means inspecting the product as it comes off the line or at major stages—defective products are thrown out or reworked, which means paying twice; paying employees to give less than quality care, then paying them to correct poor care (preventing decubiti is easier and less expensive than curing decubiti), and this does not lead to corrective actions. Quality, Deming argues, comes not from inspections but from improvement of the process, that is, keep the focus on improving the caregiving

process, not on the quality of the nurses' notes or doctors' orders, but rather on achieving an improved level of care, that is, keep focused on improving the resident's daily experience.

4. *End the practice of awarding business on the basis of price tag alone.* Buying the lowest priced often means buying low quality. The goal should be to identify a single quality supplier for any one item in a long-term relationship. For example, food vendors. The goal should be good dependable quality over a long period of time, consistently good food supplies, medical supplies, physical therapy, pharmacy supplies, and the like.

5. *Improve constantly and forever the system of production and service.* Management's job is to continually look for ways to reduce waste and improve quality, that is, don't use expensive medicine cups as water cups while doing medication rounds.

6. *Institute training.* Too often nursing assistants, licensed practical nurses, and even the directors of nursing learn their job from workers who were never trained properly. Workers are forced to follow poor instruction sets and cannot do their jobs because no one told them how.

7. *Teach and institute leadership.* The nurse supervisor or department head's job is not to tell nursing assistants what to do or punish, but to lead, (i.e., help employees do a better job), learning by objective methods who needs individual help (i.e., sort out the nursing assistants whose work is not in an acceptable range). This will pay real dividends in safer resident care and reduce risks at a facility.

8. *Drive out fear. Create trust Create a climate for innovation.* Create an atmosphere in which employees feel secure enough to ask questions, take positions, admit errors, and learn by them, not get out the "whiteout" or write an erroneous incident or accident report.

9. *Optimize toward the aims and purposes of the company the efforts of teams, groups, and staff areas.* Facility staff often compete or have goals that conflict: nursing vs. dietary, nursing vs. housekeeping (who cleans up the spill?), dietary vs. activities, vs. nursing vs. housekeeping (who is responsible for the resident's afternoon bingo?).

10. *Eliminate exhortations for the workforce.* Deming believed these never helped anybody do a good job; instead, let people put up their own slogans.

11. *Eliminate numerical quotas for production. Instead, learn and institute methods for improvement. Eliminate Management by Objectives. Instead, learn the capabilities of processes and how to improve them.* Numbers take account only of numbers, not quality or methods. Quotas

usually guarantee inefficiencies and high cost. Most Continuous Quality Improvement (CQI) programs set numerical quotas in nearly every departmental area. Employees become focused on attaining these quotas themselves. Achieving the numerical goal becomes the employees' goal and focus, not improving the resident's daily experience. Deming agrees that the "goal" of quotas is laudable, but become ends in themselves and the employee will "meet the quota" at any price, regardless of the damage to the facility (e.g., the nurse determined to pass medications at or below the prescribed error rate disregarding a small crisis that needs managing during the medication pass).

12. *Remove barriers that rob people of pride of workmanship.* People are eager to do a good job and become distressed when they can't because of misguided supervisors, faulty equipment, or defective materials. For example, too few nursing hours are provided by the facility to permit the nursing assistants or the rest of the staff to make Mrs. Jones's experience that day a good one, for example, the proverbial, "we're working short today" answer to numerous resident requests. If possible, avoid using nursing pool personnel. They don't know the residents and, all too often, don't care.

13. *Encourage education and self-improvement for everyone.* Both management and the staff will have to be educated in the new methods, including teamwork and statistical techniques.

14. *Take action to accomplish the transformation.* Deming, like most others who prescribe quality improvement programs, emphasized a need to involve top management in any quality improvement effort, but emphasized that it takes both managers and the workers for success.

Deming's 7 Deadly Organizational Diseases

1. *Lack of constancy of purpose.* Keep the focus on staying in business, including long range plans, not on making dividends next quarter or paying good dividends this year, that is, the workers need to feel the corporation is preparing for the future and will stay in the business of giving health care.

2. *Emphasis on short term profits.* Don't worry about paying a dividend.

3. *Evaluation by performance, merit rating, or annual review of performance.* These, Deming felt, destroy teamwork and nurture rivalry. Done improperly, performance ratings can build fear; leave people despondent, bitter, or beaten; and encourage mobility of management.

4. *Mobility of management.* Job hoppers don't understand the facility and are not there long enough to follow through on long-term changes needed for quality and productivity (e.g., three directors of nurses in 1 year, three administrators in as many years).
5. *Running a company on visible figures alone.* The most important figures, Deming argued, are unknown and unknowable, for example, resident satisfaction. Point: The achievement of a nursing facility's staff cannot be reduced to numbers alone.
6. *Excessive medical costs.* (What more should be said on this issue?)
7. *Excessive costs of warranty, fueled by lawyers who work on contingency fee.* Successful malpractice suits against nursing facilities continue to raise the cost of required insurance.

To prescribe Deming's diagnosis for all corporations is like a physician writing the same prescriptions for all their patients regardless of the stages of the various diseases the patients present. Deming was prescribing corrections to organizational illnesses he felt existed in the United States. Essentially, he was pointing to excesses—good ideas originally, but taken too far, or becoming mindless rules in themselves. What's right and what's wrong with organizations changes over time and resemble the swings of a pendulum, as does Deming's list of deadly organizational diseases. But Deming has some enduring messages for U.S. industry and the nursing facility, powerful reminders of how difficult it is for the facility to keep the importance of the resident constantly in focus. Others have other diagnoses and have written their own prescriptions to assist organizations to achieve and maintain quality. The Centers for Medicare and Medicaid Services (CMS) certainly have, and the CMS prescribed ways of operating the facility dominate every participating facilities daily actions.

Benchmarking

Benchmarking is a management tool by which an organization seeks to improve its business practices by comparing them with the best practices of other organizations (Argenti, 1994, p. 60; Hitt et al., 2001, p. 212; Robbins & Coulter, 2007, p. 243). The Westinghouse Corporation uses benchmarking as a quality control tool within its Total Quality Improvement Process for "identifying best practices, wherever they exist, implementing and communicating those practices throughout Westinghouse to improve competitive performance and preserve our core competencies" (Argenti, 1994, p. 61).

A Five-Step Description

Benchmarking studies not only the very best practices of other corporations, but also seeks any clearly better practices as sufficient to justify a benchmarking effort. One writer describes benchmarking as consisting of five steps:

1. Deciding what to benchmark
2. Forming a team
3. Identifying benchmark partners
4. Collecting and analyzing the benchmarking information
5. Implementing the new methodology (Spendolini, 1992, p. 48).

Benchmarking is a measuring process resulting in comparing performance measures, but it also describes how the superior performance is attained. The practices that lead to exceptional performance are called enablers. Benchmarking, then, results in two types of outputs: (a) measures of comparative performance, and (b) enablers, the theory behind the more successful process being benchmarked.

A Four-Step Description

Another writer describes benchmarking as a four-step process (Argenti, 1994, pp. 61–62):

1. Selecting and defining the process to be studied. What should we benchmark? Who should we benchmark?
2. Gather as much information as possible about the process, then communicate with the organization being benchmarked through telephone surveys, written questionnaires, and/or on-site visits.
3. Analyze the information gained to determine the magnitude of the performance gap, and identify the process enablers that facilitated the performance improvement at the organization chosen as a benchmark.
4. Adapt, improve, and implement the benchmarked process in one's own organization.

For example, most major nursing home chains strive to serve a predominantly private-paying and Medicare eligible clientele. One chain has consistently achieved this to a far greater extent than most. Chains that, despite their goals, have low census of private paying and Medicare residents might seek to "benchmark" the successful chain, that is, study and learn the process by which that one chain achieves its desired resident mix noticeably more successfully than the rest.

Benchmarking at St. Judes: Nursing homes might benefit from the "benchmarking" effort of St Jude's Hospital in Southern California. Concerned that their admissions area might be discouraging patients by its complexity, cold attitudes, long waiting periods, and confusing directions once inside, the hospital managers benchmarked hotels—the true professionals on admissions. Out of this benchmarking effort came plans for a door person, a bell person to carry bags, a concierge to advise about the hospital itself, and computerized admissions. Larger signs were installed in the lobby, which was freshly painted, and music now greets the incoming patients.

Deming warned that it is a hazard simply to copy, that it is necessary to understand the theory of what makes the benchmarked process more successfully. He cautioned: Adapt, don't adopt. The process enablers that result in high private census in the more successful nursing home chain reflect a specific business environment and corporate culture. It may or may not work when introduced into a different chain seeking to raise its own private paying census.

Total Quality Management / Continuous Quality Improvement

The earliest quality and quality control publications that led to the current total quality management (TQM) literature may have been initiated by Walter A. Shewhart at Bell Telephone Laboratories in the 1920s (*Economic Control of Quality Manufactured Product,* 1931; Hitt et al., 2001, p. 175; Melum & Siniotis, 1992, p. 347). An extensive literature on TQM has emerged and is explored in depth in the American Hospital Association book *Total Quality Management: The Health Care Pioneers* (Melum & Siniotis, 1992).

Definitional Difficulties

Total Quality Management (TQM) is difficult to define precisely, because it is a philosophy of total organizational involvement in improving all aspects of quality of service. There is no single set of steps that has gained broad acceptance as the TQM methodology. However, the basic concept is similar to Deming's fifth, point which is "improve constantly and forever the system of production and service." This view is that it is too expensive to maintain quality by inspections and more efficient to produce quality in the first place.

Quality at the Source

To achieve this, responsibility for quality is ultimately placed with the workers who actually produce the service or product. This is sometimes called quality at the source. In this scheme the quality departments are focused on training employees in quality control and implementing the quality control concepts throughout the organization (Noe et al., 2000, p. 55). Employee empowerment in decision making, the use of teams in the organization, the use of individual responsibility for services, and customer service are characteristics of most TQM efforts (Johns & Saks, 2001, pp. 225, 264).

Continuous Quality Improvement

According to Melum and Siniotis (1992), TQM is a customer-driven approach that applies the scientific method to improve organizations' systems. In their view, the focus on quality is total, including every aspect of an organization—its services, products, suppliers, business procedures, management systems, and human resources. To them, TQM is a process of continuous improvement—a process of continuously striving to exceed customer expectations. Problems in the organization are viewed as problems of processes used, not of individuals, within the organization—processes that can be improved using TQM approaches.

J. M. Juran

J. M. Juran (1988), another important figure in the managing for quality movement, summarizes the process of managing for quality as three-fold:

1. Quality planning: Decide who the customers are and what their needs are; develop features that respond to their needs and develop processes to respond.
2. Quality control: Evaluate the actual outputs, compare output to expected output, and act on the difference.
3. Quality improvement: Establish the needed infrastructure, identify improvement projects, and establish project teams. Train, motivate, and empower the teams to diagnose the causes, find remedies, and maintain gains.

Structure Process Outcome

When the nursing industry began to assume its present size and shape in the late 1960s quality measurements were primarily focused on structure, that is, an adequate physical plant, the proper equipment, enough trained staff, and enough income. The idea was that Medicare, Medicaid, and state nursing home inspectors should assure that the "structure" needed to give good care was in place. Structure, in the systems model we have described previously, is the inputs (Hitt et al., 2001, pp. 6, 145). The quality of care, however, remained unsatisfactorily low.

Process

Attention of the federal and state inspectors was then expanded to include both structure and process. Inspecting for process meant assuring that all the organizational arrangements believed needed were in place. Process is the portion of our systems model described earlier, appropriately enough, as the processor, that is, the work the organization accomplishes. Structure measures the capacity to give resident care. Process measures the way in which resident care is given. For example:

- Are the Minimum Data Sets (MDS) appropriately filled out?
- Is a well developed plan of care in place?
- Are all the resident assessment protocols triggered by the minimum data set appropriately filled out and being followed?

Outcome

Even after measuring for both structure and process, Congress ruled through the Nursing Home Reform Act in 1987 that inspectors must focus not only on structure (capacity to give care) and process (the giving of care), but also on the outcomes of the caregiving. Outcome, the third part of our previously described systems model, is the result of the effort made, the measurable impacts on the resident in the case of the nursing facility. Outcome focuses on measuring whether residents are in fact enjoying a high quality of life, full enjoyment of the Patient's Rights established by Congress, and receiving high quality nursing and medical care.

Some examples of outcome measurements may be in order.

- Congress, in the federal requirements, phrased these outcome measures in the following manner. §483.25 Quality of Care: Each resident must receive and the facility must provide the necessary care and services to attain or maintain the highest practicable physical, mental, and psychosocial well-being, in accordance with the comprehensive assessment and plan of care.

Other Examples:

- There follow a number of outcome measures to be enforced, for example, a resident's abilities in activities of daily living do not diminish unless circumstances of the individual's clinical condition demonstrate that diminution was unavoidable.
- This reasoning is extended to vision and hearing, urinary incontinence, range of motion, mental and psychosocial functioning, naso-gastric

tubes, accidents, nutrition, hydration, special needs, unnecessary drugs, and medication errors (Landefeld, Palmer, Johnson, Johnston, & Lyons, 2004, p. 42; Maddox & Sussman, 2001, p. 385). Regarding pressure sores, for example, the outcome requirement is that a resident who enters the facility without pressure (decubitus) sores does not develop pressure sores unless the individual's clinical condition demonstrates that they were unavoidable.

The current approach used by the CMS (Medicare, Medicaid) surveyors is to look at outcomes first. Only if outcomes appear deficient will the surveyors examine the processes by which the facility is giving care. If both outcome and processes appear unsatisfactory the surveyors will examine the caregiving structures in place.

Establishing and Judging Quality in the Nursing Facility

Nearly every nursing facility in the United States has its own mission statement with its accompanying goals for quality of resident care and resident life. Often, local facilities write their own mission statement with quality goals carefully spelled out in statements of policy and procedures for the facility.

Whose Quality Goals Matter?

In the daily life of the American nursing facility, it is the quality goals of CMS (Centers for Medicare & Medicaid Services; formerly Health Care Financing Administration [HCFA]) that ultimately matter. Administrators seldom judge their success or failure by corporate or facility standards. Rather, administrators' feelings about success or failure are dictated more by CMS's quality standards embodied in the Federal Requirements and Guidelines to Surveyors. This has come about because CMS surveys every facility on a nearly annual basis, decides whether the facility is deficiency free, and if not deficiency free may impose Civil Money Penalties of large sums (sometimes $100,000s). CMS requires that its quality judgments (survey results) be displayed prominently for all who visit the facility to see and posts survey results on the Web for everyone in the world to see! Not satisfied with that, each facility's survey results are posted on the Web at CMS's Nursing Home Compare site.

The practical reality is that CMS's judgments become, for most facilities, both the *de jure* (by law) and *de facto* (by practice) quality standards for U.S. nursing facilities. And if the surveyors are really unhappy they can put the facility on a "fast-track" to decertification (end Medicare and Medicaid eligibility) and prohibit new admissions until satisfied with the facility's plan for correcting the deficiencies. Given the razor thin operating margins of most facilities, inability to admit new residents, even for a short time, can induce traumatic economic woe.

The Federal Quality Assurance Process: Understanding and Accessing Federal Requirements

Nearly all federal requirements for nursing home facilities are available on the CMS (Centers for Medicare and Medicaid Services) Web site, www.cms.hhs. gov. By visiting this Web site the nursing home administrator can access and download necessary CMS information.

The essential information base includes the following.

Performance Measures

The primary instruments used to measure the performance of the nursing facility include the following.

Quality Measures

These vary from year to year as CMS seeks to progressively improve performance in various aspects of care. These are found on the CMS Web site under Medicare, then Nursing Home Quality Initiatives.

- The Long-Term Care Facility User's Manual
- The Minimum Data Set (MDS)
- The Long-Term Care Resident Assessment Instrument (RAI) User's Manual for the Minimum Data Set
- The Long-Term Care Enforcement Procedures

These information sets can be downloaded from the CMS Web site or purchased in paper or electronic forms from such associations as the American Health Care Association (www.ahca.com) or companies in the field such as the Briggs Corporation (www.briggs.com).

Continuous Quality Improvement at CMS

CMS quality improvement efforts are ongoing and change focus as deemed by CMS to be needed. Current quality improvements such as the DAVE (Data Assessment and Verification Program) may be assessed from the CMS Web site Nursing Home Quality Initiatives section (www.cms.hhs.gov/Nursing HomeQualityInits/).

Daily Update Information for the Administrator

In addition to frequent visits to the previously listed Web sites, the administrator may choose to receive daily update information via email by signing up on email lists at the Centers for Medicare and Medicaid Services and similar Web sites.

Some Common Acronyms and Definitions

The following are some common acronyms and definitions of terms associated with assessing residents and setting the payment level for each Medicare/Medicaid resident.

Case Mix. A measure of the intensity of care and services used by a group of residents in a nursing facility. "Case" refers to the overall data collected and used regarding an individual person under study. "Used" describes the combination of variables (observations) used for classifying an observation according to distinctive characteristics on the basis of a dependent variable, such as time or costs.

Case Mix Index. Each RUG-III (or current RUG version) group is assigned a weight, or numeric score, which reflects the relative resources predicted to provide care to a resident. The higher the case mix index (weight), the greater the resource requirements are for the resident. Payment for each resident is made monthly to the facility based on the case mix index for the facility.

Centers for Medicare and Medicaid Services (CMS; formerly the Health Care Financing Administration). The federal agency that administers the Medicare, Medicaid, and Child Health Insurance Programs.

Code of Federal Regulations (CFR). The federal Congress passes laws for which implementing rules are written and enforced . . . these are the *Federal Requirements and Guidelines to Surveyors.*

Data Assessment and Verification (DAVE). A program administered by CMS designed to ensure accuracy of MDS data accomplished through data analysis, off-site review, on-site review, and provider education.

Hierarchy. A Research Utilization Group methodology of assessment classification where an assessment is placed in the first classification category (there are over 40 reimbursement categories) and where a match is found by evaluating resident conditions and services. For the RUG-III version this included seven resident groups, ordered from highest to lowest, for example extensive services, rehabilitation, special care, clinically complex, impaired cognition, behavioral problems, and reduced physical functions. These categories vary from time to time.

MDS Completion Date. The date at which the RN assessment coordinator attests that all portions of the MDS have been completed.

Medicare Data Communication Network (MDCN). A secure connection that is used to transmit MDS data to each state's repository. A user ID and password is issued for each person who requires access to the CMS MDS intranet.

Minimum Data Set (MDS). A core set of screening, clinical, and functional status elements, including common definitions and coding categories that form the foundation for the comprehensive assessment for all residents of long-term care facilities certified to participate in Medicare and/or Medicaid.

Omnibus Reconciliation Act of 1987 (OBRA). A law that enacted reforms in nursing facility care and provided the statutory authority for the MDS.

Prospective Payment System (PPS). A payment system developed for Medicare for skilled nursing facilities that pays facilities an all-inclusive rate for all Medicare Part A beneficiary services. Payment is determined by a case mix classification system (RUG-III or current version)

Quality Initiative Survey (QIS). CMS intends to move surveys in the facility to a process of doing surveys on laptops using wireless technology. This will enable the surveyors to communicate with each other via laptop throughout the survey process itself.

Resident Assessment Instrument (RAI). The designation for the complete resident assessment process mandated by CMS, including the comprehensive MDS, RAPS, and care planning decisions.

Resident Assessment Protocol (RAPS). A problem-oriented framework for organizing MDS information and additional clinically relevant information about an individual's health problems or needs. Checking certain boxes or combination of boxes upon filling out the MDS form trigger the requirement for that resident's care plan to address condition(s) identified as in need of special attention.

RUG-III. Version III, or current version, of the Resource Utilization Group, a resident classification system that identifies the relative resource use of providing care for different types of residents in nursing facilities based on their resource use.

State Operation Manual (SOM). The title given to the current set of requirements and guidelines to surveyors. Current edition with changes in red can be downloaded from the CMS Web site, www.cms.gov.

Federal Standards: Minimum or Maximum?

The literature, and, often, surveyors themselves describe the federal requirements as minimum standards. They *were* minimum standards when *only*
structure was evaluated by federal surveyors. Now, after 30+ years of intense
federal continuous quality improvement efforts, federal standards, if achieved,
can be maximal, state of the art. If all federal requirements for favorable outcomes are achieved, a remarkably high quality of care is being achieved. It is
an ongoing process. Minimum Data Set (MDS) 1.0 was followed by MDS 2.0,
followed by MDS 3.0, with continuous quality improvements to come.

Quality of Care: 1993–2006

In Table 1.2 an overview shows that on most of the federal tags (each "tag"
has an "F number" and spells out a specific federal requirement) the quality of
care achieved was very high, and in most categories exhibit improvement, for
example, reduction of unnecessary drugs from 16% in 1993 to 11% in 2006.
It is on the more subjective tags that the degree of compliance was judged by
CMS to have declined: F309 Quality of Care and F324 Accident Prevention,
in particular. On most tags facilities were in compliance well over 90% of the
time. As can be seen in Table 1.3 the number of deficiencies issued to facilities citing failure to provide quality life decreased in most quality measures
between the years 1993 and 2006.

Figure 1.4 reveals that a remarkably high 17% of facilities had no deficiencies in 1999 and a similarly remarkably low 5.7 average number of deficiencies
per facility. When one considers the approximately 330 federal requirements
on which deficiencies are given, 5.7 per facility represents 1.72% deficiency
level among the 330+ possible deficiencies per facility. The percent of facilities
reporting no deficiencies in the United States increased from 11.4% in 1993
to 17.5% in 1999. This was a 54% increase during the period. The percent
of facilities with no deficiencies varied by state from 1.5% in Washington to
48.5% in New Jersey in 1999. By 2006 even fewer facilities were receiving
deficiencies (9.1%) and fewer deficiencies were being issued (8.0%).

It may be no surprise that the number of deficiencies per facility began
rising in 1998. The federal government implemented a "crackdown" on
nursing homes at the behest of the president and consumer organizations
at the same time federal funds to facilities were being decreased due to the
draconian reductions required by the Balanced Budget Act of 1997 (see table
on page 94).

Surveyors follow guidelines in Appendix Q of the State Operations Manual
to determine immediate jeopardy, which is defined as "A situation in which

TABLE 1.2.   Percent of Nursing Facilities in the U.S. With Deficiencies for Quality of Care, 1993, 1999, and Number and Percent 2006

PERCENT DEFICIENCY IN NURSING FACILITY QUALITY OF CARE
DEFICIENCY GROUP = QUALITY OF CARE

		1993 %	1999 %	2006 %	Facilities
F309	Provide Necess Care for Well Being	11.3	21.0	27.17	4,328
F310	ADLs Do Not Decline Unless Necess	8.3	2.1	1.17	186
F311	Resident Given Appropriate Treatment	5.6	6.4	3.54	564
F312	ADL Care Provided for Dependent Res	7.6	14.0	11.45	1,824
F313	Res Receive Treatment for Vision/Hearing	0.5	0.7	0.63	100
F314	Proper Treatment for Pressure Sores	18.0	18.0	16.51	2,630
F315	Resident Not Catheterized Unless Necess	1.1	1.3	15.85	2,526
F316	Incontinence Care	11.8	11.5	0.00	0
F317	No Reduction in Range of Motion	0.7	0.9	0.36	57
F318	Range of Motion Treatment and Services	8.3	9.7	5.89	939
F319	Approp Treatment for Mental/ Psychosocial	4.5	2.6	1.66	264
F320	Not Develop Mental Problems	0.3	0.2	0.11	18
F321	No NG (Feeding) Tube Unless Necess	0.3	0.1	0.04	7
F322	Proper Care for Res with NG Tube	5.2	5.3	5.86	933
F323	Facility is Free of Accident Hazards	19.7	18.7	21.46	3,419
F324	Supervision/Devices to Prevent Accidents	6.2	17.3	20.81	3,316
F325	Residents Maintain Nutritional Status	9.4	9.9	6.80	1,084
F326	Res Receives Therapeutic Diet When Req	5.6	2.2	2.35	375
F327	Facility Provides Sufficient Fluid Intake	3.6	5.3	3.56	567
F328	Proper Treatment/Care for Special Needs	5.2	4.4	6.38	1,017
F329	Drug Regimen Has No Unnecessary Drugs	16.1	11.6	11.42	1,820
F330	No Antipsychotic Drugs Unless Necess	2.4	0.8	0.67	107
F331	Gradual Dose Reduction of Antipsychotics	2.6	1.0	1.28	204
F332	Medication Error Rates of 5% or More	8.3	7.4	11.19	1,783
F333	Res Free From Significant Med Errors	4.8	3.6	3.90	622

Source: DHHS, 2006b.

TABLE 1.3.   Percent of Nursing Facilities in the U.S. With Deficiencies for Quality of Life, 1993, 1999, and Number and Percent 2006

	DEFICIENCY GROUP = QUALITY OF LIFE: F 240–F258	1993 %	1999 %	2006 %	Facilities
F240	Facility Promotes Quality of Life	1.4	0.2	0.41	65
F241	Dignity	19.1	16.3	15.96	2,542
F242	Self-Determination—Res Makes Choices	2.6	2.6	2.37	378
F243	Res Right to Participate Res/Family Group	0.9	0.6	0.28	44
F244	Facility Must Listen to Res/Family Group	1.4	0.3	1.01	161
F245	Right to Participate Social/Relig/Communi	0.2	0.1	0.10	16
F246	Accommodation of Needs and Preferences	17.1	9.4	8.19	1,305
F247	Res Receives Notice Before Room Change	0.6	0.2	0.17	27
F248	Activity Program Meets Individual Needs	12.0	8.6	6.45	1,028
F249	Qualifications of Activities Director	1.1	0.5	0.51	81
F250	Medically Related Social Services	8.8	7.8	6.50	1,036
F251	Qualifications of Social Worker	0.9	0.3	0.19	31
F252	Safe/Clean/Homelike Environment	15.5	7.3	5.45	868
F253	Housekeeping and Maintenance Services	19.5	15.3	20.51	3,267
F254	Clean Linens in Good Condition	3.6	1.7	0.82	131
F255	Private Closet Space in Each Room	1.0	0.1	0.04	7
F256	Adequate and Comfortable Lighting Levels	2.2	0.5	0.41	65
F257	Comfortable and Safe Temperature Levels	1.7	0.9	0.82	130
F258	Comfortable Sound Levels	2.4	1.7	1.26	200

Nursing Facilities, Staffing, Residents and Facility Deficiencies, 1993–1999
Department of Social & Behavioral Sciences
University of California San Francisco

the provider's noncompliance with one or more requirements of participation has caused or is likely to cause, serious injury, harm impairment or death to a resident (see Code of Federal Regulations, 2006). Certain surveyor findings trigger immediate jeopardy such as a failure to protect from abuse, failure to prevent neglect or failure to protect from psychological harm (see Code of Federal Regulations, 2006).

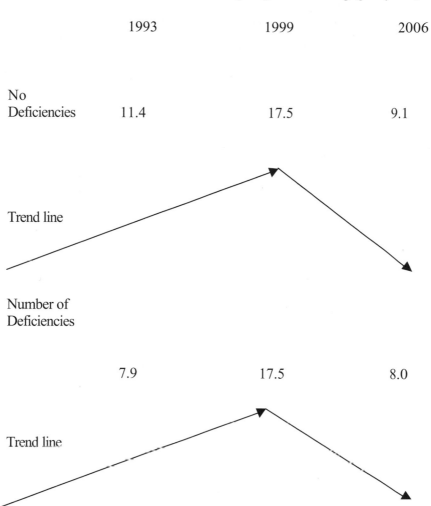

FIGURE 1.4 Trends in average number of deficiencies and percent without deficiencies of U.S. nursing facilities, 1993, 1999, and 2006.
Source: Centers for Medicare and Medicaid, 2007.

Scope and Severity Levels for Deficiencies Issued by Surveyors

	ISOLATED	PATTERNED SCOPE	WIDE-SPREAD	
More Severe	**Scope & Severity = J** Isolated—Immediate jeopardy to resident or safety	**Scope and Severity = K** Patterned—Immediate jeopardy to resident health or safety	**Scope and Severity = L** Widespread—Immediate jeopardy to resident health or safety	
	Scope & Severity = G Isolated—Actual harm that is not immediate jeopardy	**Scope and Severity = H** Patterned—No actual harm that is not immediate jeopardy	**Scope and Severity = I** Widespread—Actual harm that is not immediate jeopardy	(level G and above carry severe consequences
SEVERITY	**Scope & Severity = D** Isolated—No actual harm with potential for more than minimal harm that is not immediate jeopardy	**Scope and Severity = E** Patterned—No actual harm with potential for more than minimal harm that is not immediate jeopardy.	**Scope & Severity = F** Widespread—No actual harm with potential for more than minimal harm that is not immediate jeopardy	
Less Severe	**Scope & Severity = A** Isolated—No actual harm with potential for minimal harm	**Scope & Severity = B** Patterned—No actual harm with potential for minimal harm	**Scope & Severity = C** Widespread—No actual harm with potential for minimal harm	Levels A, B, and C deficiencies are the more typically issued.
	ISOLATED	**PATTERNED SCOPE**	**WIDE-SPREAD**	

1.8 Innovating

The effective manager is always an innovator. *Innovating* is the process of bringing new ideas into the way an organization accomplishes its purposes.

The process of innovating is the result of the administrator's study of the changes that are constantly occurring in the organization itself and the environment in which it functions. Innovating is an act of leadership. It is the manager's role to be the sensor of the organization for those external and internal changes that will have an impact on its well-being (Hitt et al., 2001, pp. 10–11; Johns & Saks, 2001, pp. 272, 277; Robbins & Coulter, 2007, p. 374).

The manager is not necessarily the innovator, but does have the task of assuring that innovation occurs within the organization. To achieve this, the manager can develop new ideas, combine old ideas into new ones, borrow and adapt ideas from other fields, or stimulate others to develop innovations (Hitt et al., 2001, pp. 537–538).

To focus on the resident and their family/significant others is to be in constant contact with the changing needs of residents. Nearly all staff have contact with residents and their families/significant others. If practical innovation is sought from all staff, the staff must become outwardly focused adaptive sensors, listening and adapting to changing needs.

Welcoming Innovations

Change Is Hard Work

Edward Wrapp observed that "Good managers don't make policy decisions; rather, they give a sense of direction and are masters at developing opportunities" (1984, p. 8; see also Hitt et al., 2001, pp. 533–534).

Wrapp addresses the question of why the good manager shies away from very precise statements of objectives for the organization. According to Wrapp, the effective manager finds it impossible to set down specific objectives that will be relevant for any extended period of time. The external environment changes continually, he observes, and the organization's strategies have to be continually revised to take these changes into account. He concludes that the more explicit the statement of strategy, the more difficult it is to persuade the employees to turn to different goals when needs and conditions change (Johns & Saks, 2001, p. 488).

Values in Imprecision

Wrapp (1984) believes that goals or objectives are communicated over time through a consistent pattern of operating decisions. We also advise guarding against the degree of specificity in goal and policy statements that discourages changes.

All of the forces that tend to lead to organizational resistance to change are formidable enemies of the manager who is obliged to introduce changes to keep the facility in tune with the environment (Johns & Saks, 2001, p. 529). The nursing home facility administrator must keep policies precise enough to guide employee decisions and at the same time continually introduce change into the facility—not an easy task (Johns & Saks, 2001, p. 492).

Innovating

A nursing facility's staff will innovate only if the administrator intentionally introduces changes in the organization that are responses to changes perceived in the environment and encourages others to do the same. Innovation is the process of finding new solutions to creating a good quality of life for residents and staff. Not all new solutions will work; the administrator must encourage and praise new solutions that fail as well as new solutions that succeed, otherwise staff will stop suggesting new solutions.

Innovation requires being in constant touch with the new—new requirements, new employment trends, new benefits, and new resident activities. To be innovative is to respond flexibly to changes in the environment. Most organizations fight innovation. Hospitals fought the introduction of birthing suites until women arranged to be delivered outside the hospital in home-like suites.

Innovation by Memo

Tom Watson, the executive who led IBM to its position of strength in the computer field, met with great resistance in introducing new technology (Hitt et al., 2001, p. C-241). In the 1950s, he attempted to move IBM from vacuum tube technology to the new transistor technology. The Japanese, he was aware, were already using tiny transistors effectively while IBM continued to use acres and acres of large vacuum tubes to accomplish the same tasks. IBM engineers had spent their lives in vacuum tube technology and weren't about to adopt the new transistor technology. After months of unsuccessful coaxing, wheedling, and cajoling, an exasperated Watson wrote a memo in which he stated that after June 1, 1958, no more vacuum tubes would be used in IBM product development (America's Most Admired Corporations, 1995, p. 28).

Innovating is not limited to the IBMs of the world. Stodgy, large, old-line corporations are successfully using innovation. In recent years the Kellogg Company has created entire new markets (adults!) for its cereals. Who would have predicted that an obscure company with the unlikely name of Minnesota Mining and Manufacturing (3M) would be one of the most innovative U.S. corporations (e.g., Post-it™)?

Rearranging Nursing Duties

A Washington, DC facility, faced with difficulties in finding nurses and pressures on nurses' time to perform administrative functions, tried replacing the charge nurse with an assistant administrator. Initially this person made out the nurse assistant assignments; insured that supplies and linen were available to the nursing assistants and the nurses; resolved any logistical problems with transportation, dietary, and housekeeping; and coordinated any immediate and long-term maintenance and housekeeping needs for the unit. This new employee made rounds daily or more often assuring that residents' needs were being met and that nurse aides were following nursing directives (i.e., walking, turning, and repositioning residents as required). This freed nurses to concentrate more on resident assessment, medication administration, and care conferences. In this case, everyone wins. The facility enables the more expensive nurse time to be devoted to good nursing care and the residents' quality of care and level of satisfaction is improved by a unit manager who is practicing leading by walking around (LBWA).

The American health insurance industry grew out of an innovation developed by a hospital administrator in Texas. Faced with a drastically reduced cash flow in the depression because patients had little money, he devised a plan to create a regular cash flow to this hospital, Baylor University Hospital, from the one group left who had a steady income: school teachers paid from public taxes. For 50 cents a month, he offered up to 14 days of prepaid hospital care per year. The teachers bought the idea, and the U.S. health insurance was born.

An AIDS Policy Innovation

While innovation is an expected part of the job description of the chief executive of a large nursing home chain, it can occur at the local level even in highly centralized chains. AIDS patients are now routinely admitted to most nursing home facilities. During a time when no AIDS patients were being admitted in a certain state, including all facilities owned by that large chain, a local nursing facility administrator decided it was time for a new policy. She announced her determination to admit AIDS patients to her facility; persuaded corporate officials not to interfere; and orchestrated a 9-month long intensive preparation period for her staff, residents, and significant others at the end of which she began routinely admitting AIDS patients with hardly a ripple in the daily life of the facility. Her census was better, the staff were proud, the residents and their significant others were comfortable, and the corporation changed its policies.

The innovators tend to be survivors of change. The future belongs to those organizations that are successful in constantly innovating over time. The years of the 21st century hold promise to innovators in the nursing home industry.

Success today requires that, compared to your competitors, you be more creative, more customer focused, and more cost conscious.

1.9 Marketing the Long-Term Care Facility

1.9.1 THE TURN TO MARKETING

Why, one might ask, should the nursing facility administrator be concerned with marketing? The proportion of Americans who will need nursing facility care is expected to increase yearly at least through the middle of the 21st century. Resident waiting lists exist in some facilities in response to Medicare's prospective payment method (the DRGs) placing more and more pressure on hospitals to rapidly discharge acute care patients to nursing homes and, increasingly, home health agencies for periods of subacute and managed care. Even so, a number of factors are coming together that may threaten any seeming guarantee of high occupancy rates.

Forces Leading to Competition

Narrowed Profit Margins

The ability of a nursing facility to survive economically is affected by an increasing variety of pressures such as federal and state reimbursement policies, the types of services offered by the facility, and the sources of resident payment. Over the past decades government regulators who pay for care of Medicare and Medicaid residents in nursing facilities have sought ways to narrow the margin of facility profit to achieve mandated government cost savings.

At the same time, facility costs have increased in meeting the additional regulatory requirements under the nursing home reform act and subsequent amendments. Such bills as the Americans with Disabilities Act, the Family Medical Leave Act, and the more rigorous universal precautions requirements all add costs, often unreimbursed, to providing care. Increasing human resources costs, particularly as the level of acuity increases, for personnel such as nurses threatens profitability. One geriatrician has observed that if trends toward increasing acuity of care continue, nursing facilities will be forced to staff up toward hospital bed labor costs.

Reduction of Federal Influence in Shaping the Product Mix

Product design in nursing facilities, that is, the mix of services and business activities, has been heavily influenced by product and price decisions made by the Medicaid and Medicare agencies. The payment policies of the states' Medicaid offices, along with Medicare claims authorities, were predominant influences on prices charged and services offered in the industry (Hitt et al., 2001, pp. 277–279).

Survival of the average facility may depend on the administrator being able to find a niche—to identify and successfully market the offerings of the facility to defined groups of persons who need the emerging types of services now available.

Always Mess With Success

The most cogent reason to turn to marketing the nursing facility is that if you don't mess with your success, your competitor will. Conventional wisdom has advised, don't mess with success. It is easy to be blinded by one's short-term success. Whenever a facility feels it has achieved premier status as the best caregiver in the community, whenever it starts taking its success for granted, it will lull itself into complacency and slack off.

The fast moving computer world is littered with such companies. A few years ago Digital Equipment Corporation (DEC) captured a big chunk of IBM's mid-range computer sales, then rested on its laurels only to be wiped out a year later when its winning (and only) design suddenly became obsolete. IBM itself, after six decades of warding off all temptations to rest on its laurels under the leadership of Tom Watson, Sr. and Tom Watson, Jr., also declined as soon as the latter retired. Just as soon as DEC and IBM began plateauing, they began plunging.

Good isn't good enough. Good-enough nursing facilities (public opinion notwithstanding) abound. Simply doing a good job of marketing the facility will not yield the edge necessary to succeed in today's pressure-packed health care marketplace. Good only puts you with the rest of the pack.

1.9.2 THE "MARKETING" OF HEALTH CARE

Several years ago the U.S. Supreme Court ruled illegal any self-imposed restrictions by health and other professionals against advertising services or prices that have the result of keeping the public ignorant of or inhibiting the free flow of commercial information (Kinnear & Bernhardt, 1986, p. 66). As a result, over recent decades the marketing of professional health services has become an increasingly accepted practice.

Health Care Providers Begin to Market

Hospitals have turned to marketing because the occupancy rates across the United States have fallen in each of the past several years.

To increase occupancy rates, hospitals are competing with each other, introducing out-patient surgery and other service centers, nursing facilities and home health agencies for patients, attempting to distinguish themselves from their competitors (Inguanzo & Harju, 1985, p. 62).

Competition occurs, according to Kotler and Clarke, when two or more organizations seek to serve the same individual or group in an exchange process. An exchange requires (1) at least two parties, (2) that each party is offering something the other values, (3) that each party is capable of communicating and delivering what is valued, and (4) that both are free to accept or reject the offer (Johns & Saks, 2001, p. 360; Kotler & Clarke, 1987, pp. 46–47).

Competition for patients among public, not-for-profit and for-profit hospitals, is a new experience. In the face of assisted-living facilities and home health agencies increasingly siphoning off residents who, until recently, would have entered a nursing facility, administrators of nursing facilities are similarly encountering a need to "market" their services.

Definition of Marketing

The American Marketing Association defines marketing as the process of planning and executing the conception, pricing, promotion, and distribution of ideas, goods, and services to create exchanges that satisfy both individual and organizational objectives (Kinnear & Bernhardt, 1986, p. 10). The nursing facility is in the business of marketing services.

Levey and Loomba, in *Health Care Administration: A Managerial Perspective* argue that health care marketing had its beginnings in a spate of articles first appearing in 1973. They comment that the spread of marketing to hospitals and nursing facilities was inevitable, due to forces such as lowered occupancy rates and increasingly marginal net income due to lowered reimbursement rates (1973, p. 347). Marketing is currently regarded as a central consideration in health services administration. It is the effort to improve the interaction between the organization's goals and the persons whose needs the organization seeks to serve.

Why is it increasingly necessary to pay special attention to the "fit" between the goals of the nursing facility and the "needs" of the persons it seeks to serve? To assure that the facility will stay in business!

The steps in marketing are described by Levey and Loomba (1984, p. 350) as

1. The audit
2. Market segmentation
3. Choosing a market mix
4. Implementing the plan
5. Evaluation of results
6. Control

This should look familiar. It is a restatement of the management steps. Kotler and Clarke observe that marketing is a "managerial process involving analysis, planning, implementation and control" (Kotler & Clarke, 1987, p. 5).

Marketing as Managerial Thinking

Marketing employs the management techniques we have discussed and recommended, using a vocabulary developed specifically for the field of marketing. The purposes of marketing are to identify, then satisfactorily serve the institutional nursing facility needs in the community. Marketing is a useful additional vocabulary, another way of thinking about how the nursing facility can successfully identify and satisfy an expanding array of health care needs (Robbins & Coulter, 2007, p. 102).

Marketing, as a variation on managerial thinking, focuses sharply on the idea that success for the facility depends on bringing about a voluntary exchange of values (services) with the target persons.

End to the Production Orientation

Fifty years ago, the focus of health care providers was on designing a quality hospital or nursing facility, correctly assuming that if it were built, patients would fill it. This is a production orientation, which holds that the facility's task is to deliver care the health professionals know is good for the residents and that the sales task is to stimulate potential residents' interest in what the facility has decided to offer. This is "seller's" market thinking.

Angry Mothers

For decades women communicated their displeasure to hospital officials, who were in a sellers' market, about the intensely institutional atmosphere and rigid rules surrounding the delivery rooms in the obstetric departments. There being no competition, the hospitals ignored these complaints. Angry women, first in New York City, and then in other cities, established birthing centers with homelike atmospheres. With obstetric occupancy dramatically lower, reflecting both the end of the baby boom and increasing absence of long-dissatisfied women customers choosing to deliver in the rapidly growing birthing center market, hospital officials suddenly decided that the homelike atmosphere of the birthing centers could, after all, be provided in the nearly empty hospitals. Hospitals now routinely compete with each other and the birthing centers to see who can provide the most pleasing accommodations and flexible birthing rules.

Kotler and Clarke commend the market orientation now taking hold in health care facilities. In this approach the main task of the provider is to discover the needs and desires of potential customers and satisfy them through product design and price, delivering appropriate and competitively viable services (Kotler & Clarke, 1987, p. 30; Star, 1989, p. 149). This is market-centeredness, focusing primarily on customer needs, wants, perceptions, preferences, and satisfaction. They advocate a responsive organization: one that makes every effort to understand, serve, and satisfy the preferences and needs of its residents and their sponsors within the constraints of budget and good clinical practice (Kotler & Clarke, p. 41). Satisfaction is defined as a state felt by a resident when a service has fulfilled his or her expectations (Kotler & Clarke, p. 72). Health care services are increasingly a "buyer's" market. Long-term customer satisfaction with the manner in which the facility is being run is one of the major factors in keeping a nursing facility at or near capacity (Peters & Austin, 1985, p. 77).

Special Context of Nursing Facility Marketing

Local residents want people they know and to whom they can entrust Mom and Dad's care. The administrator who is visibly active and creates a presence in the community can create an atmosphere of trust through such networking.

The nursing facility faces two special challenges: (1) the requirement to maintain a societal marketing orientation, and (2) public ambivalence toward the nursing facility itself. In the societal marketing orientation, the primary task of the nursing facility is to determine the needs, desires, and best interests of residents and to configure the facility to deliver satisfactions that preserve and enhance the residents, their families, and society's well-being.

Residents, both short-term and long-term, may wish to be allowed to remain in their beds, to avoid exercise, and to eat only foods they can taste (typically foods high in sugar). But society has determined through the development of nursing facility regulations that residents must be urged to get up each day, dress and move about the facility to maintain blood flow, exercise when feasible, practice good oral hygiene, and eat the balanced diet mandated by the federal and state regulations. The nursing facility is thus obligated to encourage residents to engage in behaviors society has determined are in the residents' best interest, sometimes contrary to the individual resident's preference.

A second sense in which nursing facility marketing is a special context is public ambivalence toward the nursing facility. This is a complex, little understood, but often expressed problem area. Who among us does not wish to live into healthy and robust old age in our own homes with all our senses and capabilities intact? Who welcomes the situation of the typical nursing facility resident who has three to four chronic illnesses requiring a physician's care, takes six or more medications daily, has a limited ability to perform the activities of daily living, and a need for 24-hour-a-day nursing care? There is much more approach/avoidance involved in public feelings toward the care in nursing facilities than toward hospitals where normally the patient expects (hopes) to be healed and returned to active community life. Entering new marketing areas must be done with great forethought. An improperly analyzed niche can become a new cost center rather than the hoped for new profit center.

1.9.3 DEVELOPING A MARKETING STRATEGY

Need for a Marketing Strategy

Organizations must continually adapt to changes within and outside the organization. An adaptive organization systematically monitors the external environment and revises its mission, strategies, and objectives to take advantage of emerging opportunities.

A constantly evolving marketing strategy is needed, because continuous changes occur in the demographic, technologic, regulatory, economic, political, reimbursement, and social environment leading to changing demand for nursing facility services. New competition appears, new client demands develop, and values change.

Competition for the potential nursing home client is increasing. On the acute care side, hospitals are showing increased interest in converting empty acute care wings to nursing home type beds. Some hospitals are even building new nursing homes on their grounds or near by to create a new revenue stream. From another perspective, home health care agencies are increasingly providing sophisticated nursing care such as intravenous feeding in the patient's home—previously performed mostly in hospitals and only a few nursing facilities. Thus, acute care patients may increasingly go directly home, bypassing the nursing facility. And then there are the assisted-living facilities bursting onto the scene who promise to let their residents "age in place" (read: never have to go to a nursing facility). Some assisted-living facilities are now serving sliding scale diabetics (difficult to treat diabetics) previously served by nursing homes. In addition, a large often unregulated array of multiunit senior housing facilities are being built that can also let their residents "age in place" by bringing home health care workers to these facilities.

A *marketing strategy* includes selecting a target market or markets, choosing a competitive position, and developing an effective marketing mix to reach and serve the identified customers (Hitt et al., 2001, pp. 151–152; Robbins & Coulter, 2007, p. 227).

A *market* is all the persons who have an actual or potential interest in using the facility's services. A facility may select among several market coverage strategies. It may concentrate on one market or market segment, for example, choose to serve only Medicaid residents (called market concentration). The facility may decide to offer only one service for all markets (*product concentration*), for example, serve only Alzheimer's patients regardless of their funding source. The facility may opt for a *market specialization,* that is, serve only one market segment such as persons who need rehabilitative care and are expected to return home within a specified brief period of time. Or, it may prefer to work in several product markets, for example, to serve both Alzheimer's and other brain-damaged persons of all ages (*selective specializations*).

Creating New Markets, New Niches

It is useful to distinguish between market sharing and market creation. Persons using the market-share mentality focus on how they can attain a desired share of the present market. Market creators are those who attempt to create a new market. Opening a ventilator unit in a nursing home, for example, was a recent phenomenon. To that point, ventilator care had mostly been confined to hospitals. Entrepreneurial nursing home administrators created a new long-term care market by opening ventilator units in their nursing facilities (Hitt et al., 2001, pp. 523–524). These administrators convinced third-party reimbursement officials to move ventilator patients out of hospitals and into nursing facilities, thus creating a new, larger long-term care market place. The market for nursing home ventilator beds then became saturated in several parts of the country. Time to create the next niches! Survival for both individual facilities and nursing facility chains is becoming increasingly tied to specializing in market niches in which one can gain a reputation for excellence, in order to keep census at the needed levels.

Which Niche?

Table 1.4 demonstrates that a number of possible niches exist for nursing facilities, especially in the area of respiratory therapy.

In recent years niche marketing has taken new twists. Both assisted-living facilities and nursing facilities have begun offering home care services to seniors in the community in the hope of those served moving to the facility offering home care services when a higher level of care is needed. This both offers new revenue centers for facilities and markets to a niche in the community, which might become full time in facility clients.

The number of dedicated AIDS beds was 2,002 in 1999—a fraction less than 1% of all beds in the United States, 1993–1999. The number of hospice beds was 3,121 in 1999, but this number is also less than 1% of all beds in the United States. This reflects the general trend to provide hospice care either in the home or in hospitals (Landefeld et al., 2004, p. 465). The number of hospice patients in the United States grew from 52,000 in 1992 to 105,000 in the year 2000, a trend that is expected to continue (DHHS, 2005, p. 323). Not surprisingly, more than two-thirds of hospice patients are 85 years of age and over (DHHS, 2005, p. 323).

Table 1.5 shows that 19.66% of beds were rehabilitation beds in special units in certified nursing facilities in the United States in 2006. Both

TABLE 1.4.   Percent of Residents Whose Selected Medical Conditions Were Being Treated as a Medical Condition Requiring Special Care in 2006

2006	
Respiratory therapy	12.28%
Tracheostomy care	1.03%
Ostomy care	4.54%
Suctioning	1.35%
Injections	18.36%
Hospice care	3.70%
Radiation therapy	0.10%
Chemotherapy	0.36%
IV therapy (nutrition or blood)	1.66%
Tube feeding	6.27%
Mechanically altered diet	34.46%
Assistive eating device	7.44%

Source: DHHS, 2006a, F78, F119–F123, F124–F128, F129–F132.

categories of rehabilitation beds and kidney dialysis beds in 2006 represent only about 1% of certified beds in the United States in 1999. There were also 4,726 ventilator beds reported in special care units in 1999. There were 568 dialysis unit beds surveyed.

Examining these last two tables state-by-state reveals large differences in approach among the states. Finding and establishing niches must be done carefully—what may be a great marketing tool may be cost-prohibitive in practice. Many administrators have found that, though high, ventilator reimbursements barely cover the increased costs of service!

Steps in Developing a Marketing Strategy for the Facility

Step One: The Audit

As indicated previously, the first step in developing a marketing strategy is the audit. *Auditing* is the process of identifying, collecting, and analyzing information about the external environment. Marketing human resources typically characterize a market as potential, available, qualified, served, and penetrated. The *potential market* is all the persons who express some level of interest in a defined market offer. Removing persons who are interested, but unable to pay, defines the *available market,* that is, persons who have interest, the funds, and access to the market offering. The *qualified available market* is those persons who have interest, financial means, access, and quality, that is, they meet the requirement for 24 hour per day nursing care. The *served market* is that part of the qualified available market the facility makes an effort to attract to the facility. The persons who are admitted to or served by the facility constitute the *penetrated market*—the persons actually consuming the services offered.

It is necessary to estimate the extent of demand for a service the facility might offer. Total market demand is the total volume of services that would be bought by a defined available number of persons in a specific geographic area in a defined time period in a stated marketing environment under a specific marketing program (Kotler & Clarke, 1987, p. 216). Market forces suggest the number of services the facility could expect to purchase under such a specific marketing plan.

TABLE 1.5.   Percent of Residents Whose Health Condition Was Being Treated as a Medical Condition Requiring Special Care in 2006

2006	
Rehabilitation	19.66%
Kidney dialysis	1.53%

Source: DHHS, 2006a, F78, F119–123.

In forecasting future demand, Kotler and Clarke (1987) suggest the facility examine three categories: (a) uncontrollable environment factors such as the economy, technological changes, reimbursement formula changes, and broad changes in the health care system such as the emergence of managed care; (b) new competition from other providers (e.g., new facilities, new services, new marketing budget); and (c) intraorganizational factors such as the condition of one's facility, possible new services, and promotional efforts program (Kotler & Clarke, p. 225). Forecasts may be based on what people say they will do, are actually doing, or what people have actually done in the past.

Step Two: Market Segmentation

Market segmentation is using the audit information to divide the potential persons served into identifiable subgroups. Subgroups may be longer-term residents and shorter-term residents who come for rehabilitation then return home, or groupings such as private pay patients and public pay patients. Further, a nursing home chain might segment the market it seeks by geography: region of the country, urban/rural, density, climate. Markets can be segmented by demographic characteristics such as age, family size, sex, educational level, occupation, or religion. Psychographic social classes can be used (e.g., life style, personality). Persons who are by nature gregarious and thrive on extensive personal interactions, for example, are good candidates for application to life care communities. In addition, behavior tendencies can be used to segment markets. Benefits sought (e.g., a life care community benefit set), user status (within age limits and able to pay), and readiness stage (e.g., persons over a certain age, retired, and actively seeking a caregiver) all identify market segments (Hitt et al., 2001, p. 149).

Step Three: The Market Mix

Determining the market mix consists of deciding what types of residents to approach and in what proportions. Most facilities find it useful to identify specific groups of persons being sought to serve. This is more feasible and necessary in urban settings than in rural areas where choices of whom to serve may be more limited by geography and income.

Most facilities will consciously choose a *product mix,* that is, the set of all product lines and items the facility intends to offer. A *product line* in the nursing facility setting is a set of services within the product mix that are closely related due to functional similarity, for example, being made available to the same type of persons, or marketed through the same channels. A facility may choose to serve a combination of heavy care patients from the local hospital who can expect to return home or die shortly as one group, plus another group of persons who enter as light care patients expected to remain in the facility for the foreseeable future. A *product item* is a distinct unit within a product line that is distinguishable by purpose in some other characteristic. The facility may, for example, within the heavy care group, especially solicit persons being fed intravenously or needing tracheotomy care.

Step Four: Implementing and Evaluating the Plan

Implementing the marketing plan is the process of managing organizational behaviors and outreach activities to attract residents with the identified characteristics in the proportions desired.

Creating awareness among potential consumers that the services exist, assisting them in deciding, and assuring that they are satisfied with the quality of services provided by the facility is the process of *marketing implementation*. An ongoing evaluation of the effectiveness of the marketing efforts is necessary as well.

Steps Five and Six: Evaluation and Control

Once the marketing effort is operational it is necessary to devise ways to measure the results and taking corrective action to assure that the desired results are achieved.

The Marketing of Services

Nursing facilities are primarily in the business of marketing services. A service is an activity or benefit that one person can offer to another that is intangible and does not result in ownership of anything (Kotler & Clarke, 1987, p. 318). According to Berkowitz, Kerin, and Rudelius (1986), services have four characteristics that differentiate them from durable goods (e.g., cars or television sets): intangibility, inconsistency, inseparability, and inventory.

The Characteristics of Services

Intangibility. Services cannot be touched, sat in, or driven like a car: They are intangible. Health care that the resident expects will be given in a nursing facility cannot be directly experienced before entering the facility. Nursing facilities can, however, make services appear more tangible (for example, a television advertisement portraying attentive care being given to a resident at the facility; Berkowitz, Kerin, & Rudelius, 1986, p. 609).

Inconsistency. Marketing services differs from marketing tangible goods such as an automobile because the quality of service can be inconsistent from day to day, or even shift to shift. Quality that endures over time can be built into a car through consistent assembly line procedures and quality checks, but the service received at the hands of the nurses or nursing assistants on any given day can vary widely depending on the mood of the employee.

Inseparability. A third characteristic of marketing services is that the consumer does not separate the service from the deliverer of the service or the setting in which service is given. The nursing home may be giving excellent nursing care, but if the bathrooms smell bad and are dirty the patients' and visitors' perceptions of the facility including their perceptions of quality of nursing care, are affected. The services given and the service provided are inseparably linked in the consumer's mind.

Inventory. Idle production capacity (i.e., the presence of an unoccupied bed in a health care facility), is a fourth characteristic of service marketing. Inventory carrying costs of empty nursing home beds is high: Empty beds may cost as much as 70% of the costs of occupied beds due to fixed and semi-variable costs.

In the text *Marketing Long-Term and Senior Care Services,* Midgett (1984) asserts that if a nursing facility carefully proportions the number of subsidized and private pay patients, it can provide better accommodations and services for both (p. 78). This is true, because in many states the public reimbursement rates are at or below costs, forcing providers to subsidize publicly paying patients by shifting these costs to the bills of private paying patients (Sinioris & Butler, 1983, p. 42).

Consumer Decision Making

Marketing texts typically characterize *consumer decision making* as:

1. Problem recognition
2. Information search
3. Alternative evaluation
4. Purchase decision
5. Post-purchase evaluation

Kotler and Clarke (1987) describe *consumer decision making* similarly:

1. Need arousal (trigger factors such as a hospital episode)
2. Information gathering

3. Decision evaluation
4. Decision execution
5. Post-decision assessment

The decision for a person to enter a nursing facility is often a complex one shared by several participants. The decision making unit may consist of:

- *The initiator*—the daughter, for example, who suggests looking into nursing facility care;
- *The influential friend*—for example acquaintances already in local nursing facilities or who have convalesced in one;
- *The decider*—the person(s) who ultimately forces some part of the decision, for example, the daughter who decides she cannot provide the new level of care needed;
- *The buyer*—the person(s) who will pay the bills, if not the resident themself; and
- *The user*—the person who will be the new resident or nursing home service user (Hitt et al., 2001, pp. 73–74; Kotler & Clarke, 1987, p. 275)

Consumer decisions are based on their perceptions of whether the service provided by the nursing facility will meet their needs. Research suggests that physicians typically have a major influence on patient decisions (Smith, 1984, p. 105). Recommendations from local physicians can provide the facility with a sustainable advantage (Ghemawat, 1986, p. 550). Hospital discharge planners are an important group whose image of the facility and communication with it can also provide a competitive edge program (Kotler & Clarke, 1987, p.475).

Effective Marketing Tools

A personal tour through the building that includes meeting staff and patients is one of the most effective marketing tools available to the facility. During the visit or visits the potential client(s), usually the children or close friends of the prospective resident, are gathering impressions on which they will make judgments of the facility. Often, subliminal perceptions become the key factor. Subliminal perceptions are factors of which the decision maker is not consciously aware, such as general appearance of the facility, absence of odors, friendliness of the staff, and appearance of the patients (Robertson, Zielinski, & Ward, 1984, p. 186).

One writer has argued that image is credibility (Peterson, 1986, p. 36). Numerous ways of creating a positive image for the facility in the community are available. Developing a community advisory board, hosting neighborhood open houses, publicizing enthusiastic families and volunteers, and cosponsoring community events such as local arts festivals, are but a few of the avenues available to facilities.

Advertising

Many facilities have begun to advertise their services. Advertising consists of nonpersonal forms of communication conducted through paid media with a clear sponsorship program (Kotler & Clarke, 1987, p.483). The purpose of advertising is to motivate the target audience to move through the following buyer readiness states toward actual use of facility services:

- Cognitive (aware that the facility is available)
- Affective (favorable image of facility when comparing it to alternatives)
- Behavioral (conviction, for example, ask physician to "place mother there")

REFERENCES

America's most admired corporations. (1995, March 6). *Fortune,* p. 66.

Argenti, P. A. (1994). *The portable MBS desk reference.* New York: Wiley.

Barnard, C. I. (1938). *The functions of the executive.* Cambridge, MA: Harvard University Press.

Berkowitz, E. N., Kerin, R. A., & Rudelius, W. (1986). *Marketing.* St. Louis: Mosby.

Centers for Medicare and Medicaid. (2007). Department of Health and Human Services, Washington, D.C. Retrieved from www.cms.hhs.gov

Christensen, C. R., Berg, N. A., & Salter, M. S. (1980). *Policy formulation and administration* (8th ed.). Homewood, IL: Irwin.

Code of Federal Regulations. (2006). 42 CFR Part 489.3. Washington, DC: Centers for Medicare and Medicaid.

Dale, E. (1969). *Management: Theory and practice* (2nd ed.). New York: McGraw Hill.

Demski, J. S. (1980). *Information analysis* (2nd ed.). Reading, MA: Addison-Wesley.

Department of Health and Human Services. (2005). Centers for Disease Control and Prevention, National Center for Health Statistics. Hyattsville, MD: Author.

Department of Health and Human Services. (2006a). Centers for Medicare and Medicaid Services, Oscar Form 672: F78–F132.

Department of Health and Human Services. (2006b). Centers for Medicare and Medicaid Services, Oscar Report, 18S.

DePorter, C. (2006, July). Personal interview at Division of Facilities Services, Raleigh, NC.

Evashwick, C. J. (1993, Fall). Strategic management of a continuum of care. *The Journal of Long-Term Care Administration, 21,* pp. 13–24.

French, J. R. P., Jr., & Raven, B. H. (1960). The bases of social power. In D. Cartwright & A. Zander (Eds.), *Group dynamics: Research and theory* (2nd ed.). Evanston, IL: Row, Peterson.

George, C. S., Jr. (1972). *The history of management thought* (2nd ed.). Englewood Cliffs, NJ: Prentice Hall.

Ghemawat, P. (1986). Sustainable advantage. *Harvard Business Review, 64*(5), pp. 53–58.

Gordon, G. K., & Stryker, R. (1983). *Creative long term care administration.* Springfield, IL: Charles C Thomas.

Harrington, C. H., Carrillo, M. S., Thollaug, S. C., Summers, P. R., & Wellin, V. (2000). *Nursing facilities, staffing, residents, and facility deficiencies, 1993 through 1999.* San Francisco: University of California at San Francisco, Department of Social & Behavioral Sciences.

Hamel, G., & Prahalad, C. K. (1994). *Competing for the future.* Boston, MA: Harvard Business School Press.

Hitt, M. A., Ireland, R. D., & Hoskisson, R. E. (2001). *Strategic management: Competitiveness and globalization* (4th ed.). Cincinnati, OH: South-Western College Publishing.

Inguanzo, J. M., & Harju, M. (1985, January 1). Creating a market niche. *Hospitals, 59,* pp. 62–67.

Jackson, J. (1960). The organization and its communication problems. In A. Grimshaw & J. W. Hennessey, Jr. (Eds.), *Organizational behavior: Cases and readings.* New York: McGraw Hill.

Johns, G., & Saks, A. (2001). *Organizational behavior* (5th ed.). Toronto: Addison Wesley Longman.

Juran, J. M. (1988). *Juran's quality control handbook* (4th ed.). New York: McGraw Hill.

Katz, D., & Kahn, R. L. (1967). *The social psychology of organizations.* New York: Wiley.

Keen, P. G. W., & Woodman, L. A. (1984). What to do with all those micros. *Harvard Business Review, 84*(5), pp. 142–150.

Kinnear, T. C., & Bernhardt, K. L. (1986). *Principles of marketing* (2nd ed.). Glenview, IL: Scott, Foresman.

Kodner, D. L. (1993, Fall). Long term care 2010: Speculations and implications. *Journal of Long Term Care Administration, 21,* pp. 82–86.

Kotler, P., & Clarke, R. N. (1987). *Marketing for health care organizations.* Englewood Cliffs, NJ: Prentice Hall.

Kotter, J. P. (1982). *The general managers.* New York: Free Press.

Kriegel, R. J. (1991). *If it ain't broke.* New York: Warner.

Landefeld, C. S., Palmer R. M., Johnson M. A., Johnston C. B., & Lyons W. L. (2004). *Current geriatric diagnosis & treatment.* New York. Lange Medical Books/McGraw-Hill.

Levey, S., & Loomba, N. P. (1973). *Health care administration: A managerial perspective.* Philadelphia: Lippincott.

Levey, S., & Loomba, N. P. (1984). *Health care administration: A managerial perspective* (2nd ed.). New York: Lippincott.

Maddox, G. L., & Sussman, S. W. (2001). *The encyclopedia of aging* (3rd ed.). New York: Springer Publishing Company.

Meal, H. C. (1984). Putting production decisions where they belong. *Harvard Business Review, 84*(2), pp. 102–111.

Melum, M. M., & Siniotis, M. K. (1992). *Total quality management: The health care pioneers.* Chicago: American Hospital Publisher.

Midgett, M. (1984). Skilled nursing facility marketing. In W. J. Winston (Ed.), *Marketing long-term care and senior care services* (pp. 77–81). New York: Haworth.

Miller, D. B. (Ed.). (1982). *Long term care administrator's desk manual.* Greenvale, NY: Panel.

Mintzberg, H. (1979). *The structure of organizations: A synthesis of the research.* Englewood Cliffs, NJ: Prentice Hall.

Molloy, G. E. (1994, October). Quality is the administration job #1. *Nursing Homes, 54,* pp. 36–39.

Noe, R. A., Hollenbeck, J. R., Gerhart, B., & Wright, P. M. (2000). *Human resource management: Gaining a competitive advantage* (3rd ed.). Boston: McGraw-Hill Companies, Inc.

Omnibus Budget Reconciliation Act (OBRA). (1991, September 26). *Medicare and Medicaid.* Federal Register, 56(187), 48825–48922.

Peters, T. (1987). *Thriving on chaos.* New York: Harper and Row.

Peters, T. (1985). *A passion for excellence: The leadership difference.* New York: Random House.

Peterson, S. (1986). Take note: Image is as image does. *Provider, 12*(11), 36–39.

Robbins, S. P, & Coulter, M. (2007). *Management* (9th Ed.). New York: Pearson / Prentice Hall.

Robertson, T. S., Zielinski, J., & Ward, S. (1984). *Consumer behavior.* Palo Alto, CA: Scott, Foresman.

Robey, D. (1982). *Designing organizations.* Homewood, IL: Irwin.

Shackle, G.L.S. (1957). *Uncertainty and business decisions: A symposium* (2nd ed.). Liverpool, England: Liverpool University Press.

Shewhart, W. A. (1931). *Economic control of quality of manufactured product.* Van Nostrand, Co.

Simon, H. A. (1960). *The new science of management decision.* New York: Harper and Row.

Sinioris, M. E., & Butler, P. (1983, June 1). Basic business strategy: Responding to change requires planning, marketing, and budgeting strategies. *Hospitals, 57,* p. 57.

Smith, S. M. (1984). Family selection of long-term care services. In W. J. Winston (Ed.), *Marketing long-term and senior care services* (pp. 101–113). New York: Haworth.

Spendolini, M. J. (1992). *The benchmarking book.* New York: American Management Association.

Star, S. H. (1989). Marketing and its discontents. *Harvard Business Review, 89*(6), 148–154.

Swiss, J. E. (1983). Establishing a management system: The interaction of power shifts and personality under federal MBO. *Public Administration Review, 43*(3), 238–245.

Tannenbaum, R., Wechsler, I., & Massarik, F. (1961). *Leadership and organization.* New York: McGraw Hill.

Terry, G. R. (1969). *Principles of management.* Homewood, IL: Irwin.

Webster's new world dictionary. (1968). New York: World.

Welch, J. F. (1993, December 13). A master class in radical change. *Future, 83,* p. 83.

Williams, S. J., & Torrens, P. R. (1980). *Introduction to health services.* New York: Wiley.

Withington, F. G. (1966). *The use of computers in business organizations.* Reading, MA: Addison-Wesley.

Wrapp, H. E. (1984). Good managers don't make policy decisions. *Harvard Business Review, 84*(4).

PART II

Human Resources

2.1 Organizational Patterning of the Nursing Facility and Its Staff

Complexity of the Staff's Organizational Tasks

The goal of total quality management (TQM) is that human resources in every unit arrive at a level of daily performance reflecting a passion for quality (Hitt, Ireland, & Hoskisson, 2001, pp. 175, 212; Johns & Saks, 2001, pp. 190–194, 537–540; Robbins & Coulter, 2007, p. 222). This goal is more easily articulated than accomplished. The multitude of regulations to be obeyed can seem overwhelming (see Allen, 2006). It is often said, only partly in jest, that the nursing home industry is the second most regulated industry, nuclear power is first. Even that may no longer be true. The nuclear power industry is being deregulated while legal constraints on the nursing home industry are being tightened.

Remembering the array of requirements to be met by each facility is beyond the capacity of a single person. As regulations continue to proliferate, the average nursing home administrator must increasingly depend on department heads and their staffs to be the experts in each area.

The decision on how to staff a nursing facility depends on many variables. An overarching consideration is the level of medical complexity of care to be delivered. Changes in case mix will normally result in altered staffing patterns. Admission of several medically complex residents may lead to employment of an additional experienced registered nurse and the retraining of most of the floor nurses (Maddox & Sussman, 2001, p. 166). Admission of several lighter care residents may call for additional aides rather than additional registered nurses. In the following sections we present options in organizational forms and a staffing pattern that the administrator of a 100-bed facility with an average level of intensity might consider.

Organizational Pattern for a 100-Bed Facility

Figure 2.1 shows the organizational pattern and staffing levels for a 100-bed facility recommended in the federal government regulations.

ADMINISTRATOR
Asst. Administrator (0-1)
Administrative Assistant (0-1)
Secretary (1 FT)
Receptionist (1 FT)

Medical Director (PT)→↑ ←Human Resources (0-FT)

Resident Council→↑

↑	↑	↑	↑
MEDICAL SERVICES DEPTS.	**NURSING**	BUSINESS DEPT Bookkeeper, **A/R clerk**	QUALITY ASSESS-MENT
	DON		
ALLIED HEALTH Dentist, podiatrist	ADON	MEDICAL RECORDS (1 FT)	
	MDS		AN
PHARMACIST (PT or contract)	**COORDINATOR (key to finances!)**	ADMITTING (1 FT or part-time)	INFECTION CONTROL PROGRAM
THERAPY		DIETARY Food service supervisor	
	THREE SHIFTS:	(consulting dietitian if not	PHYSICAL
PHYSICAL		RD)	PLANT
OCCUPATIONAL	RN'S, LPNs,		HEALTH
SPEECH	CNAs		AND
(in-house or		(Sufficient supervisors,	SAFETY
contract)	(enough to meet the	cooks, saladmakers,	PROGRAM
	care needs of	dietary aides)	
LAB, X-RAY	residents in		
	building)	SOCIAL SERVICES (1 FT)	
		ACTIVITIES (1 FT)	
		HOUSEKEEPING (Director, enough staff)	
		LAUNDRY (in-house or contracted)	
		MAINTENANCE (1 FT, staff or contracts)	

FIGURE 2.1 Organizational pattern for a 100-bed facility.

Various Configurations

In actual practice, these 17 "departmental" areas can be, and routinely are, given different titles and combined variously. Nevertheless, however configured, these areas must be accounted for in the typical nursing facility organizational plan.

In Figure 2.1 each position within the 17 departments or functional areas (e.g., admissions) is depicted, along with the number of its staff and whether they are full time or part time.

Emergence of the "MDS" Coordinator

In recent years the minimum data set (MDS) coordinator role has become central both to the quality of care in the nursing facility and the reimbursements received by nursing facilities. The MDS is the federal effort to both define and control quality of care within nursing facilities that are Medicare or Medicaid certified.

The upper area in Figure 2.1 reflects the administrator, their immediate staff, and advisory roles (indicated by the arrows) of the medical director and resident council. The first column includes the medical and allied health professionals essential to the facility (e.g., physicians, dentists, pharmacist, occupational and physical therapists). The nursing service with its three shifts is the second column. Areas in the third column are also necessary to the functioning of a facility (e.g., the business office, dietary, social services, activities, housekeeping, and maintenance). In the final column are activities mandated by the federal requirements.

Workable Variations

Numerous workable variations on the model exist. In this one, line authority is given to the administrator leading to the several functional areas or departments. The administrator has responsibility, directly or indirectly, for all the functions of the facility.

A variant of this model, more suited to a larger facility of perhaps 200 residents, is to group several of these functions under middle-level managers who report to the administrator. One such arrangement is to appoint several middle-level managers (Johns & Saks, 2001, pp. 20–21; Noe et al., 2000, p. 115) who are directors of:

- Resident services (e.g., volunteers, transportation, barbers, beauticians)
- Administrative services (e.g., admissions, business office, clerical staff and human resources)
- Therapy services (e.g., physical, occupational and speech therapy)
- Nursing services (all nursing activities)
- Supportive services (housekeeping, laundry and maintenance)
- Dietary services

The more common model is depicted in Figure 2.1 where all department heads report directly to the administrator. In the typical 100-bed nursing facility eight or nine department heads will report directly to the administrator.

We turn now to consideration of the organizational work to be accomplished by each department and their staffing requirements.

The Administrator's Office

The administrator is responsible for assuring that all work is accomplished according to policy at an acceptable level of quality.

Administration

To summarize briefly, consider the following as an initial description given in no particular order of priority. It is the charge of administration to:

- assure a satisfactory quality of care and of life for residents and staff
- advocate for the residents and, as needed, staff and the facility
- monitor and control all the subsystems in the facility
- develop and manage the budget
- manage the interface between the facility, its many constituencies, and the world outside
- monitor and manage the human resources functions
- coordinate or assure coordination of the work of all departments and functions in the facility
- lead and provide stimulus on a daily basis to activities that implement the facility's goals and mission
- forecast and lead the facility to a successful future
- assist all staff and residents to understand the nature and value of change
- interface with owners, inspectors, ombudspersons, third-party insurers, hospitals, fire departments, and the myriad of other persons, groups, and functions necessary to the survival of the facility
- communicate with staff, residents, and others
- empower department heads and staff to accomplish their work
- facilitate the functioning of the facility by walking around and similar management approaches
- set the tone for the facility in matters of dress, taste, compassion, and concern by word and behavior
- settle territorial and jurisdictional disputes among staff, residents, and owners

The effective administrator does whatever it takes to have effective control of resident care in the facility. In recent years a number of facility administrators have utilized some variation of a daily department head meeting. Some call it "stand-up" and meet for plus or minus 10 minutes each morning, others call it "stand-up" and sit down for plus or minus 30 minutes each morning and review every resident, others meet with department heads only once a week or less often.

In addition, the administrator is, more than any one else in the facility, responsible for resident rights. Table 2.1 demonstrates 97%+ conformance with the exceptions of being able to provide F157, the 30-day notice of changes; F167, the subjective areas of privacy and confidentiality; and F164 personal privacy/confidential records.

In Table 2.2, 97.6% to 100% compliance was achieved with the exception of 84% compliance for clinical records—a difficult area as records are increasingly being transitioned from 100% paper to plus or minus 5% paper and 95% electronic.

Assistant Administrator / Administrative Assistant

An assistant administrator has line authority to represent the administrator, can make decisions on their behalf, and is usually assigned some area to oversee. An administrative assistant, on the other hand, has no line authority, cannot make decisions for the facility, and does not represent the administrator except in an information gathering, or processing manner. The administrative assistant is a staff position.

In the typical nursing facility of 100 beds there tends not to be enough "organizational room" for an assistant administrator; 300 or more beds would call for an assistant administrator. The appointment of an assistant administrator and administrative assistant depends on the personality of the administrator.

Secretary and Advisory Functions

Generally, the facility secretary works in the administrator's office, in an area shared with the receptionist/telephone operator/manager. The receptionist needs to know all the employee application procedures if applicants are to feel welcome. The receptionist needs to be in the communication loop. The receptionist is key. If relatives walk in at 11:00 A.M. and the receptionist cheerily asks, "Are you here to see Uncle Don?" and the family informs her that he died an hour earlier … "Oh, I'm sorry, I didn't know."

As a rule, the administrator has several advisory persons or groups, represented in Figure 2.1 by arrows. The medical director and resident council often fit into this slot. Other consultants, such as the pharmacist

TABLE 2.1.   Percent of Nursing Facilities in the U.S. With Deficiencies for Resident Rights, 1993, 1999, and Percent and Number in 2006

DEFICIENCY GROUP = RESIDENT RIGHTS

		1993 %	1999 %	2006 %	Facilities
F151	Resident exercises rights, is free of coercion	1.4	1.1	0.83	133
F152	Surrogate exercises incompetent res rights	1.7	0.9	1.08	172
F153	Access to records, ability to purchase rec	0.5	0.1	0.15	24
F154	Res informed of health and med condition	2.6	1.1	1.01	161
F155	Right to refuse treatment/research	1.5	1.0	1.61	257
F156	Inform res of services/charges/legal rights	12.5	3.1	4.02	640
F157	Inform of accidents/significant changes/transfer	6.2	7.9	9.43	1,502
F158	Resident manage own financial affairs	0.2	0.1	0.08	13
F159	Facility management of res funds	8.7	2.4	2.77	442
F160	Conveyance of res funds upon death	1.5	0.8	1.09	173
F161	Surety bond or other assurance	3.1	0.7	1.39	221
F162	Limitation on charges to personal funds	0.7	0.4	0.20	32
F163	Resident may choose a personal physician	0.2	0.2	0.09	14
F164	Personal privacy/confidential records	7.7	7.2	9.64	1,536
F165	Voice grievances without reprisal	0.5	0.3	0.19	31
F166	Facility resolves resident grievances	3.6	3.5	2.99	477
F167	Survey results readily accessible to res	6.8	3.6	3.78	603
F168	Res receive info/can contact advocates	0.2	0.2	0.10	16
F169	Residents' right to work/refuse to work	0.3	0.0	0.01	2
F170	Res can send/receive unopened mail	0.4	1.3	1.59	254
F171	Resident has access to stationery, etc.	0.0	0.0	0.05	8
F172	Res access to secretary, physician, etc.	0.3	0.2	0.10	16
F173	Allows ombudsman to examine res rec	0.0	0.0	0.01	1
F174	Access to telephone with auditory privacy	4.1	1.4	1.36	217
F175	Right to share a room	0.1	0.0	0.04	7
F176	Self-admin of drugs if deemed safe	3.3	2.5	4.39	699
F177	Res right to refuse certain transfers	0.4	0.2	0.03	4

Source: DHHS, 2006b.

TABLE 2.2. Percent of Nursing Facilities in the U.S. With Deficiencies for Other Activities, 1994, 1999, and Percent and Number in 2006

		DEFICIENCY GROUP = OTHER ACTIVITIES			
		1994 %	1999 %	2006 %	Facilities
F514	Clinical records meet prof standards	13.5	10.2	16.20	2,581
F516	Facility safeguards clinical records	0.6	0.6	0.73	117
F517	Plans to meet emergencies/disasters	0.7	0.4	0.89	142
F518	Train employees, emergency proc/drills	3.3	2.4	2.89	460
F519	Transfer agreement with hospital	0.0	0.0	0.03	4
F520	Facility maintains qual assurance comm	0.7	1.0	2.86	455
F521	Quality assurance activities	3.1	1.9	0.00	0
F522	Disclosure of ownership requirements	0.0	0.0	0.03	4

Source: DHHS, 2006b.

(see American Society of Consultant Pharmacists—www.ascp.com) or dentist, and any other advisory committees might appear here. The administrator's office is responsible for keeping on file the original of several types of information, for example, reports of the state facility inspection teams, department reports, and other important documents.

Medical and Allied Health Functions

Patterns of Physician Care

As a rule, the typical 100-bed facility does not require the services of a full-time medical director. The medical director is normally paid a contractual monthly fee to provide medical supervision. It is desirable to have the medical director be a member of the American Medical Director Association (www.amda.com), which keeps the facility medical director up to date with federal guidelines and current geriatric clinical practice.

The Open Medical Staff

The predominant pattern for nursing facilities of approximately 100 to 200 beds is to allow any physician licensed to practice in the state to admit residents to the facility and to provide their medical care while they reside there (no one can reside in a nursing facility without physician admitting orders and continuing physician supervision). Under this pattern the part-time medical director tries to assure that the medical needs of the residents are met as they arise. The medical director often substitutes for the personal physician who fails to visit the patient on a timely basis or perform the annual physical periodically as required by federal or state regulations. People prefer to talk with those of equal rank, thus a vital role played by the medical director is to visit on a peer basis with physicians who are not meeting the actual care needs or making the required visits to patients in the facility. Because there is normally no organized medical staff, the medical director advises the administrator of the facility concerning the quality of its physician and nursing care and assists the director of nursing to assure that a good quality of resident care is delivered. The medical director may or may not admit and care for residents in the facility, but usually does so for some of them. This has the functional value of allowing the medical director to be in the facility frequently "walking around," seeing their patients. New guidelines for medical directors, requiring greater involvement, were published in 2006 (see National Association of Directors of Nursing Administration/Long-Term Care—www.nadona.org).

The Closed Medical Staff

A second model of medical direction is the *closed medical staff*. This means that only physicians who have been approved by the organized medical staff of the facility may admit or treat its patients. An organized medical staff is the closed group of physicians who provide all the primary care to the patients. Initially, the board or governing body appoints one or more physicians to organize a medical staff, elect a medical director, and write by-laws to govern the medical care given in that facility, functioning much like the medical staff in an organized hospital.

Closed medical staffs are more feasible for larger facilities of perhaps 300 or more residents. In this situation the physicians, usually 5 or 6 for a facility of 500–600 residents, divide care of the residents among themselves. Numerous variations are possible. A closed medical staff has several advantages. One of them can be on duty (or immediate call) at all times and can attend to patients needing medical care, but whose assigned physician is not immediately available. Some or all of the physicians may be full time, but most are part time. Continuous care is thus available and, because the staff physicians have some economic dependency on the facility, the administrator has the required services available. Under the open staff model considerable energy must often be devoted to gain conformity of medical services on the timely basis mandated by the federal (and state) requirements.

As demonstrated in Table 2.3, a 97% to 99.6% compliance rate is achieved.

With the 2006 new medical director requirements issued by the Centers for Medicare and Medicaid, physician availability is improving. In 1975, about

TABLE 2.3.   Percent of Nursing Facilities in the U.S. With Deficiencies for Physician Services, 1993, 1999, and Percent and Number in 2006

DEFICIENCY GROUP = PHYSICIAN SERVICES

		1993 %	1999 %	2006 %	Facilities
F385	Residents' care supervised by a physician	1.0	0.4	0.38	61
F386	Physician responsibilities during visits	4.2	1.5	2.10	334
F387	Frequency & timeliness of physician visit	2.1	1.9	2.57	409
F388	Visits by physician/physician assistant	0.2	0.2	0.27	43
F380	Emergency physician services 24 hr/day	0.1	0.1	0.08	13
F390	Physician delegates tasks	0.2	0.1	0.04	7

Source: DHHS, 2006b.

which time nursing homes were required to employ a medical director, there were 13.5 doctors of medicine in patient care. By 2003, that number had increased to 23.5 (Department of Health and Human Services [DHHS], 2005, Table 105, p. 342). In 2003, there were 736,211 doctors of medicine who were professionally active (DHHS, 2005, p. 344.)

Dental Care

Dental care is a major, often neglected, aspect of services delivered in the nursing facility. Local dentists normally do not own the portable equipment costing $2,000–$15,000 and more to give dental care inside a nursing facility. Beyond this lack is perhaps the dental practitioner's insecurity about functioning outside their office and dealing with the complex medical histories of patients whose medical records are a few inches thick. Finally, the dentist is reimbursed at approximately half the traditional office fee.

The need for periodic dental care does not change because one enters a nursing facility. Yet, no one in the typical facility is trained in oral care. The mouth is not included in any significant way in the nursing curriculum, and physicians do not focus on the mouth.

Formerly, the majority of current residents in nursing facilities had dentures. The introduction of fluoride and other dental care technologies after World War II is resulting in increasingly larger proportions of residents having teeth rather than dentures. By 2006, it has been estimated that as few as 5% of residents arrive with dentures thus presenting a full mouth of teeth needing care. For as long as any patients/residents have dentures, the use of an inexpensive denture label kit will simplify life for the residents and staff of the facility.

Solutions to the lack of continuing dental care will vary, but any successful one will likely include the appointment of a local or area dentist who specializes in geriatric dental care as the Dental Director, paid a monthly retainer fee of perhaps $2.00 to $4.00 per patient resident (just as one pays to have a part-time medical director). This dentist will make monthly visits, perform needed care, and bill third-party payers for care given.

It is customary for the Dental Director to assist the facility in hiring a dental hygienist who will make rounds seeing residents on a monthly basis or more often, and train the nursing staff to observe and meet the residents' oral needs. One approach is to train oral care aides, a regularly employed nurse's aide, who assumes responsibility for maintaining the daily oral health care of residents in the facility.

Table 2.4 suggests a 99% compliance rate.

However, surveyors are for the first time focusing on making dental services for facility residents equivalent to dental care among the general population. Deficiencies for dental services can be expected to increase as this trend continues.

Foot and Eye Care

There is need for a *podiatrist*—a trained professional, who is not a medical doctor, concerned with care of the feet. Podiatric care includes clipping of toenails for diabetics and others and ailments such as corns and bunions.

As the nursing facility population becomes less and less able to make health care visits outside the facility, a periodic visit by a podiatrist, who normally brings an assistant, is becoming a routine need of resident care. The podiatrist and assistant may arrange their work area in a room or even a secluded hallway on a monthly basis and provide care to a large portion of the residents over the course of a morning or afternoon. The number of practicing podiatrists has increased only slowly during the decades 1980 to 2000, increasing

TABLE 2.4.   Percent of Nursing Facilities in the U.S. With Deficiencies for Dental Services, 1993, 1999, and Percent and Number in 2006

	DEFICIENCY GROUP = DENTAL SERVICES	1993 %	1999 %	2006 %	Facilities
F411	Dental services in SNFS	0.4	0.5	0.84	134
F412	Dental services in NFS	0.0	0.4	0.43	68

Source: DHHS, 2006b.

from 7,780 to 12,242. Nevertheless, caring for elderly in the nursing facility setting is one of the major professional foci of podiatrists, because a single nursing home visit can result in serving multiple clients in a single setting (DHHS, 2005, Table 108, p. 346).

Eye care needs are similar to those for teeth and feet. As the nursing home population's mobility becomes more and more restricted, arrangements for a local optician to make periodic visits is becoming a routine health care need.

Pharmaceutical Services

The consulting or the facility pharmacist is responsible at the minimum for assuring that:

- all medications are available as ordered,
- all medications are within expiration date and properly labeled and handled,
- all reorders and stop orders are implemented,
- each resident's medications are reviewed monthly for possible adverse reactions and interactions, and
- appropriate pharmacy policy and procedures are followed.

The consulting pharmacist is responsible for reviewing the drug regimen including observing medication passes and recording and reporting drug error rates and any other problems observed. While the federal requirements require the consultant to report to the attending physician and the director of nursing, the administrator would be wise to stipulate in the consultant contract that the pharmacist also keep the administrator fully informed either individually or at a meeting attended by the administrator and staff.

Besides receiving the required reports the administrator can talk with the pharmacist, the nurses, the physicians, and the residents to learn in greater depth how the system is functioning. If drug reorders are not arriving on time, the nurses will be ready to share this information with the administrator. If the residents are not getting the medicines they believe they depend on, they will be quite willing to report it. But in this, as every such case, both the resident and staff must be queried.

Table 2.5 suggests good compliance in general, with the need for better compliance in the areas of pharmaceutical services, labeling, and procedures for storage. The computerization of medications is an area of rapid change.

TABLE 2.5.   Percent of Nursing Facilities in the U.S. With Deficiencies for Pharmacy Services, 1993, 1999, and Percent and Number in 2006

	DEFICIENCY GROUP = PHARMACY SERVICES	1993 %	1999 %	2006 %	Facilities
F425	Facility provides drugs & biologicals	51.2	1.23	31.96	
F426	Facility provides pharmaceutical services	3.7	5.6	10.35	1,649
F427	Licensed pharmacist provides consultation	1.5	0.7	1.43	228
F428	Res drug regimen rev monthly by pharm	2.4	1.0	0.80	128
F429	Pharmacist reports irregularities	5.7	3.0	3.23	514
F430	Reports of irregularities are acted upon	0.0	2.0	2.49	397
F431	Proper labeling of drugs and biologicals	2.3	2.2	4.61	735
F432	Drugs stored in locked compartments	4.3	5.2	7.54	1,201

Source: DHHS, 2006b.

Physical Therapy (PT) / Occupational Therapy (OT) / Speech Therapy (ST)

A facility of 100 residents may or may not have in-house physical, occupational, and speech therapy services. While there has been a continuing debate over whether to do physical therapy in-house (employ your own physical therapist) or to hire an outside physical therapy group the reimbursement data are now indicating that hiring outside physical therapists is more cost effective inasmuch as there is little or no "down time" for outside physical therapists who also bill more effectively for reimbursement services provided.

The number of physical therapists active in the United States increased from 50,000 in 1980 to 196,000 by the year 2000 due, in part, to high Medicare reimbursement rates for physical therapists (DHHS, 2005, p. 346).

These therapists' work is not fully accomplished unless the nursing and other staff are involved in the process of helping the residents achieve the desired level of function in their activities of daily living and not merely during the therapy period. This implies cooperation between the specialized rehabilitative staff and the regular staff who, in effect, are doing "habilitative" therapy for the residents all the time.

A method of bridging the potential gap between the physical therapist's work and the nursing staff is to establish a restorative nursing program, usually undertaken by a nurse who specializes in this area. The restorative nurse works directly with both the therapy staff and the nursing staff to assure that efforts by the therapists are successfully integrated into the activities of daily living of the residents.

The administrator may want to assure that a rehabilitative team approach is being implemented. This can be accomplished by studying one or two residents' rehabilitation plans, then casually observing the extent to which they are being implemented by the involved staff members.

As indicated in Table 2.6, a remarkable 98%+ compliance rate is achieved.

Laboratory and Other Diagnostic Services

On a physician's order, laboratory and X-ray or other diagnostic services must be provided. These may be on the premises or contracted for in a local hospital or private office. Portable X-ray and, increasingly, additional diagnostic services are generally available on an on-call basis to provide services when a fall or other event occurs that might have injured a resident.

Delayed or inaccurate laboratory work is often a concern among nursing and medical staff. Telephone calls placed or other inquiry modalities inquiring by frustrated nurses about results that should have been received may indicate need for examining the current procedures and contracts to emphasize the need for timely communication.

Table 2.7 demonstrates high compliance in the less subjective tags, a 94.5% compliance in F502, providing and obtaining lab services.

For information about how to read and understand lab reports try accessing these Web sites.

TABLE 2.6.   Percent of Nursing Facilities in the U.S. With Deficiencies for Rehabilitative Services, 1993, 1999, and Percent and Number in 2006

DEFICIENCY GROUP = REHABILITATIVE SERVICES

		1993 %	1999 %	2006 %	Facilities
F406	Facility provides specialized rehab services	1.6	0.8	1.24	197
F407	Rehab services ordered by physician by qual	0.4	0.1	0.14	23

Source: DHHS, 2006b.

TABLE 2.7.   Percent of Nursing Facilities in the U.S. With Deficiencies for Laboratory Services, 1994, 1999, and Percent and Number in 2006

	DEFICIENCY GROUP = LABORATORY SERVICES	1994 %	1999 %	2006 %	Facilities
F502	Facil provides/obtains lab services	1.1	2.0	5.48	873
F503	Lab services provided by fac/referring specim	2.6	0.4	0.09	14
F504	Lab services only when ordered by physician	0.2	0.2	0.60	96
F505	Physician promptly notified of lab results	0.2	0.7	1.23	196
F507	Lab reports are filed in clinical record	0.1	0.1	0.41	66
F508	Facility provides/obtains radiology services	0.1	0.2	0.38	61
F513	Reports of X-rays/diag services filed in record	0.0	0.1	0.11	17

Source: DHHS, 2006b.

- College of American Pathologists: www.cap.org
- The Doctor's Doctor: www.thedoctorsdoctor.com
- Lab Tests Online: www.labtestsonline.org

Nursing Services

Nursing Department Tasks

The nursing service has among others the following responsibilities:

- providing nursing care to residents as ordered by the physician
- completing the Minimum Data Set, any required protocols triggered by the Minimum Data Set, creating, implementing, and updating the comprehensive plan of care
- administering medications to the residents
- keeping patient records
- monitoring residents for changes in condition and notifying the responsible physician—in short, serving as the physician's eyes and ears on a 24-hour basis
- achieving optimal quality of care and quality of life for residents
- making certain that every resident is functioning at the highest possible level
- playing a coordinating role with other staff, for example, assuring that planned physical therapy, activities, physician office visits, and the like take place

In short, nursing is involved in a myriad of activities such as ⬛ assessments ⬛ wound care ⬛ starting IVs ⬛ tube feeding ⬛ oxygen therapy ⬛ range of motion ⬛ toileting ⬛ feeding ⬛ counseling ⬛ friendship ⬛ comfort ⬛ ambulation ⬛ transfer ⬛ assistance with the activities of daily living ⬛ changing the diapers and sheets ⬛ turning patients ⬛ use of assistive devices ⬛ bathing ⬛ toileting ⬛ dressing ⬛ ambulating ⬛ cleaning up spills ⬛ washing hands ⬛ room tidiness ⬛ ice water ⬛ hospice ⬛ discharge planning ⬛ recruiting ⬛ training ⬛ disciplining ⬛ evaluating staff ⬛ interfacing with the other departments ⬛ observing the universal precautions ⬛ interfacing with physicians ⬛ pharmacists, numerous health care professionals ⬛ counseling ⬛ reassuring families and significant others ⬛ washing hands ⬛ coping with volunteers ⬛ cooperating with the police, the fire department ⬛ doing infection control ⬛ working short ⬛ conducting inservices ⬛ charting ⬛ charting ⬛ charting ⬛ bowel and bladder programs ⬛ fire safety ⬛ disaster preparedness ⬛ answering call bells ⬛ checking on the residents hundreds of times each day ⬛ participating in lengthy care planning sessions ⬛ afternoon and evening snacks ⬛ getting food substitutes from dietary ⬛ settling battles among residents ⬛ washing hands ⬛ coping with Alzheimer's, extensive dementia ⬛ learned helplessness ⬛ death and dying ⬛ emergencies ⬛ morticians, ⬛ endless admissions ⬛ discharge planning ⬛ lost clothing ⬛ lost teeth ⬛ lost jewelry ⬛ running out of bed pads ⬛ hazardous waste rules ⬛ inspectors from everywhere for days at a time ⬛ electrical outages ⬛ failing equipment ⬛ room transfers ⬛ roommate dissatisfaction ⬛ refusal to eat ⬛ broken bed rails ⬛ restraint issues ⬛ missing oxygen tank wrenches ⬛ snippy staff ⬛ arrogant physicians ⬛ dissatisfied residents ⬛ troublesome visitors ⬛ unresponsive decubitus ulcers ⬛ unresponsive medical directors ⬛ the on-call nurse or physician don't return calls for 45 minutes ⬛ overflowing linen bins ⬛ broken wheelchairs ⬛ epidemics among staff and residents ⬛ out-of-uniform staff ⬛ missing name tags ⬛ wandering patients ⬛ pool (contract) personnel who don't know or don't care ⬛ misplaced charts or efiles ⬛ emergency carts that were used and not restocked ⬛ constant phone calls ⬛ late lab reports ⬛ physicians who don't sign orders or visit on a timely basis ⬛ and this is only the tip of the iceberg. Nursing is the quintessential embodiment of the reality that if it can happen it will.

With this myriad of duties, it is not surprising that some things don't get done as acceptably as desired. In Table 2.8, indications are that while the vast majority of nursing duties are successfully carried out, success in achieving acceptable levels in the areas of performing comprehensive assessments and care plan, accuracy of assessments, and services by qualified personnel still present a challenge in about 15% or more of the nation's facilities.

TABLE 2.8.   Percent of Nursing Facilities in the U.S. With Deficiencies for Resident Assessment, 1993, 1999, and Percent and Number in 2006

DEFICIENCY GROUP = RESIDENT ASSESSMENT

	1993 %	1999 %	2006 %	Facilities
F271 Admissions orders	.3	.2	.23	37
F272 Comprehensive assessments	37	13	12	1,864
F273 Frequency	2.3	.7	.8	140
F274 Change in condition	7.6	3.6	3.5	557
F275 Annual assessment	1.5	.6	.8	137
F276 Review of assessments	6.1	4.4	2.8	447
F278 Accuracy of assessments	15.5	5.2	11.01	11,754
F279 Comprehensive care plans	30.5	16.1	18.7	2,978
F280 Dev/Prep/Review of comp care plan	9.8	6.0	11.8	1,890
F281 Services provided meet profess. standards	6.7	12.8	26.34	4,196
F282 Services by qualified persons in accord with care	6.7	12.8	12.4	1,977
F283 Discharge summary: recapitulation/final	7.5	1.1	.98	156
F284 Post discharge requirements met	3.6	.7	.98	107
F285 Pre-admission screening PASARR	.5	.2	.7	98

Source: DHHS, 2006b.

Subacute Care Nursing

When nursing homes admit subacute care patients, their nurses must become proficient in tasks heretofore considered the expertise of hospital nurses. Additional high-tech nursing skills are required. Among them are the use of implanted ports (a vascular, i.e., blood vessel, access that remains in place for an extended period of time), mid-line catheters (placed in the arm for a 3–4 week period of IV therapy), central line catheters (the area surrounding the heart), and epidural lines (just outside the spine usually to administer pain medicine). Most nursing facility nurses are skilled in administering epidural medications (i.e., situated upon or outside the dura mater, which is the outermost, toughest of the three meninges of the brain and spinal cord), but are not skilled in what is known as category two activities, which are more invasive.

In 2006, under 2% (1.62%) of nursing home residents were receiving IV therapy (nutritional or blood; DHHS, 2006a, F78–F93).

In addition, in 2006, nursing staff were responsible for:

• Respiratory therapy	12%
• Tracheotomy care	1%
• Ostomy care (feeding through an incision in the stomach)	4.52%
• Suctioning	1.38%
• Injections	17.85%

Pain management, prescribed for one of every four residents in 2006 (24.84%) is a growing area of responsibility for nursing because it often involves nursing judgments about when to give pain medication if the medication is not prescribed on a fixed dosage (DHHS, 2006a, F78, F133–F139).

Nursing service responsibilities are spelled out in some detail in §483.30 Nursing Services of the federal requirements. Figure 2.2 demonstrates nursing homes' response to the increasing acuity of residents being admitted during these years. The total nursing hours (RNs, LPN/LVNs, and NAs) per resident rose from 2.9 in 1993 to 3.2 by 1999, and to 3.6 in 2005, representing a steady increase in the acuity level being treated.

Average Nursing Hours Per Resident Day

Figure 2.3 breaks out the division of nursing hours among RN hours, LPN/LVN hours, and nursing aide hours. The main change over 1993 to 2005 was

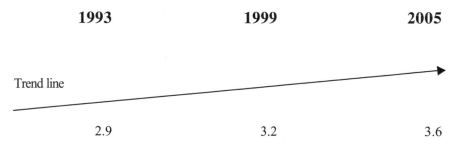

FIGURE 2.2 Trend in total nursing hours per resident day in facilities with Medicaid and Medicare beds in the United States, 1993, 1999, and 2005.
Source: The State of Long-Term Health Care Sector 2005, Reimbursement and Research Department American Health Care Association, August 29, 2006 and Department of Social & Behavioral Sciences, University of California, San Francisco.

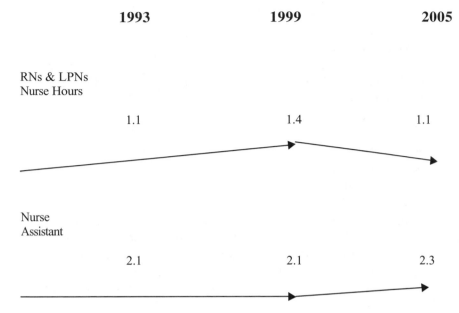

FIGURE 2.3 Average nursing hours per resident day in all certified U.S. nursing home facilities, 1993, 1999, and 2005.
Source: The State of Long-Term Health Care Sector 2005, Reimbursement and Research Department American Health Care Association, August 29, 2006 and Department of Social & Behavioral Sciences, University of California, San Francisco.

to slightly decrease the more expensive RN time and slightly increase reliance on nurse assistants.

Quality of Resident Life

There are unwritten dimensions to care performed by the nursing service. It is not possible, and perhaps not desirable, federal efforts notwithstanding, to set them all down, for many of the nursing acts that increase the quality of life cannot be fully spelled out in policy statements. The quality of life enjoyed is directly proportional to the quality of the effort given by the nursing staff.

Dr. William Thomas' Eden Alternative movement should cause alarm bells to sound. Dr. Thomas observes that the majority of nursing home resources are spent on the war against disease when the real need is to address loneliness, helplessness, and boredom. The typical current nursing home is the creation of government regulations founded on a hospital model. Edenizing is the process of combining nature, hope, and nursing homes. A nursing home can be more nearly a human habitat when it is "Edenized." That is, when it has birds, cats, dogs, fish, rabbits, chickens, children, plants, and gardens to walk in and eat from (Thomas, 1996, pp. 1–180). The Eden concept places an emphasis on intergenerational contact (Maddox & Sussman, 2001, p. 555, 798).

Nurse Availability

While there has seemed to be a chronic shortage of good nurses, the total number of active registered nurses increased from 1.2 million in 1980 to 2.2 million in 1999 (DHHS, 2005, Table 108, p. 346). An unchanging 6.3% of all RNs reported working in nursing homes and extended care facilities during the years 1998 through 2004 according to the Seasons Seminars 2004 National Sample Survey of Registered Nurses (www.seasons-seminars. com).

Increasing Dependency on the Nursing Assistants

The nursing home population is heavily dependent on the nursing staff, especially the nursing assistants. The five essential activities of daily living are:

1. Eating
2. Dressing
3. Toileting
4. Bathing
5. Transferring (e.g., from bed to chair or bed to toilet)

In 2003, for all persons in the United States aged 65–74, 26% had limitation of activities caused by chronic conditions while for all persons in the United States aged 75 and over the limitation rises to 44% (DHHS, 2005, p. 243). Limitations among the nursing home population are dramatically more debilitating.

The average nursing home resident is dependent on nursing staff for nearly 4 (3.94) of these daily activities (DHHS, 2006a, F78–F93).

Eating: Half are independent (49.16% in 2006) while 33.6% require assistance and 17.25% are dependent on staff, a total dependence of 50.82% of all residents (DHHS, 2006a, F78–F93).

Dressing: 11.42% of residents can dress themselves independently. Of the 88.58% needing assistance, 60.24% require some assistance and 28.34% are fully dependent on the nursing staff (DHHS, 2006a, F78–F93).

Toileting: Only 18.08% of residents can successfully toilet themselves, 50% require assistance, and 32% are wholly dependent on staff assistance. Thus 82% of the typical facility's residents need assistance in toileting (DHHS, 2006a, F78–F93).

Transferring: 22.45% can move from bed to chair or bed to bath without assistance. Half (52.21%) require assistance while one-fourth (25.34%) are wholly dependent on staff (DHHS, 2006a, F78–F93).

Bathing: Fewer than 5% (4.57%) of residents can bath themselves independently. Six of each 10 (59.29%) require assistance, and over one-third (36.14%) must be bathed by staff (DHHS, 2006a, F78–F93).

Organizational Interdependencies

Organizational interdependencies between nursing and virtually every other area exist within the facility. Nursing is dependent on dietary, housekeeping, laundry, maintenance, the business office, the social worker, and the allied health professionals, to mention a few. In sum, for nursing to do its tasks properly, nearly every other department and functional area within the organization must also be doing its tasks in a cooperative manner.

Staffing

Three nursing shifts, 24 hours a day, 365 days a year offer a staffing challenge. The proportional ratios between registered nurses, licensed practical nurses, aides, and even geriatric nurse practitioners will vary with the staffing philosophy of the facility administrators and the patient profile. As acuity level increases in many facilities, the proportion of professionally trained nurses increases. Research by Patchner and Patchner (1993) suggests that permanently assigning nurses and nursing assistants to sets of residents leads to improved care through enabling holistic care and becoming personally involved in and vested in their duties (p. 37). In 1999, administrators were 99.1% successful in providing the required number of registered nurse hours, but only 95% successful in providing sufficient nursing staff, as judged by the nation's surveyors (Harrington, Carrillo, Thollaug, Summers, & Wellin, 2000, p. 122).

Administrative Observations

Just as the director of nursing services is expected to make daily resident rounds, the administrator may decide to emulate nursing. The administrator must decide to what extent they wish to receive daily reports on admissions, discharges, changes in resident conditions, accidents, incidents, transfers, deaths, and the like as part of their information system. The reports are not a satisfactory substitute for the administrator's personal observation, on a daily basis, to learn by wandering around what is actually taking place in the facility. Also, one has to be on the scene to be the coach, energizer, or communicator of one's vision for the facility.

The Business Office

In a typical 100-bed facility one full-time and often an additional part-time employee staff the business office. Briefly, the business office

- keeps financial records
- manages accounts receivable and accounts payable
- maintains vendor files
- assists in monitoring the budget
- prepares the payroll
- keeps required records and makes financial reports
- deals with third-party payers, Medicare, Medicaid, and others
- safeguards and controls resident funds
- often acts as receptionist and answers the telephone

New Key Role for Business Office: CMS Accuracy

Neither the MDS coordinator nor the team members who sign their portions of the MDS are necessarily business / reimbursement oriented. Because CMS now bases Medicare and Medicaid payments on the boxes checked on the MDS, nearly two-thirds of the total revenue of the average nursing facility depends on which boxes are checked. The business office must now understand the MDS scores and resulting RUG (resource utilization groups) as a matter for full understanding and careful attention to correctness of resident assessments for business purposes just as the nursing, social service, dietary and other staff must master the MDS and RAPs to assure competent resident care.

Medical Records

A full-time employee must, by federal requirements, be assigned to keep the medical record service up to date. Usually this person is called a ward clerk. Facilities are required to keep a great number of records, among the most important of which is the medical record. If medical records are not complete and current, federal and state inspectors will normally issue a directive that it be corrected within a specified time period. Increasingly, medical records require a full-time person operating a computer. A professional therapist with 25 years experience in several facilities in the same chain observes that within a 1-year period she worked in two facilities each actually providing equally good resident care. One facility kept excellent records and received very few deficiencies, the other equally good facility kept poor records of the good quality care it was providing and received numerous serious deficiencies. Documentation truly counts.

Admissions

In states where first-come-first-served rules do not exist, the person(s) in charge of admissions influences the case mix of the facility. Usually a person with a social work background is employed as the admissions coordinator. Often a single employee will head both admissions and social work. Sometimes the director of nurses does admissions. In most cases, the admissions process is shared jointly by the director of nursing and the admissions director. In any case, admissions have profound effects on the facility work load, atmosphere, ability to achieve its goals, and ability to provide appropriate care. Who is admitted from where and with what care needs and reimbursement rates are the lifeblood of the facility.

The admissions person(s) must find, screen, process, facilitate, and manage case mix, keeping financial, light vs. heavy care, good will of the hospital discharge planners, managed care, or other source elements all balanced. The admissions person(s) is an important promoter of the facility, marketing to all the relevant world, for example, hospital discharge planners, the local physicians, third-party payers, managed care organizations, Worker's Compensation insurance, insurance companies, and the like. A daily fax to local hospitals showing bed availability can maintain a presence and lead to admissions.

Consider having an admissions application that can be filled out and submitted on your Web site. Your federal survey results are online for potential applicants to review, so let them also be able to apply online after they review your surveyor reports. The Web is becoming a major source of referral to facilities. Make sure that your listing is correct on such Web sites as www. seniorstreet.com, an online senior health care facility directory where consumers search for long-term care facilities.

Make It Easy for the "Customer"

- Greet the customer
- Listen to the customer

- Identify the needs of the customer
- Ask for the business of the customer

"In your opinion, do you believe we can serve your mother?"
Every "lost" admission can be a $90,000 loss to the facility.

Admission to a nursing facility is a major life transition for both the new resident and that resident's significant others. A caring staff will always make sure someone—the administrator, the head nurse, the admissions director—calls the significant others after the first night with a full report on how the resident is doing.

Dietary Department

The Food Standard

Food is an essential ingredient in the quality of resident life. Satisfaction with the facility is as often influenced by the food as by the quality of nursing care. Some families feel they may not have enough medical background to judge the adequacy of nursing care, but most do consider themselves experts in the matter of food. Tasty food is important to a satisfactory quality of life. Hospital food, eaten for a relatively short period of time, can be tolerated. Nursing home food, consumed for much longer periods, is subject to much greater scrutiny by both residents and their families/significant others.

The Food Standard: Can It Be Met?

The dietary manager in the typical nursing facility (one with 70% Medicaid, 15% Medicare, 10% private pay, 5% other) is permitted to spend about $4.00 to $5.00+ per day for raw food costs. The typical life care community (one with nearly 100% private pay) spends $12.00+ per day for raw food costs. While the nation's nursing facilities maintain good nutritional status for residents 90% of the time, it is of concern that surveyors believe that nutritional needs are not met 10% of the time (Harrington et al., 2000, p. 105). A more realistic raw food budget for the nation's facilities would help. Surprisingly, the nation's surveyors believe that 99.8% of the time nursing facilities provide a well-balanced diet (F360).

The dietary department's influence extends 24 hours a day. The availability of bedtime snacks, or midnight snacks for insomniac residents is as much a part of the ambiance of the facility as the availability of continuous nursing services. This department is heavily interactive with nursing services (e.g., refreshments at social activities) and with most other departments. The food service depends on other departments as well: laundry for linens and maintenance to keep the kitchen functioning. Some facilities contract for food service with outside vendors. In this situation, the head of dietary may be an employee of the food service contractor.

According to Table 2.9, the major area needing improvement is sanitary conditions and food properly prepared and palatable.

The administrator can monitor food services in a number of ways. Daily, random walks through the kitchen, eating with residents in the dining hall, and assisting with feeding in resident rooms and in the dining rooms (if properly qualified to do so) are productive ways to monitor. Much can be learned by getting a tray and eating its contents under circumstances similar to those experienced by the resident.

Achieving the nutritional diet prescribed by the physician and developed by the registered dietitian or registered dietitian consultant, assuring tasty food at the right temperature, doing nutritional assessments, monitoring weight gains and losses, monitoring I/O (input and output), providing food substitutes as requested, catering for facility functions and its many visiting groups, and maintaining the dietary area according to cleanliness standards are but a few of the critical functions of dietary.

TABLE 2.9.   Percent of Nursing Facilities in the U.S. With Deficiencies for Dietary Services, 1993, 1999, and Percent and Number in 2006

	DEFICIENCY GROUP = DIETARY SERVICES				
		1993 %	1999 %	2006 %	Facilities
F360	Well-balanced diet	.6	.2	.3	54
F361	Qualified staff	1.5	.5	.7	112
F362	Sufficient staff	1.6	.8	.6	99
F363	Menus and nutritional adequacy	15	5	6	939
F364	Food properly prepared, palatable	14	8	7	1,172
F365	Meet individual needs	2.2	2.4	2.5	408
F366	Food substitutes	4.7	1.3	1.1	183
F367	Therapeutic diets	1.1	1.1	3.5	569
F368	Frequency of meals/intervals between meals	5.7	4.7	3.6	621
F369	Assistive devices	.9	.8	.9	150
F370	Food from approved sources			.9	6
F371	Store, prepare food under sanitary conditions	30	26	34	5,445
F372	Dispose garbage properly	3.5	3.0	3.4	535

Source: DHHS, 2006b.

Consider Whether the Administrator Has a Role in Diets Served in These Two Facilities

Facility A diets served		Facility B diets served
Regular	45% of residents	High Fiber
Low-Salt	18% of residents	High Protein
Low-Fat	10% of residents	High Protein/High-Calorie
Mechanical Soft	17% of residents	No Sugar Added
Puree	10% of residents	No Added Salt/No Concentrated Sugar
		Strict No Added Salt/Soft
		Honey Thick
		No Concentrated Sugar/High Calorie
		No Concentrated Sugar/High Protein
		No Concentrated Sugar/No Added Salt/Low Calorie
		High Protein/High Calorie/Nectar Thick
		Nectar Thick
		High Protein/No Concentrated Sugar
		No Added Salt/High Calorie
		No Added Salt/High Protein/High Calorie
		No Added Salt/High Protein/Hi-Calorie/Low Fat
		No Concentrated Sugar/1400cc FL
		High Protein/High Calorie/Honey Thick
		No Added Salt/Honey Thick/High Protein/High Calorie
		No Concentrated Sugar/High Calorie
		Strict No Concentrated Sugar/No Added Salt
		No Concentrated Sugar/1500 cc
		No Concentrated Salt/Nectar Thick, PurMeat, Soft
		No Added Salt/No Sugar/Nectar Thick, Finger
		Thin Puree/High Calorie/High Protein/ Nectar Thick
Likely efficacy	High	Extremely High
Achievability	High	Extremely Low
Likely deficient practice	Low	Extremely High

These are two actual facilities. In short, the likelihood that dietary will be able to successfully serve the diets prescribed is inversely proportional to the number and complexity of diets prescribed by the physicians and registered dietitians. In this case, more may be less.

In 2006, 7.84% of residents experienced unplanned weight loss/gain (DHHS, 2006a, F78–F142). Eating is important (see National Association of Nutrition and Aging Services Programs—www.nanasp.org).

> *Eating:* Half are independent (49.16% in 2006) while 33.6% require assistance and 17.25% are dependent on staff, a total dependence of 50.82% of all residents (DHHS, 2006a, F78–F93).

The level of complexity in providing the physician prescribed diets for nursing home residents is high. Of residents in 2006, 6.41% required tube feeding, 34.74% required mechanically altered diets, 19.21% required eating rehabilitative programs, and 7.39% used assistive eating devices.

While the need for qualified nutritionists in nursing facilities has been increasing, the number of active nutritionists in the United States has increased from 32,000 in 1980 to 90,000 in 2000 (DHHS, 2005, Table 108, p. 346).

Social Services

Social services is concerned not only with the resident's initial adjustment to the facility, but also their continuing accommodation to the environment. The social worker is also responsible for monitoring each resident's socio-psychological experiences and orientation in the facility (DHHS, 2005, p. 29; Gordon & Stryker, 1983, p. 178).

It is the social worker who is often most directly in contact with the resident's family or significant others. This staff member is the one involved in assisting residents who have current or approaching financial needs that will be met by a public agency. In short, the social worker functions in the nursing home in a manner similar to social workers employed by the local Department of Social Services. Maintaining the quality of each resident's social well-being in a facility is a complex function.

Significantly assisting each resident to meet their various social, psychological, physical, environmental, family, financial, and related needs is never achievable by the social worker alone. The social worker must stimulate the various other staff members to participate in this process. A typical problem to which the administrator must be attuned is a tendency for responsive residents to receive the lioness's share of the social worker's time and attention. The less responsive and unresponsive have needs, also.

Activities / Recreation

Nursing services primarily address the medical needs of the residents, and in that process partially meet their social and interpersonal requirements.

The activities coordinator's task is to assure that the physical, social, and mental well-being of each resident is included in each comprehensive resident assessment and the required comprehensive plan of care. For the nearly comatose, disoriented, or agitated patients, this assignment is indeed a challenge. The activities director and the social services worker are assigned primary responsibility for attention to the quality of psychosocial life that exists within a facility. It is difficult to imagine a more complicated undertaking in shaping the quality of the resident life.

In 1993, according to federal surveyors, 88% of facilities satisfactorily provided activities for residents. By 1999, 91% of facilities were meeting activities goals (Harrington et al., 2000, p. 91).

Housekeeping

Importance of "Good Housekeeping"

Not only do federal and state inspectors make intuitive value judgments about a facility based on its cleanliness and physical appearance, so also will most of the residents themselves and their significant others. Dirty floors and walls, empty toilet paper holders, yellowing toilets and lavatories, and offensive odors associated with them communicate a message to the residents, staff, and visitors revealing what the facility thinks about itself. Inattention to housekeeping details leads inspectors and the public alike to wonder to what extent it carries over into resident care, sanitation in food preparations, and cleanliness of the residents themselves.

The head of housekeeping may have excellently designed job assignments for the four to eight housekeepers. The administrator can tell how effective these schedules are simply by walking around the facility. On these tours the administrator must be able to "see" dirt.

There is a surprising amount of regulation surrounding the housekeeping area such as the required Material Safety Data Sheets for all chemicals to which the head of housekeeping and the administrator must give attention.

In 1993, federal surveyors were satisfied that 80% of facilities were meeting housekeeping requirements. By 1999, 85% of facilities were satisfying federal surveyors that facilities were providing a sanitary, orderly, and comfortable environment (Harrington et al., 2000, p. 93). Table 2.10 illustrates that what is considered good housekeeping was achieved only 80% of the time in 2006.

TABLE 2.10. Percent of Nursing Facilities in the U.S. With Deficiencies for Housekeeping, 1993, 1999, and Percent and Number in 2006

DEFICIENCY GROUP = HOUSEKEEPING AND MAINTENANCE SERVICES				
		1993	1999	2006	Facilities
F253	Housekeeping and maintenance services	19.5	15.3	20.5	3,267

Source: DHHS, 2006b.

Laundry

Clean linens, clean resident clothes, the availability of linens and clothes when needed, and safe and sanitary handling techniques for both soiled and clean linen are areas of responsibility of the head of laundry. Whether it is better to do laundry in-house or to contract with a linen service (known as outsourcing, the purchasing of portions of services from outside providers) is a subject of continuing debate. Whatever the decision, there will be procedures for handling linens that the administrator can observe for conformity to regulations and to facility policies.

Maintenance Department

Distinguishing between maintenance and housekeeping responsibilities is often an issue. If a wall has a hole in it, it is clearly maintenance's job to fix the hole. If that same wall is only dirty and needs washing, it is probably housekeeping's job. Each facility must designate through established policies the respective responsibilities of these two functions. The repair and upkeep of physical systems is clearly the responsibility of maintenance.

Preventive maintenance, anticipating when a piece of equipment will need servicing or risk ceasing to function, is a complex task requiring experienced judgment. A well-trained maintenance director can do much to anticipate troublesome, unnecessary breakdowns of equipment. The administrator can participate in the maintenance process by occasionally assuming a "maintenance mindset," then walking though the facility touching, feeling, and judging the state of repair of all they encounter.

Some Areas Requiring Special Teamwork Attention From the Administrator

- patient care planning and implementation of resident care plans
- pain management as prescribed by the physicians

- successful billing, from recording supplies consumed to required "wording" for claims
- housekeeping vs. maintenance
- dietary/nursing coordination in getting food to residents on a timely basis, at the right temperature, attractively presented with attention to accommodating resident preferences
- differentiating between activities functions and the social worker function—dangers of persons' needs falling between the cracks
- discharge planning
- resident advocacy to the staff and families
- nursing / housekeeping / laundry coordination

2.2 Identifying the Human Resources Functions

Managers in organizations have always performed certain basic human resources functions.

Human Resources Functions

Human resources functions are a range of activities that can include record keeping, employee recruitment and selection, training and development, compensation management, performance evaluations, and often labor relations (Noe et al., 2000, p. 5; Robbins & Coulter, 2007, pp. 327, 342).

- **Record Keeping**—assuring that all necessary information is in the employee's file and that it is kept confidential. This is becoming increasingly complicated as files are computerized.
- **Recruitment**—assisting department heads in finding employees for vacant positions.
- **Selection**—assisting department heads in interviewing and assessing job applicants.
- **Training and Retaining Employees**—assisting department heads in employee orientation, inservice training, and continuing education.
- **Compensation Management**—assisting department heads and payroll office in administering salary and the other benefits offered by the facility.
- **Performance Evaluation**—assisting managers in conducting employee evaluation in conformity with the facility human resources policies.
- **Labor Relations**—assisting managers in creating a favorable work environment.
- **Health and Safety**—drug testing and monitoring employee health status, for example, assuring Hepatitis B and Tuberculosis immunizations are provided as required and kept current.

Human Resources Management as an Occupation

In its rudimentary state, human resources was the responsibility of each department manager. (In a 100-bed nursing facility, this tends to be true today. Usually, the department mangers do initial interviewing, perhaps bringing the administrator in on the final selection.) Chruden speculates that, historically, as the department supervisor's job became more complex, the responsibility for certain human resources activities, for example, hours worked and payroll, were taken over by a clerical assistant. From this initial record-keeping activity, the responsibilities were gradually broadened until individuals began making a full-time career in what is now called human resources administration (Johns & Saks, 2001, pp. 248–250; Noe et al., 2000, p. 15.).

Human resources managers do not "manage" employees except for those who work under them in the human resources department, if there is more than one employee in that unit. Human resources management is a staff function; it has no line authority in the organization. All the employees in the organization are directly managed by their department supervisors, who hold line authority. It is the line managers who, in fact, are responsible for performing most of the human resources functions for the employees under them. The department heads do the actual hiring, require inservice training and development, give performance evaluations and promotions, award raises, and discipline, suspend, and discharge their staff.

The role of the human resources manager and staff is to assist the line supervisors, for example, the department heads in the nursing facility, to carry out human resources responsibilities according to policies set by facility ownership. Thus, human resources staff make an important contribution to overall employee satisfaction by assuring that human resources policies are carried out as consistently as feasible from one department to another.

In a facility of perhaps 100 to 150 residents, no full-time human resources director is usually hired. However, some of the typical "human resources department" functions are usually given to one employee who, in effect, serves as a part-time personnel staff in the facility. This person is sometimes designated staff development coordinator or a similar title. Alternately, assisting the department managers with personnel matters such as record keeping and assuring that employees are tested for tuberculosis and are offered Hepatitis B vaccinations (as required by the Bloodborne Pathogens regulations), may be assigned to an assistant administrator, an administrative assistant, a staff nurse, or an employee in the business office.

Emerging Human Resource (HR) Management Techniques

Technologies now being utilized by HR staff include interactive voice technology, the Internet, client-servers, relational databases, imaging, and specialized software (Noe et al., 2000, p. 582).

These technologies will facilitate:

- employee control over their training and benefit package
- paperless employment offices
- computer access to employee records (no more 1" thick folders locked in a steel file)
- 24-hour access to files and changing files
- closer surveillance of employee performance
- a growing rash of privacy issues (Noe et al., 2000, p. 583).

Interactive Voice Technology

Computer-based voice-activated systems will allow employees to access their files and accounts such as retirement accounts, vacation taken, and the like.

The Internet and the World Wide Web

Employees in any facility can communicate with employees in any other facility to compare opinions in open chat rooms and the like. Employees' blogs can influence facility image in the community.

Networks and Client–Server Architecture

A network of desktop computers can share databases on employees and HR information. Employee data can be accessed by multiple users. A client-server can hold multiple databases about employees, for example, financial, employment, and health records databases can be accessed singly or multiply. Relational databases with fields such as employee name, serial number, social security number, job classification, and immunization status can enable HR (and other!) personnel to quickly produce HR information, for example, a list of employees needing to be retested for TB in the next month.

Imaging

Using scanners allows for information, for example, application, disciplinary actions, evaluations, health records, and the like to be stored electronically and printed out on an as needed basis. Paper will have a reduced role in HR management.

CD-ROM *and Laser Discs*

These devices are recreating the training programs of facilities. A nurse's aide might, for example, complete a CD-ROM or Laser Disc course on infection control and document this in their required inservice record.

Groupware

Electronic meeting software will allow multiple users to share and work on the same document simultaneously. Not everyone might have to come to a lengthy resident care planning meeting to update a Minimum Data Set form due.

Needless to say, access to and the uses of these databases create privacy concerns. Just as nearly every American's debt status is instantly available to anyone in a computer-based credit report, complete information about every employee (and resident) may be only a keystroke away (Noe et al., 2000, pp. 582–592).

2.3 Planning Employment Needs: Writing Job Descriptions

Each facility needs to break down all work to be accomplished (the processor portion of the systems model) into a set of activities that can be performed by one person. Several definitions provided by the U.S. Employment Service (USES) and the U.S. Office of Personnel Management may be useful to review at this point (Ivancevich, Szjlagyi, & Wallace, 1977, p. 98).

Job Analysis

The process of defining a job in terms of tasks or behaviors required and specifying the qualifications of the employee to be placed in that job (Noe et al., 2000, p. 117; Robbins & Coulter, 2007, p. 326).

Job Description

Information about the job that results in a statement of the job to be done, usually including a list of duties and responsibilities in order of importance. Usually a job description includes (a) the title, (b) the qualifications, (c) to whom the worker is primarily responsible, and (d) the duties or specific expectations (Argenti, 1994, p. 234; Noe et al., 2000, p. 127; Robbins & Coulter, 2007, p. 462).

Job Specification

A statement of the skills, education, and experience required to perform the work. This is derived from the job description (Robbins & Coulter, 2007, p. 326).

Job Titles

Job titles, or job classifications, distinguish one job from all others. Job titles may also indicate the occupational level of the job (e.g., nurse supervisor indicates a higher position, administratively at least, than registered nurse) or the level of authority of seniority of a job, for example, registered nurse levels 1, 2, and 3.

Task

A coordinated and aggregated series of work elements used to produce an output (e.g., making beds).

Position

The responsibilities and duties performed by one individual. There are as many positions as there are employees.

Job

A group of positions that are similar in their duties, for example, laundry, housekeeping, and grounds (Robbins & Coulter, 2007, p. 461).

Job Family

A group of two or more jobs that have similar duties, for example, the duties of the registered nurse and licensed nurse practitioners (Ivancevich et al., 1977, pp. 98, 100; Johns & Saks, 2001, pp. 176–177; Noe et al., 2000, p. 127; Robbins & Coulter, 2007, p. 462).

All the work to be accomplished in operating a nursing facility must be broken down into a series of tasks. Tasks are grouped together so that they can be performed by one individual.

Job Analysis

The process of grouping a series of related tasks into a position. Each position can be described in terms of the tasks and behaviors involved and of the education and training needed to perform the job successfully.

Potential Problems With Job Descriptions

The federal government examines job descriptions and specifications for possible discriminatory effects. Each of the requirements for a job must be necessary for the adequate performance of that job. If, for example, a nursing facility in an area with an unusually large number of available job applicants required 2 years of college for applicants for the nurse's aide position, it must be able to demonstrate why this is essential to perform the job, that is, that the requirement has proven validity. This is a higher educational requirement than usual; therefore, the facility would be obliged to prove that it did not serve to discriminate against members of a particular group on the basis of sex or ethnic origins (Noe et al., 2000, p. 131).

Once job descriptions have been written and the expected workload of the facility estimated, future employment needs can be forecast.

2.4 Forecasting Future Employment Needs

The planning process begins with a projection of the number of residents and the expected levels of medical complexity the facility expects to serve over a period of time, usually during the next 1 to 5 years. This forecast can then be translated into specific personnel requirements for the future period (Noe et al., 2000, p. 146; Robbins & Coulter, 2007, p. 240).

Taking a Manpower Inventory

Numerous factors must be taken into account in projecting the present and future availability of qualified personnel in sufficient number. This is the process of taking a manpower inventory.

Several sources of employment information exist. The Employment Security Commission and the Department of Labor gather data that are useful in estimating the future availability of needed employees (Noe et al., 2000, p. 147).

Identifying Trends

Data such as those mentioned help to identify trends. A number of trends are of potential importance.

Competition for Human Resources

It is practical to take an inventory of present and planned health and related facilities that are or will be competing for similarly qualified personnel. For example, if no acute care hospital exists in the geographic area, but a large for-profit hospital is expected to be constructed within 2 years, competition may increase dramatically. Or, similarly, if the local hospital is one of the several local hospitals that are downsizing or closing their doors each year, the labor pool may be suddenly increased (Hitt et al., 2001, pp. 187–190; Robbins & Coulter, 2007, p. 323). One result of worker shortages in various functional areas within the nursing facility is increasing dependence on outsourcing, that is, having services performed by an outside organization, such as having laundry done off-site (Noe et al., 2000, p. 156).

Job Security

Companies no longer guarantee their employees job security. Over the past two decades employment has ceased to be a lifetime commitment by companies to their workers. Employees of today increasingly perceive themselves as individuals who manage their personal career over their lifetime, which increasingly involves several employers. Companies are decommitting to their employees, and employees are decommitting to their companies (Noe et al., 2000, p. 21).

In-Migration or Out-Migration Patterns in the Labor Supply

Knowledge of whether the worker pool from which employees must be chosen is shrinking or enlarging is important. Statistics are usually available on the local unemployment rate. Unfortunately, for the nursing facility a low local unemployment rate can have the effect of a noticeable reduction in the quality of applicants, level of job interest, and longevity for positions such as nurses' aide, housekeeper, and grounds person (Noe et al., 2000, p. 149).

Wage Scale Movements in the Area

An increasing worker pool may reduce wage scales, while a shrinking worker pool may cause the wage scale to rise. The perceived widespread nursing shortage in recent years resulted in rapid increases in nursing salaries during those years. As the nursing shortage eased nurses' wages began to trend slightly downward. Nursing "shortages" are increasingly cyclical.

Expected Impacts of Educational Institutions

Educational institutions such as local community colleges are becoming major sources of training for manpower needed by nursing facilities. Any expected increase or decrease in training activities, for example, the addition or closing of a licensed practical nurse program in the local community college, could dramatically affect the availability of labor, especially trained nurse's aides.

Knowledge of these trends can assist planners to take action before an anticipated employment crisis. If a shortage is foreseen, the facility might join with other local health care providers in a program to attract additional health-related personnel to the area.

2.5 Recruiting Employees

Once the forecast of the resident profile expected to be served has been translated into specific personnel requirements for the facility, they become the basis for the recruitment and selection program. The forecast assists the facility in determining the number and types of employees it will need to recruit as well as the sources for recruitment (Noe et al., 2000, p. 160).

Influence of Affirmative Action and Americans With Disabilities Act

Since the passage of the Civil Rights Act in 1964, the process of seeking new employees has become more public. Prior to that time, facilities could choose employees without scrutiny by government agencies with regard to possible job discrimination based on age, sex, race, marital status, religion, national origin, or handicap.

Today government agencies can review for possible legal violations by examining the following: (a) the facility's list of recruitment sources for each job category, (b) recruitment advertising, and (c) statistics on the number of applicants processed by personal category (e.g., sex, age, race) level and type of disabilities, and by job category and level (Johns & Saks, 2001, pp. 178–181).

The government may require a nursing home chain or an individual facility to recruit qualified employees whose group is not proportionately represented in their present staff. If, for example, there are no African American nurses on the staff and the government ascertains that the facility does not advertise its job openings at African American nursing schools or in newspapers or other sources normally used by African American persons seeking jobs, the government may require that a governmentally defined Equal Employment Opportunity program be used by the facility or chain.

Many employers are under governmental pressure to increase the number of minority members and women employed in the facility, especially at the higher levels from which these groups have traditionally been excluded.

Requiring a facility to increase the proportion of minority persons is called *ratio hiring*.

While it has not been a matter of Office of Civil Rights enforcement, disproportionately few male nurses tend to be hired, probably out of deference to the mostly female (usually three-quarters) nursing facility population and availability of male nurses.

In general, it is functional to seek a workforce that is diversified and representative of the community that the facility serves.

The Americans with Disabilities Act has also influenced the hiring process in a number of ways.

Influence of the Labor Market

The *labor market* is the geographic area from which applicants are to be recruited. Recruitment for a new administrator or director of nurses may be national in scope and today may be done via Web searches. The new administrator may be willing to move across the country. When staffing for jobs requiring little skill, the scope of the labor market will tend to be a relatively small geographic area surrounding the facility. The new janitor or nurse's aide is unlikely to be willing, or economically able, to move across country to accept a position at the facility.

If there is a surplus of labor at recruiting time, the facility may be flooded with applications. If there is a shortage, on the other hand, such as during the nursing shortage, it may take considerable initiative to find and hire well-trained staff. In today's employment arena each facility needs its own Web site with an employment application that can be filled out over the Internet.

Impacts of Transportation

The ease with which employees can commute to the facility will have a direct impact on the geographic area from which the facility can recruit. The absence of an efficient public transportation system, especially for evening and night workers, will oblige the facility to hire only persons who have access to automobiles, or can walk to work.

Nursing facilities in the central city face special problems in finding suitable employees. Population migration to the suburbs traditionally leaves less-qualified persons living in the center city, a place to which suburbanites are little inclined to commute. Some larger institutions have arranged special transportation to and from work for suburban employees in an effort to attract competent staff.

Recruitment Sources

A number of sources for recruitment exist, both within and outside the facility. Present employees may be an excellent source.

Present Employees

The current employees of the facility can be a primary source for filling vacancies. Hiring from among present employees is a policy decision to promote from within. There are a number of advantages to such a policy (Noe et al., 2000, p. 161).

Career Ladders

Career ladders are paths along which the employee can hope to progress. They constitute a major source of employee incentive and satisfaction. Persons entering the facility are encouraged to stay if there is reasonable expectation that, when openings occur, there will be advancement possibilities from within the organization. This practice stimulates employees to develop skills that will be necessary to qualify for promotion (Noe et al., 2000, p. 319).

Job Posting and Job Bidding—on the Bulletin Board or the Internet

A job that becomes available is literally posted on appropriate bulletin boards, and employees are encouraged to bid, or apply. Through this device employees become more aware of the actual requirements of positions and the selection processes for filling vacancies. Such information can be placed on the facility Web site. Advancement of present employees has the obvious advantage of recognizing and rewarding successful workers. It also has benefits for the facility by placing a person who already has some understanding of the organization and is loyal to its policies.

However, invariably hiring from within may measurably slow the process of introducing persons with new ideas and fresh approaches into the facility. There are times when the management may purposely seek to bring in an outsider who will be expected to reorganize or reengineer a department or work area.

Outside Sources

Unless it is planned to reduce the size of the staff, every vacancy presents the organization with an option to promote from within or hire from without.

A promotion from within might trigger a series of promotions. If the nursing supervisor is promoted to director of nursing, the charge nurse may be moved up to nursing supervisor, and the senior registered nurse to charge nurse, thus creating an opportunity for several moves up in seniority or level and eventually opening a beginning registered nurse position (Noe et al., 2000, p. 164).

Any vacancy, if filled from within, will eventually result in hiring a new person from an outside source. Some of the more common outside sources are discussed in the following paragraphs.

Referrals

Employees, residents, and their significant others are good sources of referrals. Satisfied employees, residents, and their significant others constitute a valuable asset for the recruiting effort (Noe et al., 2000, p. 164).

Employee referrals can be especially beneficial. When a staff member's recommendation is accepted, they are receiving special recognition by the facility. In addition, the employee will have a vested interest in assisting the recruit to adjust to the environment and to be productive. However, the facility must be careful to avoid referrals that lead to nepotism (favoring one's family members) or to the formation of closely knit groups or cliques composed of persons who have close outside ties and tend to exclude others. Employee, resident, and family referrals are, in essence, word-of-mouth recommendations that reflect the reputation of the facility within the facility.

Advertisements

Advertisement in appropriate media, such as newspapers, professional and trade journals, and on the Web, is one of the most common methods for contacting prospective applicants. For registered nurses, the professional journal may be an appropriate medium; however, local newspapers are the most used source. For nurse's aides and maintenance staff, the local newspaper will also be an appropriate medium (Noe et al., 2000, p. 165).

Public Employment Agencies

State governments operate local public employment agencies using federal payroll tax rebates from the USES. Public employment agencies can provide lists of individuals who are unemployed and currently drawing unemployment insurance benefits (Noe et al., 2000, p. 166).

Private Employment Agencies

Agencies in the private sector offer specialized services, more closely matching the needs of the potential employer and employee. Fees are charged.

Most often the employee pays the agency. However, the employer sometimes shares in the fee and occasionally pays it altogether. The facility may also sign a contract with a private employment agency over a period of time. In this case, the contract should be carefully reviewed to avoid unwanted or unintended commitments, such as a fee to the agency for all new employees, whether found by the agency or the employer (Noe et al., 2000, p. 166).

Search Firms

Search firms generally focus their efforts on middle- and upper-level management positions. Clients for search firms normally are employers who agree to pay the search firm for finding a suitable candidate. The search firm operates in a more far-flung geographic area than is normally possible for the employer (although the Internet is changing even this), and it is able to offer a nationwide inventory. These firms can save employer time and energy by providing extensive screening before any candidate is recommended.

Professional and Industry Organizations

Many professional and industry groups, such as health care facilities associations and nurses associations, may maintain rosters of their members who are seeking employment, which they publish in their journals and post at meetings. Much interviewing, both formal and informal, occurs at association meetings for job openings. For nursing home administrators, the American College of Healthcare Executives publishes *Career,* a monthly employment newsletter. The American College of Healthcare Administrators offers its members access to employment openings through Job Bank USA. Company Web sites may list job openings.

Educational Institutions

Accredited schools are an increasingly important source for nursing home personnel. Community colleges and technical institutes are training students not only to be licensed practical nurse positions but also to be nurse's aides (Noe et al., 2000, p. 167).

Unsolicited Applications

A number of unsolicited employment inquiries will arrive at the facility by mail or in person. Although the proportion of such applicants who are suitable may be low, there are nevertheless important reasons for careful attention to them. It is good public relations practice to extend courteous treatment to applicants who approach the facility on their own initiative and to deal with them candidly about the likelihood of employment with the organization.

Some administrators report a tendency for long-term care and hospital employees to seek a change of job every few years. They may be entirely competent people who periodically look for a new work situation while remaining within their field. Such individuals may submit unsolicited applications simply to let a facility know of their availability.

Electronic Recruiting and Screening

Computer recruitment networks and videoconference interviews allow employers to search for employees over a wide geographical area without having to leave the facility (Noe et al., 2000, p. 168). Search firms often use a video interview as a first step in screening persons for positions; the facility can do likewise.

2.6 Hiring Staff

Recruitment is the process of locating prospective staff. *Personnel selection* is the process of deciding which of the applicants best fits the requirements of the job for which they are being considered. Often, however, this prospective staff member is evaluated not only for one of several positions the organization has open at that moment, but simultaneously for anticipated slots expected in the near future. Nurses with extensive acute care experience, for example, will be interviewed and kept in mind by a facility moving toward offering subacute care.

Through experience, employers have learned that when individuals are carefully selected for clearly defined positions, the result may be faster adjustment to the position, greater job satisfaction, and a minimum number of misfits between applicants and job needs in the organization (Johns & Saks, 2001, pp. 110, 178–181).

Measuring the Impacts of Legislation

Employers are directing greater attention to the job selection process. This is because of the often intense scrutiny given employers by the government enforcers of the Civil Rights Act of 1964, the Equal Employment Opportunity Act of 1972, and more recently, the Americans With Disabilities Act, which was passed in 1990.

The Civil Rights Act of 1964 prohibits discrimination in employment practices on the basis of race, color, religion, sex, or national origin. This Act uses the Equal Employment Opportunities Commission (EEOC), which was created by the Wagner Act in 1935, to implement the provisions of the Civil Rights Act. A later amendment, known as the Tower Amendment to Title 7, permitted the use of ability tests in employee selection procedures. Subsequently, the courts and the EEOC have made numerous rulings that determine the construction and use of ability tests (Maddox & Sussman, 2001, p. 348).

The Equal Employment Opportunity Act of 1972 is an amendment to Title 7 of the Civil Rights Act of 1964 and is intended to cover all employers of 15 or more persons and numerous other groups, such as educational institutions. Enforcement machinery was authorized and subsequently set up. Today human resources policy is shaped by these acts as well as court decisions and regulations instituted by authorized governmental agencies. They affect such employment practices as retirement rules and considerations during pregnancy.

In 1987, four federal agencies jointly published a far-reaching document titled *Uniform Guidelines on Employee Selection Procedures* (EEOC, Civil Service Commission, Department of Labor, & Department of Justice, 1987, pp. 38,295–38,309), establishing the standards by which federal agencies determine the acceptability of validation procedures used for written tests and other selections.

The guidelines require the employer to be able to demonstrate that the selection procedures used are valid in predicting or measuring employee performance in a specific job. They define discrimination as adverse impact:

> The use of any selection procedure which has an adverse impact on the hiring, promotion or other employment or membership opportunities of members of any race, sex, or ethnic group will be considered to be discriminatory and inconsistent with these guidelines, unless procedure has been validated in accordance with these guidelines. (EEOC, Sec. 3A)

Adverse impact is defined as occurring whenever the selection rate for any racial, ethnic, or sex group is less than 80% of the rate of the group with the highest selection rate.

If 200 of 1,000 white applicants are selected (a selection rate of 20%), at least 16% of the minority applicants must be selected. Several court rulings, such as Griggs v. Duke Power Company, have already clearly established the principle that all human resources tests and activities must avoid having any discriminatory effect, whether intended or unintended (Noe et al., 2000, p. 88).

The "Uniform Guidelines" have, in effect, become a handbook for decision making in human resources matters. The human resources selection process must now be reported to state and federal compliance agencies, usually on EEOC forms that require accurate data on the actual hiring results of the nursing facility. As Noe has observed, what used to be the exclusive concern of the facility administrator and human resources officer can now be carried into the courtroom (Noe et al., 2000, p. 80).

The Federal Equal Employment Opportunity (EEO) poster should be prominently displayed in an area accessible to both staff, applicants, and residents. All advertising must announce the facility's position as an Equal

Opportunity Employer. For facilities that receive revenues through the Veterans Administration (VA) contracts, all job openings for positions involving more than 3 days' duration and with a starting salary of $25,000 annually or less must be listed with the local state employment agency.

Matching Facility Human Resources Needs and Applicants

Taking on the right person for a position is a complex task. The employer understandably wants to find out as much about the applicant as possible to determine their likelihood of success if hired for a position in the facility (Johns & Saks, 2001, pp. 454–455; Robbins & Coulter, 2007, p. 67).

Methods of Obtaining Information

There are several methods for learning about applicants. Most organizations use written application forms, interviews, and background checks. The search for a new administrator or director of nurses may involve appointing a committee, lengthy exploration, extensive interviewing, obtaining of departmental employee input, and the final selection. Filling a vacancy for a nurse's aide is much less complicated. But in both cases it is important that all the information solicited be demonstrably job related or predictive of success in that position (Noe et al., 2000, p. 169).

Reliability and Validity of Information

Information that is valid and reliable is necessary for making an informed decision about an applicant's skills, knowledge, aptitudes, level of motivation, and likely fit with the organization (Johns & Saks, 2001, p. 125; Noe et al., 2000, p. 180; Robbins & Coulter, 2007, p. 330).

Reliability of the tests, interviews, and other tools used in selecting among applicants refers to the consistency with which the same results are obtained over a period of time and when used by different testers (called inter-rater reliability).

In measuring applicants' abilities, reliability means that an applicant will achieve the same or nearly the same score or results when taking the test at different times, for example, a week or two apart. If a test were to give differing results from week to week it would be unreliable, just as a set of scales used to weigh produce in a store must reliably give the same weight week after week every time produce of equal weight is placed on it. Reliability also requires that different applicants with the same skills score the same on the test. If word-processing skill is being measured, applicants with the same level of skill must score the same on the test.

A test or selection procedure provides validity when it actually measures what it is intended to measure and does it well. In essence, *validity* is a measure of how effectively an instrument does its job (Noe et al., 2000, p. 181; Robbins & Coulter, 2007, p. 331).

Two Types of Validity

Personnel experts have relied on at least two types of validity for several years: content validity and construct validity. Content and construct validity are used by governmental agencies in judging the results of a facility's hiring program (Noe et al., 2000, p. 184).

Content Validity

Content validity is the degree to which a test, interview procedure, or other selection tool measures the skills, knowledge, or performance requirements actually needed to fill the position for which the applicant is applying. As more and more facilities begin to offer medically complex care, a nursing position may require the ability to administer drugs intravenously (IVs). A test establishing that the applicant can perform IVs skillfully has content validity.

Construct Validity

The extent to which a selection tool measures a trait or behavior perceived as important to functioning in a job is construct validity. Intelligence is an abstract construct that is established through putting together answers to a series of different questions that together yield a measure of the theoretical construct called intelligence.

The following is an example of construct validity: A nursing home administrator's requirement of a "friendly facial expression" toward residents is an example of a construct (trait) that the administrator believes is needed for the position.

To validate a friendly facial expression as a job requirement the administrator would have to identify the work behaviors required for the position; identify the constructs, for example, smiling, that are required; and then show by empirical evidence that this selection requirement is truly related to the construct.

It is of real importance for a nursing facility to require that all staff treat residents in a cheerful or friendly manner, although this directive may be difficult to achieve. In a Fort Worth, Texas case a federal judge ruled that American Airlines had the right to discharge an otherwise good flight attendant because he did not smile enough. The flight attendant had sued the company, contending that he was a good employee and met all requirements of the job except for the smile. The federal judge upheld American's policy of requiring a friendly facial expression as "essential in the competitive airline industry."

Application Forms—Pre-Employment Questions

Employers must avoid questions that might be construed as violating the Civil Rights Act, Title 7, or the Americans With Disabilities Act. Before hiring a person, questions should be avoided that relate to age, sex, race, national origin, education, religion, arrest and conviction records, marital status, credit rating (Title 7), or disabilities (Americans With Disabilities Act and Title 7). The interviewer must review any unsolicited requests for reasonable accommodation under this Act. If the applicant is a minor, that is, under 18 years of age, federal and state child labor laws may specify hours of work, type of work, machinery to be operated, and supervision requirements. In recent years, about 1,500 complaints based on religious discrimination alone were filed annually (Noe et al., 2000, p. 91).

Table 2.11 gives a list of subject areas about which one is permitted, or not, to ask questions on application forms or in the pre-employment interviews under Title 7.

Handicap-Related Questions

The Equal Employment Opportunities Commission issued a 49-page notice (915.002 on May 19, 1994) with the goal of clarifying what questions employers may ask that might be related to handicap as viewed under the Americans With Disabilities Act. This 49-page notice made it clear that an employer may ask an applicant about the nature of any need the applicant may have for adjustment to a handicap only after making a job offer. It is only at this point that the employer may consider what a reasonable accommodation might be. Prior to offering a job it is unlawful to ask questions such as, "Do you need a reasonable accommodation to perform the essential functions of the job? If so, what kind?"

In an attempt to clarify what pre-employment interview questions are permissible and which are not, the EEOC Notice offered the following as examples.

Lawful	Unlawful
1. Do you drink alcohol?	How much alcohol do you drink per week?
2. How well can you handle stress?	Do you ever get ill from stress?
3. Are you currently illegally using drugs?	Have you ever been treated for drug problems?
4. Do you regularly eat three meals per day?	Do you need to eat a number of small snacks at regular intervals throughout the day in order to maintain your energy level?
5. How did you break your leg?	How did you come to use a wheelchair?
6. Do you have a cold?	Do you have AIDS?

Interviewing Applicants

Interviews are used extensively in evaluating job applicants. Each organization will develop its own style and identify its varying information needs as it conducts interviews (Noe et al., 2000, p. 192).

Preliminary Interviews

One approach is to use a preliminary approach that generally consists of having the applicant fill out a short questionnaire, after which there is a brief conversation with the applicant based on the questionnaire. This serves to screen out unsuitable candidates, using a minimum of time and organizational resources.

Telephone/Video Interviewing/Screening

The person who will interview candidates for positions can elicit a good bit of information before the interview, such as:

- present employment
- why looking for a position, what kind of next position is being sought
- candidate's salary requirements
- why candidate left previous positions, past salaries
- persons supervised, if a manager, and their job functions
- give candidate information about your facility
- set up an interview if, after the above explorations, mutual interest exists

TABLE 2.11.   Suggestions for Interviews

Inquiries before hiring	Lawful	Unlawful*
1. Name	Name	Inquiry into any title that indicates race, color, religion, sex, national origin, handicap, age or ancestry.
2. Address	Inquiry into place and length of current address	Inquiry into foreign addresses that would indicate national origin.
3. Age	Any inquiry limited to establishing that application meets any minimum age requirement that may be established by law.	A. Requiring birth certificate or baptismal record before hiring. B. Any other inquiry that may reveal whether applicant is at least 40 and less than 70 years of age.
4. Birthplace or national origin		A. Any inquiry into place of birth. B. Any inquiry into place of birth of grandparents or spouse. C. Any other inquiry into national origin.
5. Race or color		Any inquiry that would indicate race or color.
6. Sex		A. Any inquiry that would indicate sex. B. Any inquiry made of members of one sex, but not the other.
7. Religion-creed		A. Any inquiry that would indicate or identify religious denomination or custom. B. Applicant may not be told any religious identity or preference of the employer C. Request pastor's recommendation or reference.
8. Handicap	Inquiries necessary to determine applicant's ability to substantially perform specific job without significant hazard.	Any other inquiry that would reveal handicap.

(Continued)

TABLE 2.11. Suggestions for Interviews (Continued)

Inquiries before hiring	Lawful	Unlawful*
9. Citizenship	A. Whether a U.S. citizen. B. If not, whether applicant intends to become one. C. If U.S. residence is legal. D. If spouse is a U.S. citizen. E. Require proof of citizenship after being hired.	A. If native-born or naturalized. B. Proof of citizenship before hiring. C. Whether parents or spouse are native-born or naturalized.
10. Photographs	May be required after hiring for identification purposes.	Require photograph before hiring.
11. Arrests and convictions	Inquiries into conviction of specific crimes related to qualifications for the job applied for.	Any inquiry that would reveal arrests without convictions.
12. Education	A. Inquiry into nature and extent of academic, professional, or vocational training. B. Inquiry into language skills such as reading and writing of foreign languages.	A. Any inquiry that would reveal the nationality or religious affiliation of a school. B. Inquiry as to what mother tongue is or how foreign language ability was acquired.
13. Relatives	Inquiry into name, relationship, and address of person to be notified in case of emergency.	Any inquiry about a relative that would be unlawful if made about the applicant.
14. Organizations	Inquiry into organization memberships and offices held, excluding any organization, the name or character of which indicates the race, color, religion, sex, national origin, handicap, age, or ancestry of its members.	Inquiry into all clubs and organizations where membership is held.
15. Military service	A. Inquiry into service in U.S. Armed Forces when such service is a qualification for the job. B. Require military discharge certificate after being hired.	A. Inquiry into military service in named service of any country but the United States. B. Request military service records. C. Inquiry into type of discharge.

(Continued)

TABLE 2.11.   Suggestions for Interviews (Continued)

Inquiries before hiring	Lawful	Unlawful*
16. Work schedule	Inquiry into willingness to work required work schedule.	Any inquiry into willingness to work any particular religious holiday.
17. Other	Any question required to reveal qualifications for the job applied for.	Any nonjob related inquiry that may reveal information permitting unlawful discrimination.
18. References	General personal work references not relating to race, color, religion, sex, national origin, handicap, age, or ancestry.	Request references specifically from clergymen or any other persons who might reflect race, color, religion, sex, national origin, handicap, age, or ancestry of applicant.

I. Employers acting under bona fide Affirmative Action Programs or acting under orders of Equal Employment law enforcement agencies of federal, state, or local governments may take some of the prohibited inquiries listed above to the extent that these inquiries are required by such programs or orders.

II. Employers having Federal defense contracts are exempt to the extent that otherwise prohibited inquiries are required by Federal law for security purposes.

III. Any inquiry is prohibited that, although not specifically listed above, elicits information as to, or that is not job related and may be used to discriminate on the basis of, race, color, religion, sex, national origin, handicap, age or ancestry in violation of law.

* Unless bona fide occupational qualification is certified in advance by the State Civil Rights Commission.

Reprinted with Permission from Panel Publishers. Miller, 1982, pp. 2059–2061.

Interviewing Methods

Interviewing methods vary, but can be generally classified into three types according to the degree of structure used: the nondirective, the in-depth, and the patterned interview.

In the *nondirective* interview the interrogator refrains from influencing the applicant's remarks. This allows the applicant maximum freedom to ask questions and give information. The interviewer's task is to pay special attention to attitudes, values, or feelings that may be exhibited by the candidate (Johns & Saks, 2001, p. 108).

This approach maximizes the amount of information the applicant may reveal and is often called an open-ended interview technique. The interviewer asks only broad general questions such as "Tell me about what you did and how you liked your last job," or "What is it about working in a long-term care facility that attracts you?" or "Where do you want to be in your career in the next 5 years?" There is no prescribed set of questions.

An *in-depth* interview provides more structure in the form of specific question areas to be covered. This is sometimes called a directed interview. Examples of questions appropriate to the in-depth interview are:

- What do you consider your most important skills for this job?
- Tell me about your last job.
- Under what type of supervision techniques do you function best?
- What did you like most about your last job? What are your feelings toward older people? What do you like most and dislike most about older persons?

The *patterned* interview allows the least amount of freedom to both the interviewer and the applicant. All questions are sequential and highly detailed. Generally a summary sheet must be filled out by the interviewer interpreting the results of the encounter.

In every case, do anything you can to make the interviewee comfortable. And be on time for the interview.

Some Approaches

- Avoid forming strong impressions during the early minutes of the interview.
- Allow the candidate to do most of the talking.
- Don't clue the candidate into precisely what you are looking for early in the interview.
- Ask specific questions about past job behavior.
- Probe for all the information needed.
- Take notes, but not on the application form.
- Use second and third interviews when appropriate.

General Areas for Questions

One major nursing home corporation suggests the following areas as appropriate.

Professional Maturity

- What has been the toughest assignment you have ever had and how did you handle it?
- What would you do if (name an adverse situation that an employee in that job might encounter)?
- What actions have you taken if you disagreed with a supervisor's decision?
- What is the impact or role of your department on your current facility's objectives?

Skill Level

- What are your present job responsibilities?
- What results were achieved in terms of successes and achievements?
- What do you feel you can learn from this position?
- What are your greatest strengths? What areas need improvement?
- What was the biggest contribution you made to your current position?
- How would your references rate your technical competence?
- The ability to solve problems is critical to this position. Please provide an example of how this ability has been important to your success.
- What important trends do you see in your profession?

Character

- What do you consider the most important aspects of a job?
- Where do you see yourself in 2 years? 5 years? 10 years?
- What have you liked best about your present (recent) supervisor(s)? liked least?
- Why should we hire you?
- How successful do you think you have been so far in your career? How long would it take you to make a meaningful contribution to this facility?

Accumulate a Reference List?

Increasingly facilities "raid" each other. One might say, "I've got two jobs in this category. Do you know another person?" Then also hire the people referenced—excellent workers don't normally walk in the front door!

Research Findings on the Use of Interviews

A good deal of research has been conducted on the reliability and validity of interviews as a tool for judging job applicants. Some of the major findings include the following:

- Structured interviews are more reliable than unstructured interviews.
- When there is a greater amount of information about a job, inter-rater reliability is increased, that is, several interviewers are more likely to come to the same decision.
- Interviews can explain why a person would not be a good employee, but not why they would be a good one.
- Factual written data seem to be more important than physical appearance.
- Interpersonal skills and level of applicant motivation are best evaluated by an interview.
- Allowing the applicant time to talk provides a larger behavior sample. Also, one can learn more from listening than by talking.
- An interviewer's race affects the behavior of the person being interviewed. (Chruden & Sherman, 1980, p. 134)

Responding to the Market

While the previously described processes may serve well when there is a large applicant pool for jobs in the facility, the reality is that nurses, nurses' aides, and similar facility employees often change jobs. The applicant may have taken the afternoon off to find a new job. Making such applicants feel welcome and offering an interview at the point of application may increase a facility's ability to have first choice in obtaining needed new hires.

Background Investigations

If the interviewer decides the candidate is of interest to the organization, background information can be sought.

It is advisable to obtain from applicants a signed request for references. Increasingly, former employers are reluctant to put any recommendations into writing for fear of lawsuits. Many will only provide information about the date of hire, position(s) held, and date of separation.

Background Checks

Background checks are increasingly important. Grant and Kemme (1993) recommend that despite most employers' adoption of a neutral policy on employment, for example, revealing only name, job, title, and dates of employment, it is important to persevere. They recommend a screening process consisting of (a) background checks: trustworthiness, honesty, gaps in employment, required licenses, relevant background, for example, for a driver; (b) drug tests (the Americans with Disabilities Act does not protect drug users); and (c) criminal background checks (which may be mandatory). Here the so-called Business Necessity Rule applies. Employers must consider all job-related circumstances around a conviction to determine if the person would be a safe employee in the facility. Some allowable considerations are (1) time of conviction, (2) nature of conviction, (3) number of convictions, (4) facts of each case, (5) job-related-ness, (6) length of time between conviction and application, and (7) efforts at rehabilitation (Grant & Kemme, 1993, p. 13). Generally, any person convicted of substance abuse becomes a high risk for the facility. Reference requests should be obtained on at least two jobs, preferably the two most recent, or for the past 3 years (whichever is longer). For applicants with no work experience, school, volunteer, or personal references can be used. For nurse's aide applicants, two basic checks need to be made:

- the state registry to verify current certification and whether the applicant has met training and competency requirements,
- the substance abuse registry in every state in which the facility has reason to believe the applicant has worked as a nurse's aide to determine whether any record of resident abuse or neglect or misappropriation of resident property has occurred, and
- sometimes criminal background checks must be made.

The Privacy Act of 1974 (Public Law 93–579) gave federal staff the right to examine their human resources records, including letters of reference, unless they waived this right when they requested the letter. Although not mandated by federal law, the Privacy Act of 1974 seems to have led to a trend for employers to permit staff to review and change their human resources files.

Negligent hiring lawsuits can be minimized by gathering as much pertinent information as possible about applicants. Discrimination charges can be minimized by focusing on job-related criteria.

Credit Reports

Under the federal Fair Credit Reporting Act (Public Law 91–508), the employer must advise applicants if credit reports will be requested. If the candidate is rejected because of a poor credit report, they must be so informed and given the name and address of the reporting credit agency. The Internet makes credit checks nearly instantaneous.

Physical Examination

All facility staff must have periodic health examinations to ensure freedom from communicable disease. The practical impact of this stipulation is to seek a pre-employment physical to assure that this is met by new staff. There is debate as to whether requiring a physical before offering a job is permitted or whether one must offer the job, then require a physical before the employee begins work. In essence, all applicants must be informed that a condition of employment will be the pre-placement health exam following the conditional job offer.

There are several practical reasons for a physical examination. It establishes the physical capability of the applicant to meet the job requirements (a delicate proceeding given the tenor of the Americans With Disabilities Act). It provides a baseline against which to assess their later periodic physical exams. The employment-related physical examination is especially valuable in determinations of claims of work-associated disabilities under Workers' Compensation laws. The laboratory analyses that are part of the exam can detect the presence of illicit drugs in the applicant and may detect communicable disease to which the residents should not be exposed (Noe et al., 2000, p. 198).

If the physician determines that the new employee cannot perform the essential functions of the job due to a disability under the definition of the Americans With Disabilities Act, the facility must follow policy on Reasonable Accommodations for Individuals with Disabilities. If the physician determines the employee cannot perform the essential functions of the job, but does not have a disability under the definitions of the Americans With Disabilities Act, the employee is notified that they are not qualified for the position.

Normally the health file is not considered part of the human resources file due to its confidential nature; only authorized persons may have access to the employee's health record on a "need to know" basis.

Family and Medical Leave Act of 1993 and Americans With Disabilities Act

These are discussed elsewhere.

Compliance With the Immigration Reform and Control Act

Passed in 1986, this act determines which individuals are legally eligible to work in the United States.

The Decision to Hire

Who should decide which applicant to hire? Not the human resources staff. Generally, the final decision to hire is given to the head of the department in which the recruit will work. The administrator of the facility can define a role for themselves in the final decision making or leave it entirely up to the department head.

Two Approaches to the Hiring Decision

The hiring decision itself is complex. Two basic approaches have been identified in the literature: the clinical and the statistical.

In the clinical approach the decision maker reviews all the information in hand about the match of the applicant and the job and then decides.

In the statistical approach the decision maker identifies the most valid predictors, then weights them according to complicated formulas. This method has been shown to be superior to the clinical approach. However, few facilities will normally have enough staff time available to make this practical. A compromise would be for the decision maker to rate each applicant for a position on several dimensions, such as test score results, education, experience, apparent interest level, and the like, assigning numerical scores on each dimension to each candidate. The results can provide a systematic set of comparison data for reaching the final decision.

Achieving Construct Validity for Hiring Nursing Home Staff—Heart Behind the Numbers

It is not enough to establish that an applicant has the technical skills needed for a job. Staff must realize that successful caring for frail, elderly nursing home patients is often less dependent on the technical knowledge of the staff than on their compassion for others. Knowing the technique for gait training for a disabled person is useless if the staff member cannot encourage the person to leave the chair. As the nursing home population becomes more medically complex, *both* caring and technical skills becomes increasingly important. Sensitivity, compassion, and caring have construct, as well as technical competence, which will increasingly have validity as hiring criteria in the nursing home setting of the 21st century.

It is not just the administrator or director of nursing who need passion—all staff in the facility need to be passionate in carrying out their tasks.

Passion Index

Drawing a vertical line down his flip chart on the left side he listed basic skills and competencies such as knowledge of the tasks to be performed, being well informed about what competing facilities were doing, having a good employment record, experience in long-term care—all the usual requirements.

On the right side of the chart he wrote "Fire in the heart" commenting that if he had to choose he would chose someone with fire than one well trained and well recommended. Staff who have fire, he felt, are more motivated, will work harder, go the extra mile and are more resourceful at meeting resident or facility needs. Nurses and nursing assistants who have drive and enthusiasm for caring for the resident can be taught technical skills they lack. Applicants who lack fire in their hearts or passion for their work are not so easily taught.

Counting Grades

How much do grades count? Do the highest grade point averages in nursing school or the nursing assistant test point consistently to the best candidates? Consider the following findings. Over half of the Fortune 500 companies chief executive officers had a B or C– average in college. Two-thirds of U.S. Senators come from the bottom half of their class. Three-fourths of U.S. presidents were in the lower half of their school classes. More than half of millionaire entrepreneurs didn't finish college (Kriegel, 1991, p. 11).

Offering the Job

Once the successful candidate is chosen, they should be informed. Information such as proposed salary, job title and level, starting date, and any other relevant information should be communicated. Normally, a period of time during which the offer may be considered is specified. In every case, the candidate needs to be informed about starting date, pay rate, where and when to report, and the name of their supervisor, at the very least.

It is useful to include the human resources handbook with the offer if the applicant has not yet received one. The handbook (discussed later in detail) describes facility policy on a number of matters about which the prospective employee should be made aware as part of their own evaluation of the proposed position. It is useful to set a 3-day time limit for the newly hired staff member to complete all paperwork.

Unsuccessful applicants should be informed by letter as soon as the job is filled.

Persons Employed and Percent Distribution in Selected Health Care Sites in the United States, 2004

	MILLIONS	PERCENT DISTRIBUTION
Nursing care facilities	1.8	13.4
Residential care facilities without nursing	.6	4.5

Home health care services	.9	7.1
Hospitals	5.7	41
Offices and clinics of physicians	1.7	12.5

(DHHS, 2005, p. 341).

One out of every 10 employed U.S. civilians (9.9%) work in the health field. Nursing facilities hire nearly as many health care workers as all physicians offices and clinics.

2.7 Training Staff

Orientation

First Day on the Job

Orientation is the foundation for employment. The unoriented employee is a serious liability.

The first day on the job will potentially leave a lasting impression (Johns & Saks, 2001, pp. 250–251; Noe et al., 2000, p. 203). It is an opportunity for the facility. The new employee traditionally brings an initial reservoir of goodwill toward the facility. Enthusiasm and anxiety characterize the first day. A sensitively managed orientation program can help the new employee reduce anxiety and begin to build positive images of the new work environment.

Typical first day activities can include:

Official welcome to the new employee.
Introduction to as many of the staff as is appropriate.
Tour of the facility, including location of lockers for safekeeping of personal effects, staff lounges, restrooms, and parking arrangements.
Instructions on use of any time clock.
Safety rules, such as infection control and emergency procedures, especially those concerning fire and staff assignments in case of fire.
Explanation of residents' rights.
Discussion of contents of the human resources handbook. (Rogers, 1980, p. 23)

There is only one "first day on the job" for each new employee. Whether the orientation is for the director of nurses or a nurse's aide, it is equally important to the success of the organization. If the place is organized to take notice of the new employee and attempts to meet their needs on the first day, this latest member of the staff will be more likely to assist the facility in meeting its needs during the following months and years.

Facilities of 300 beds are as capable of a personalized orientation program as those with only 80. In practice, by having a properly constituted human resources process, the larger organization may have a functional advantage over the smaller, where orientation may be left to chance and good intentions without assigned responsibility for this introduction.

Using a Checklist

Precisely because orientation is both an important and complex task, use of a checklist is valuable. Those charged with familiarizing the new staff member with the organization are thereby less likely to overlook any element of the employee's new responsibilities as they review each item on the list (Scott, 1983, p. 898). One researcher suggests that the use of a checklist may help reduce employee turnover by assisting each new employee to gain an initial realistic and clearer set of expectations about the new positions. Turnover is always expensive (Johns & Saks, 2001, p. 119; Robbins & Coulter, 2007, p. 389). Estimates vary from $1,000 to more depending on the position and the length of training needed before the person is functioning efficiently.

Others consider it advisable that both providers and receivers of the orientation be required to sign each activity on the checklist. This maximizes the probability that the orientation will be successfully completed. When this document is placed in the employee's human resources file, the signed orientation form becomes a legal basis for establishing that the information was received. Responsibility for the orientation and its documentation can be vested in a single staff member, who is thus accountable for its successful completion from introduction to signed checklist.

The Human Resources Policy Handbook

The human resources policy handbook, often called the employee's handbook or the staff manual, is a compilation of the facility policies that directly relate to work conditions. Whereas a job description relates to only one job, the human resources policies are general in nature and cover the entire staff.

Each facility will have its own handbook. Chains generally have sets of policies that apply to all their staff, allowing local facilities to add their own policies within the broader policy guidelines and any requirements specific to state or local government regulations.

The main elements most often included in such a handbook are a statement of general policies, followed by details of benefits and general information relevant to the conditions of employment. The human resources handbook can be considered the rules, or terms under which staff are hired and carry out their work. Note that employee handbooks have been a subject of concern to management in recent years because some courts have held the handbooks to be an enforceable contract between the employer and the employee. Entering disclaimers in the handbook has not prevented staff from successfully suing in court. Following is an example of points that should be covered in the handbook.

A. Introduction and welcome to the facility

B. History or background of the facility / mission statement / handbook disclaimer

C. General employment policies

1. Equal opportunity employment (conforming to the Civil Rights Act) / sexual harassment policy, age discrimination policies (Argenti, 1994, p. 30; Johns & Saks, 2001, p. 400).
2. Classification of staff into full time and part time by number of hours worked per week; working hours of the facility.
3. Confidentiality of information about residents and facility matters.
4. Resident's rights statement.
5. Employee's records—confidentiality, employee access policy, usual contents: (1) application for employment; (2) pre-employment checks, letters, records of phone calls; (3) credit checks; (4) performance evaluations, promotions; (5) federal and state withholding certificates; (6) correspondence; (7) disciplinary actions; (8) grievances; (9) attendance; (10) signatures for receipt of human resources policy manual, orientation activities, and inservice attendance records; (11) health-related materials such as annual physical results, hepatitis B vaccination records (Bloodborne Pathogens requirements), annual tuberculosis tests results, records of injuries or other medically related matters; (12) license or certificate verification; and (13) other relevant materials.
6. Reporting policies—required call-in times prior to shift if unable to come to work.
7. Discipline system—whether a progressive system, and if so, a listing of each rule with a statement of disciplinary action, that is, the number, if any, or oral and written warnings before dismissal. For example, failure to follow a dress code may allow an oral warning and one or more written warnings before dismissal, whereas physical abuse of a resident could bring immediate suspension/investigation and, if appropriate after investigation, dismissal.
8. Uniforms / appearance.

9. General conduct expected, for example, respect, vulgarity, courtesy, attendance and punctuality, working quietly, absenteeism, visitors to staff, outside work.
10. Gifts (not permitted from patients/their families or significant others or sponsors).
11. Eating, drinking, smoking, kitchen traffic rules.
12. Use of alcohol and illegal drugs.
13. Parking, mail, rest breaks, meal breaks, lost and found, phone calls to staff (a never ending concern), smoking and use of tobacco policy, employment of relations, search of staff (package and purse inspection).
14. Destruction of nursing home property.
15. Suggestion box, permitted uses of bulletin boards, solicitation/distribution of literature rules.
16. Probationary period, use of anniversary or other dates for human resources reviews, seniority policies.
17. Health requirements and physical examinations.
18. Employee debts, garnishment of wages.
19. Performance ratings, promotion policies and interdepartmental transfer policies, job posting.
20. Wages and salaries, time cards, pay plan, date procedures for determining payroll calculations, payrolls, deductions, overtime policy, severance pay.
21. Grievance procedures.
22. Hospitalization and first-aid treatment.
23. Facility position on unions.
24. Resignation notice and procedures, exit interview.
25. On-the-job injuries policies.
26. Inservice education requirements.
27. Reimbursement for specified expenses, for example, travel, meals, memberships.
28. Confidentiality of company affairs / nondisclosure of information.
29. Family and Medical leaves, Workmen's Compensation Insurance.
30. Fire and disaster/evacuation plans.
31. Incident reports.

D. Benefits

1. Holidays.
2. Vacations, leave-accumulation policies.
3. Leaves of absence: sick leave, funeral leave, military leave, maternity leave, jury duty, extended leave.

4. Health benefits, dental benefits.
5. Tax deferred savings plans (e.g., 401K plan; Keough plan, etc.).
6. Stock purchase plan (if any) known as Employee Stock Option Plans (ESOPs).
7. Retirement benefits.
8. Insurance: life insurance, unemployment compensation, occupational disease insurance, workers' compensation insurance, disability insurance (Noe et al., 2000, p. 457), long-term care insurance, other.
9. Shift differential (if paid).
10. Other, for example, child care benefits, meals at work, and so forth.
11. Group rates: chains and groups of facilities can negotiate reduced rates on a variety of items such as accident insurance, life insurance, liability policies, and the like.

Training

As we have noted, directing is the task of assuring that each work role is successfully communicated to the employee. Directing is the process of (1) communicating to the staff what is to be done, then (2) assisting them to perform their role successfully (Givnta, 1984, p. 19).

Purpose

The purpose of the orientation program is to provide an initial introduction to the new employee. The purpose of training is to communicate the organization's needs to the staff and assist them in meeting those needs. This is a continuous process, beginning formally the first day on the job, but extending for the duration of the employee's association with the facility. Each employee will have their own learning curve (Argenti, 1994, p. 254; Noe et al., 2000, p. 210).

Steps in Establishing Training Needs

Staff members responsible for establishing the nursing facility's training program normally analyze three elements in planning for this course: (a) the organization, (b) the tasks, and (c) the person carrying out the work (Chruden & Sherman, 1980, p. 181; Johns & Saks, 2001, p. 336; Noe et al., 2000, p. 211; Robbins & Coulter, 2007, p. 334).

Organizational analysis consists of examining the facility's goals, resources, and internal and external environments to determine where training efforts need to be focused. A number of inservice topics are mandated for the various departments over the course of each year. These can form the initial framework for training needs (Noe et al., 2000, p. 212).

Task analysis involves review of job descriptions and activities essential for performing each job. The emphasis of training programs can then be placed on certain tasks that are judged to be inadequately carried out or simply in need of reinforcement because of their importance to the facility, such as fire drills and disaster preparedness. Additionally, whenever a facility begins accepting more medically complex residents, training for new techniques for the nursing staff is often in order.

A person or employee *skill analysis* can be made to arrive at the skills, knowledge, and attitudes required in each position. Person analysis means interpreting each position in terms of the personal attributes or behaviors necessary for performing the job acceptable (Maddox & Sussman, 2001, p. 105).

Once the goal of a training program has been determined, the following steps can be taken: (1) formulate instructional objectives, (2) develop instructional experiences to achieve theses objectives, (3) establish performance criteria to be met, and (4) obtain evaluations of the training effort (Chruden & Sherman, 1980, p. 180; Johns & Saks, 2001, p. 336).

On-the-job training is conducted by a staff member assigned to assist a new or continuing employee to acquire the abilities needed in a position in the facility. Ideally, on-the-job training permits the trainee to be an additional or extra worker for the first few days, allowing observation and progressive involvement in performing the tasks and behaviors required (Noe et al., 2000, p. 236).

Inservice training refers to employee education offered throughout the work career of the employee. Normally, inservice education consists of small seminars for groups of staff. All types of educational techniques are used including flip charts, films, lectures, videos, role playing, case discussions, and the like (Ruhl & Atkinson, 1986, p. 66). In many busy facilities three or more inservice training programs occur every week.

The nursing facility is a training site for numerous educational programs. Most facilities participate as training sites for nursing schools, physical therapy programs, pharmacy programs, and similar allied health training programs in nearby colleges and training programs (Noe et al., 2000, pp. 216–219).

New Methodologies

Increasingly, videos covering many training needs are available along with Web-based training being offered by the national long-term care associations (Noe et al., 2000, p. 239).

Evaluating Training

Evaluation of training efforts can be difficult. While it is true that tests can be devised to measure memorization, the nursing home is seeking to assess something more complex: changes in employee behavior. To quantify behavioral changes, it is useful to state learning objectives as behavioral objectives (Johns & Saks, 2001, p. 43).

Behavioral objectives can be measured by observing whether staff, in carrying out their duties, exhibit the behaviors sought as the objective of the training. Usually the goal is to have the employee acquire a skill or change an attitude (Noe et al., 2000, p. 232). Using performance centered behavioral objectives can assist evaluation.

For example, performance-centered objective in a nurse's aide training program might be (a) to be able to demonstrate proper procedures for turning a resident who is suffering from decubitus ulcers (pressure sores; Maddox & Sussman, 2001, p. 814), and (b) to consistently greet any patients encountered in the hallways using a pleasant tone of voice.

Both of these are performance-centered objectives. Proper techniques for turning a resident who has a decubitus ulcer can be physically demonstrated by the aide in training, and the aide's demeanor toward residents encountered in the hallways can be monitored by the trainer or other staff members (Noe et al., 2000, pp. 242–245).

Diversity Training

The composition of the nursing facility staff reflects the changing demographic landscape. Diversity training is designed to change employee attitudes about diversity and developing skills need to work in teams with employees of, for example, differing values, gender, ethnic, racial and religious backgrounds, and sexual preferences. Employees can gain an appreciation and acceptance of cultural differences among themselves (Noe et al., 2000, p. 255; Robbins & Coulter, 2007, p. 78).

2.8 Retaining Employees

2.8.1 WHAT THE FACILITY NEEDS FROM THE EMPLOYEE

We have argued that the facility needs employees who have a passion for their job and will consistently make decisions in conformity with its policies. This is possible to the extent that each staff member can be characterized as having the following:

- a high degree of interest in the job—a willingness to make every effort;
- a genuine dedication to the well-being of the residents and their quality of care and quality of life—passion for the work;
- a strong positive self-image permitting employees to see beyond their own needs and to be concerned, rather, with those of the residents and their significant others;
- skills, both technical and interpersonal, in communication and human relationships;
- the capacity and willingness to make decisions in accordance with the best interest of the facility, every act contributing toward providing the highest quality of life for the residents, their significant others, the facility staff, and the community;
- the ability to be self-starting, reliable, creative, and able to exercise positive appropriate leadership—a fire in their heart; and
- career commitment to the facility.

Obviously, this is the description of an ideal employee. Few staff members will be able to embody fully all of these qualities. If, however, these characteristics can be constantly encouraged and developed among the employees, the quality of life enjoyed by the residents and staff should be high.

2.8.2 WHAT EMPLOYEES NEED FROM THE FACILITY

What employees require of the facility can be divided into five areas: (a) social approval; (b) self-esteem; (c) security; (d) use of power, accomplishment, service, and exercise of leadership; and perhaps most important (e) to work for an organization with a vision that allows the employee to participate in a larger meaning, giving them a sense of purpose and pride in their accomplishment (Johns & Saks, 2001, p. 279).

The degree to which any one individual might seek satisfaction from employment will vary, both among the entire staff and within the same member as their personal situation changes over time.

Social Approval

Most people rely on a network of approval and satisfying social interrelationships. Whether or not they express it openly, many of them enjoy engagement in activities sanctioned by significant others—persons to whom an individual looks for favorable regard of behavior patterns, ideas, and values. Family, members of the community, and one's social group are typical examples of *significant others*.

If the community, or significant others in the community from whom approval is sought, disapproves of the employee working at the facility, they will not have positive feelings about the job itself or feel that being a "good" employee is worth the effort.

Self-Esteem

Adequate self-esteem is essential in order to function. Individuals need a positive self-image, that is to feel good about themselves, what they are doing, and the world about them. Each person has a need for status. Most people want to be part of an organization that has a sense of purpose to which they can dedicate their energies with pride.

Economic Security

In this case we define security as the financial benefits provided by the facility. Without sufficient income for maintenance, health insurance for eventualities, vacations for refreshment, and funds to meet future retirement expenses, an employee may remain insecure.

Hygiene Factors

Hygiene factors are those such as salary, company policies, and basic working conditions. In theory, when hygiene factors are adequate they do not bring about appreciable levels of employee satisfaction. Hygiene factors, then, are the minimum work conditions (Argenti, 1994, p. 217; Noe et al., 2000, p. 279).

Additional Intrinsic Needs

Some employees expect even more of the work situation. Their intrinsic needs arise out of the essential nature of their personality (Johns & Saks, 2001, pp. 38–42). Wielding power and having authority in certain situations are intrinsic needs. Satisfaction from the process of completing their tasks, of achievement, is another such need, as is leadership. Giving service can be fulfilling behavior.

Participation in a Vision

Employees want to work for a corporation that stimulates their dreams and aspirations and touches their hearts. They enjoy collaborating with highly motivated people who are accomplishing work that matters, that has purpose and meaning—something beyond just striving to be the largest, or the best known, or the highest income company. The staff need the administrator to take a personal interest in them—to be recognized as an essential member of the team (Riter, 1993, p. 40).

2.8.3 STRATEGIES AVAILABLE TO THE FACILITY TO MEET BOTH ITS OWN AND THE EMPLOYEE'S NEEDS

Retaining high performing employees over an extended period of time is economically desirable for the facility. The financial costs of training each new staff can be high, especially if the employee participates extensively in inservice training programs offered by the facility and takes advantage of any additional on the job training for skills improvement (Johns & Saks, 2001, pp. 119–120).

In the nursing home setting, employee continuity is critical for the residents themselves, providing an important element of stability and continuity in their lives. More than in most work settings, employees in nursing homes tend to form personal relationships with the patients, often being regarded as significant friends by residents who have lost all of their family and many cherished others.

A motivated, contented staff, capable of contributing significantly to the quality of resident patient life, consists of employees who are enjoying a high level of job satisfaction and are thus enabled to provide a high level of patient care.

An administrator in a large California chain facility says he is successful because he primarily concentrates his energy on the staff. Only highly motivated, happy staff, he believes, give loving care to residents. His zest and enthusiasm and evident concern about staff enable staff to treat residents and staff in the same manner.

A Facility Philosophy of Human Resource Management

What motivates employees? Every day the administrators of the more than 16,000 U.S. nursing homes make decisions based on their assumptions of what motivates their staff. These conclusions reflect the administrator's beliefs about human resource management and may be consciously or unconsciously held. We will explore one general theory about employee motivation (Noe et al., 2000, p. 280).

Theory X and Theory Y

Douglas M. McGregor (1960), a management theorist, published a book expounding what he called Theory X and Theory Y. McGregor wrote that the behavior of administrators is strongly influenced by their beliefs. He asserted that most business managers are Theory X types who believe that the employee naturally dislikes work, prefers to receive extensive direction from superiors, wishes to avoid taking responsibilities in the organization, has little ambition, and is motivated more by a need for security than any other factor (Robbins & Coulter, 2007, p. 454). This approach requires that managers use fear or punishment to motivate employees, all of whom must be closely watched if work is to be accomplished.

McGregor insisted that Theory X is not valid and that managers should be guided by what he called Theory Y instead. Theory Y (Robbins & Coulter, 2007, p. 455), is based on the following assumptions (pp. 33–35):

1. Using energy to work is as natural as using energy to play or rest. The administrator can control working conditions to lead to work being a source of satisfaction, voluntarily performed, or to work being seen as a source of punishment and thereby avoided.
2. If individuals are committed to the organization's goals, they will exercise self-direction and self-control without need for threat of punishment or of external behavior controls.
3. Rewards for achieving organizational objectives bring employee commitment; employees can achieve personal self-satisfaction in achieving organizational goals.
4. The average employee, when properly motivated, will accept and also seek responsibility.
5. The preponderance of employees have the capability of exercising imagination, ingenuity, and creativity in assisting the organization to achieve its goals.
6. Most jobs underutilized the capabilities of employees.

McGregor's theory caused considerable discussion in management circles. One researcher doubted that most managers were Theory X types. To test this, he surveyed 259 managers in 93 companies and found that managers did not completely accept either Theory X or Theory Y. In their opinion, reality is more complicated than either theory. Not surprisingly, a few years later this led to Theory Z.

Theory Z

Several writers proposed that, on balance, Theory Y is correct, but what motivates employees changes over time and is dependent on changing societal values. They argue that administrators must constantly come up with new strategies for motivating employees. In their view a straightforward, productivity-reward system is overly simplistic. A satisfactory quality of life, both for the individual and for the group, while more complex and abstract, is the appropriate focus (Argenti, 1994, p. 339).

Personality Tests

Some facilities utilize a variety of tests to evaluate applicants and employees. The most widely known is the Myers-Briggs Type Indicator personality test (Noe et al., 2000, p. 323; Robbins & Coulter, 2007, p. 399). As many as 2 million people take this test each year in the United States (Noe et al., 2000, p. 323). The test consists of 100 questions that ask respondents how they feel or act in a variety of situations. The test places respondents into categories of introverted or extroverted, sensing or intuitive, thinking or feeling, and perceiving or judging. These characterizations are then used to place a person in one of 16 personality types. Someone whose test results show them to be extroverted-intuitive-thinking-perceiving is classed as a conceptualizer (Argenti, 1994, p. 285). This and other tests are sometimes used to classify persons into Left Brain and Right Brain categories, the theory being that left-brained persons are systematic, thorough, balanced, and ask detailed questions about each situation, while right-brained persons are more intuitive, quick, and less complex in their approach to decision making.

Meeting the Employee's Need for Social Approval

Individuals have a need to be part of an enterprise that is regarded by significant others as successful. Hence, approval of the nursing facility by significant others is important to nursing home employees.

In the community the word-of-mouth reputation of the facility is important. Persons and groups regarded as experts in the field (the local hospital, home health agency, hospice, the local physicians, the case managers at the local Health Maintenance Organizations [HMOs], Independent Practitioner Organizations [IPOs], Professional Provider Organizations [PPOs], Workers Comp, and similar groups) can be important, or significant others, whose approval is sought by the staff. Newspaper, radio, and television reports about their workplace shape employee feelings.

To cite an example, in one large city a nursing home operated by the county was for 4 years attacked in the news media and threatened with decertification for Medicare and Medicaid by federal and state officials because its sanitation and resident care were regarded as significantly substandard. During those 4 years it was difficult to hire staff. Nurses, janitors, physical therapists, nurse's aides, and maintenance people who worked there were harangued by friends, neighbors, and workers in other health care facilities. Why were they willing to work under such conditions? After a succession of three administrators in the course of 4 years, during which the home suffered constant public attacks both by the media and individuals, an improving level of care became apparent.

Employees do care about the reputation of their organization.

Meeting the Employee's Need for Self-Esteem

Why does one nurse's aide strive harder than another? Why does one registered nurse look for additional responsibilities at the same time that another seeks to avoid taking any? Why do wage incentives stimulate some individuals and not others? Why does a career advancement track within the facility stimulate some employees to strive to climb the ladder while others ignore the opportunities offered?

What motivates employees varies not only for the individual employee but, over time, for the same employee. Motivation is a difficult concept to define. It has been described as the factor that energizes employee behavior, directing or channeling such behavior, and sustaining it (Johns & Saks, 2001, p. 111; Robbins & Coulter, 2007, p. 470).

An individual's needs, desires, and expectations change. When one need or desire is achieved at a satisfactory level, the salience or strength of others is modified. For a nurse who has just been licensed to practice, acceptance by other nurses may be a priority until this recognition is achieved. At that point other needs, such as maximizing income, may take precedence.

Understanding Motives

The complexity of motives has been described by Dunnette and Kirchner (1965; see also Johns & Saks, 2001, pp. 135–136; Robbins & Coulter, 2007,

p. 357), who attempted to apply motivational psychology to the work situation. They point out the following:

1. Identifying motives is complex. Some employees will work hard to obtain more money, but why? A strongly felt need for additional money may reflect a desire for the increased status more money brings, meeting a felt need for a sense of economic security, providing a symbol of power, or simply a willingness to work harder until the car is paid off, at which point time off from work may replace the desire for more money as a primary motivation.
2. Motives are always mixed. Each individual experiences a wide range of motives that strength and weaken as their circumstances change, and some needs are met while others are frustrated.
3. The same incentive—for example, increased health insurance benefits—may generate different responses. Individuals also differ in the ease with which their needs are satisfied.
4. Some motives may recede when satisfied, for example, hunger and thirst. Others, such as a desire for increased status or more salary, may become intensified when, for example, more status or more income is achieved.

The process of giving employees increased roles in the decision-making processes of the facility is known as job enrichment, for example, to assign a nurse supervisor and aides complete responsibility for the care of a set of patients, this rather than special responsibilities such as separate nurses doing medications, others doing range of motion exercises, and the like (Argenti, 1994, p. 234; Johns & Saks, 2001, pp. 181–183; Robbins & Coulter, 2007, p. 461). Job depth refers to the extent to which an employee has power to influence decisions. When the director of nurses consults the aides on a floor as to whether they are prepared to receive a proposed admission these aides have increased job depth (Argenti, 1994, p. 234; Robbins & Coulter, 2007, p. 461).

A. H. Maslow's hierarchy-of-need concept is perhaps the most often cited human need model in the literature (see Figure 2.4; Argenti, 1994, p. 277; Johns & Saks, 2001, pp. 137–139). He theorizes that needs become salient, that is, powerfully motivating, at each successively higher level mainly after the needs at each lower level are satisfactorily met. That is, until the individual has met the needs for survival and basic security (lower level), these will dominate until met.

Once lower-level needs are met to a satisfactory degree, the individual's motivation can become more dominated by social, self-esteem, and self-actuating needs (levels 3, 4, and 5). Maslow's model is widely used. In our view, it seems to be a functional and useful explanation of some of the more basic dynamics of employee motivations.

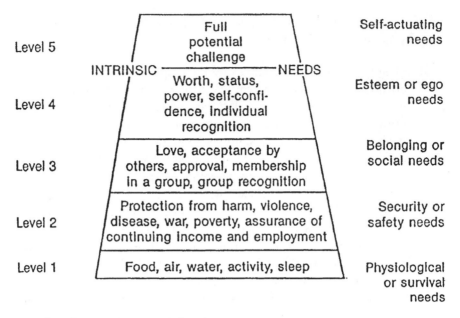

FIGURE 2.4 Maslow's hierarchy of need concept.

While the lower-level needs may decrease in strength when achieved, the higher-level needs, especially the need for self-actualization, tend to continue to grow stronger as they are being met. Examples of these types of needs or motivations are those cited previously as "additional intrinsic needs," such as being in authority, wielding power, accomplishing goals, and exercising leadership.

A word of caution: Each individual has a unique ever-changing need pattern. In our view, what motivates an individual depends on a combination of life experiences and, as scientists are suggesting more and more, on each individual's genetic and chemical make-up.

Childhood experiences such as economic deprivation may cause an employee to be anxious about financial security, no matter how much income is being earned. The social and economic class with which an employee identifies affects their perceptions of their "needs." Being raised as a male or a female also can influence the needs individuals will manifest on the job.

Personality Types: A and B

Attempts have been made to identify basic personality types. Investigators who were focusing on the causes of heart disease described two personality types. Type A are characterized as hard-driving, achievement-oriented people who strive to succeed to the highest level whatever the area of activity, whether in sports, job titles, or on-the-job productivity. Type A persons, especially those who are chronically angry, appear to be at increased risk of heart disease (Maddox & Sussman, 2001, p. 257; Robbins & Coulter, 2007, p. 402).

Type B personalities are characterized as having only moderate achievement needs, as less competitive and more satisfied with moderation, whether in sports, titles, or on-the-job productivity.

Type A employees come to the facility with a high internalized motivation level. They are overachievers in comparison with Type B persons. Why? Much has yet to be learned about motivation, genetic influences, and the influence of chemical balances within individuals.

An Exercise to Try

Supervisors' ideas about what motivates the staff and employees' ideas about what is motivating often differ significantly. The following is a list of concepts the reader can ask of a set of supervisors and employees in their facility regarding what they consider the most important aspects of their jobs:

Ask participants to rank 1 = most important, 10 = least important:

- To be treated fairly
- Consistency from management
- Job security
- Interesting work
- Full appreciation for work done
- Good wages
- Good working conditions
- Feeling "in" on things
- Promotion and growth within the facility/company
- Sympathetic understanding of personal problems
- Tactful discipline
- Management loyalty to workers

In the following section, we discuss areas available to an employer seeking to retain staff through meeting needs for approval:

- Leadership by vision
- Training programs

- Career paths
- Performance feedback and goal setting
- To err is to learn
- Recognition
- Power and control
- Respect for the creative potential of each employee—Maintaining passion
- Membership on a team
- Ninjas of joy

Leadership by Vision

Most facilities have set goals. Meetings exhorting employees to meet those goals, such as making the month's budget and keeping census up, are, in the end, limitations. Goals limit unless goals are part of and remain part of a vision. Organizations such as nursing facilities need a vision to fire up the employees, to engage their spirits, and set long-term directions for their efforts. Each department manager needs a vision of what their department can achieve, a vision to provide meaning to each employee's efforts. Kriegel (1991) argues that a vision or dreams are goals with wings (pp. 36–37). A dream or vision is an ideal state; a goal is a more real state. The dream supplies enthusiasm, vigor, and direction for the facility's efforts. Goals are short-term targets to be achieved, such as assuring that all the paperwork for admissions are completed in a timely manner and all doctor's telephoned orders signed within the time permitted. Employees want to feel they are doing more than contributing to the profit ratio. They want to be part of a movement, a compelling vision, something that grasps their imagination. Employees want to be part of a facility that has a vision, a dream about the quality of life of each resident and staff member. Business is won (or lost) on the front lines (Maddox & Sussman, 2001, p. 851).

Training Programs

Training programs increase employee skills and simultaneously communicate to them that those skills are valued by the management.

The programs themselves serve numerous functions. They demonstrate management's interest in the staff and provide an additional arena for exchange among employees, as well as an increased opportunity for feedback to the administration about the degree of skills and understanding of facility goals among employees. As these dynamics occur, the level of employee satisfaction can improve. With the new skills or insights the employee experiences an increased feeling of being in tune with the performance expectations of the organization.

Career Paths

Offering a career path means providing upward mobility within the organization. In a freestanding nursing home, creating career mobility is more difficult than within a chain that owns and operates 400 facilities.

Making career paths available within the facility communicates to the employee that the organization wants to meet their desires to succeed and progress in job level and income. For the nursing aide, a career path might include facility support through released time and or tuition assistance. This makes more feasible enrollment at a local technical institute to become a licensed practical nurse or a registered nurse.

The charge nurse might receive support to participate in a program to become a geriatric nurse practitioner. The kitchen worker might be assisted in attending classes that lead to qualifying as a dietetic service supervisor.

The labor market can be an influencing factor. If the home is freestanding, in a rural area with a limited number of persons in the potential pool of nurse's aides or kitchen workers, career assistance may lead to an undesirable depletion of the worker pool.

On balance, however, providing career paths that create upward mobility appears to increase worker satisfaction and improve employee retention rates. Not all of the aides will aspire to become licensed nurses, because they are not all similarly motivated. However, the availability of a career program can improve workers' attitudes. Those who choose not to participate have the satisfaction of knowing the option is available and that they may choose to exercise it if they wish. In general, the mere presence of options is important to employees.

Performance Feedback and Goal Setting

Employees receive informal feedback on their job performance on a daily basis. Formal reaction and the formal process of goal setting for an individual employee occurs under more structured circumstances. This is known as the performance evaluation, which normally includes establishing goals for the employee to achieve until the next scheduled performance evaluation (Johns & Saks, 2001, p. 149; Noe et al., 2000, p. 284; Robbins & Coulter, 2007, p. 534).

To Err Is to Learn

The facility administrators' attitude toward errors and failures is critical to success—as Kriegel (1991), has observed, failure is a good place to start. Failure itself is not a crime. The problem, really, is failure to learn from failure. It is not whether the medication nurse will make mistakes, it is what the nurse does after making the mistake that determines how good that nurse is.

Mistakes are inevitable. Mistakes are both inevitable and an opportunity to learn. If facility's managers show that they understand this the employees will respond with more openness about their mistakes. Cover-up of mistakes by employees takes lots of energy and usually leads to more lies to shore up the initial one. The mistake concealer is a problem for the facility. The employee who comes into the department manager's office and says, "I screwed up," is an employee with whom there is good communication, and an opportunity to learn has been created. In short, management needs a positive attitude toward mistakes. Employees prefer to work in an open honest atmosphere in which management helps them to learn from their mistakes.

Recognition

Employees want to be thanked. Most employees seek recognition for their work. Much of their behavior can be interpreted through *expectancy theory,* pioneered by Victor Vroom in the 1960s (Argenti, 1994, p. 178; Johns & Saks, 2001, p. 143; Noe et al., 2000, p. 422; Robbins & Coulter, 2007, p. 465). Expectancy theory holds that the level of motivation to perform (make an effort at work) is a mathematical function of the expectation individuals have about future outcomes multiplied by the value the employee places on these outcomes. Vroom defines expectancy as a "momentary belief concerning the likelihood that a particular act will be followed by a particular outcome" (Vroom, 1964, p. 170; see also Johns & Saks, 2001, p. 48).

The charge nurse who believes that working long hours and asserting herself on the job will lead to quick promotion to nurse supervisor is an example of an expectancy. It serves as a guideline for the charge nurse in seeking promotion to nurse supervisor. The charge nurse expects the behavior to be rewarded. Recognizing employees' expectancies can help a supervisor understand how they are motivated.

If the charge nurse's long worked hours and assertiveness lead to promotion, the expectation is reinforced. According to reinforcement theory, behaviors depends on reward (Johns & Saks, 2001, p. 46). When rewards follow performance, performance improves (Johns & Saks, 2001, p. 49). Conversely, when rewards do not follow performance, performance deteriorates. If the charge nurse had not been promoted, performance might have deteriorated (Noe et al., 2000, p. 423).

In *reinforcement theory* the outcome reinforces the employee's response either positively, leading to repeating the response, or negatively, leading to reduction of its use. Influencing employee behavior through reinforcement is called *operant conditioning,* literally influencing working behavior by conditioning the employee's response through rewarding (or punishing) the behavior (Noe et al., 2000, p. 422).

When employees perform in a desired manner and are given praise and recognition for that behavior, the manager is engaging in what may be called behavior modification (Johns & Saks, 2001, pp. 56–60; Maddox & Sussman, 2001, p. 117). Behavior modification involves using operant conditioning, usually through rewards, praise, and positive recognition when an employee performs as desired by the facility.

One theorist (Rotondi, 1976, pp. 22–28) suggests the following as a pattern for modifying employee behavior to conform to facility goals:

- Maintain a consistent work environment
- Consciously identify the desired behaviors of employees
- Decide on the rewards to be used
- Clearly communicate to the employees both the desired behaviors and the rewards
- Reward desired behaviors immediately
- Scale rewards to the behavioral achievement attained, that is, vary the rewards and minimize the use of punishments

Power and Control

Nursing facility administration needs to define policies to govern their decision making. However, this has both positive and negative aspects. The positive aspect is that the staff is given guidance and an appropriate framework within which to make decisions for the organization. The negative aspect is that deciding beforehand, through policy making, can substantially deprive the employee of a feeling of personal involvement in decision making for the organization (Johns & Saks, 2001, p. 279).

Feelings of Powerlessness

Christopher Argyris (1972) is a behavioral scientist who has observed a tendency for organizations to overlook a desire that he believes most employees have to function in a mature, adult manner. In the literature this is referred to as the *immaturity–maturity theory,* which holds that most organizational designs treat employees as immature, thus frustrating their need to function as responsible adults.

Argyris believes that the typical organization tends to ignore individual potentials for competence, for taking responsibility, for constructive intentions, and for productivity. He feels that in the typical lower-level job of the nurse's aide, the laundry worker, or the housekeeper, staff members are treated as immature. This, he argues, alienates and frustrates these workers, leading them to feel justified in rejecting responsible behavior and tempting them to defy the organization by allowing the quality of their work to deteriorate.

He sees the same problems among managers who work within organizational structures that create environments hostile to trust, candor, and risk taking. In such situations, the attitudes actually encouraged are conformity and defensiveness, which tend to be expressed by producing detailed substantiation for unimportant problems and invalid information for critical issues. Argyris (1972, p. 7) asserts that this leads to ineffective problem solving, poor decisions, and weak commitment to any decisions that are made.

Argyris is pointing to the converse of a coherent set of policies to cover all decision making in the facility: Little significant role in decision making is left to the employee. This may lead to a high level of frustration among those affected.

Common reactions to frustration can be selecting an acceptable substitute goal that is attainable or engaging in behavior that is maladaptive. An employee barred from making any meaningful decisions at the facility may cease trying and may concentrate energies on a leadership role in an outside voluntary organization. Or the employee relieves their frustration through aggressive or abusive behavior toward other employees or the residents.

Combating Powerlessness: Employees as "Owners"

You don't wash a rental car because you don't own it. A solution to this problem is to attempt to make everybody an "owner." Giving all employees a sense of ownership in the facility means treating each employee as a member of the team (Argenti, 1994, p. 375). This can be accomplished by allowing them some control in their work and giving them information about what the facility is attempting to accomplish. Peters and Austin advocate this approach in their book A Passion for Excellence. They call the approach "all people as 'businesspeople' " (Peters & Austin, 1985a, p. 23).

Ownership implies that all employees exercise some real portion of control in the facility. Of course, each employee does exercise some fraction of control over the workplace. It is up to the individual staff member to decide whether to give care pleasantly or in an "I don't care," or a "you don't deserve my respect" manner when alone with the resident.

"Businesspersons"

Peters & Austin's belief is that if the organization treats every employee as a "businessperson," the employees will respond as "businesspersons" fully engaged in the facility's goal of giving quality care and adequate income and committed to its success. A sense of ownership is accompanied by a feeling of control over what happens. This is sometimes accomplished by job enlargement, increasing the number of tasks an employee performs so that they find increased satisfaction through involvement in a process from start to finish (Argenti, 1994, p. 234).

An industrial psychologist gave the subjects in a study some difficult puzzles to work and some boring proofreading to do. While they were attempting to accomplish these tasks, the psychologist played a loud tape recording of one person speaking Spanish, two speaking Armenian, and a copy machine in use.

Half of the subjects were given a button to push to stop the noise. The other half had no control over the noise. Those with buttons to push solved five times as many puzzles and had one-fourth fewer errors in proofreading, although never once did any subject with buttons to push ever push the button! Those who perceived that they had control over their situation clearly outperformed those who felt they had little or no control. In numerous repetitions the same results were obtained.

In the field, the same results were achieved: Workers who were given buttons to push achieved superior results for the company. The Ford Motor Company plant in Edison, New Jersey, gave every worker on the assembly line a button to push that shut down the assembly line. The Ford workers shut down the assembly line 30 times the first day and an average of 10 times a day thereafter. After the first day the shutdown lasted an average of 10 seconds—just time to make this or that small adjustment, turn a bolt, or the like.

What happened at the plant? Production remained steady. Three other factors changed significantly. The number of defects dropped from 17 per car to less than 1. The number of care requiring rework after coming off the line dropped by 97%. A backlog of union grievances plummeted. Why? Because the line workers felt they had some meaningful control in their jobs; they had a sense of ownership in the plant. Employees who have a sense of ownership in the facility will try to do what is best for it. The nurse's aide with this perception is more capable of meeting their social needs such as self-esteem, self-acceptance, and status.

How can nurses' aides be given ownership in the facility? One director of nurses accomplished it by consulting the aides before admitting a patient to their area. When the aides told the director of nurses that the care load was too great at one particular juncture, the director of nurses refused the proposed admission.

These aides had a sense of control over their work situation. They worked harder than they had previously and exercised their control judiciously to make sure the quality of resident care was not compromised by over admitting. These nurse's aides had a button to push. They never pushed it without a good reason.

Nurse's Aide "Ownership"

Why should nurse's aides be involved in running the facility? Ford Motor Company has a practice of soliciting input from all hourly workers. The assembly line workers are asked to comment on the manufacturability of parts and are members of advance design teams. Hourly workers offered 1,155 suggestions for changes in design or production for three small trucks. More than 700 of these suggestions were adopted.

The nursing home administrator is commonly conceived to have at least three immediate constituencies: the staff, the residents, and the residents' significant others. We argue that one of the administrator's major tasks is to create and enforce as many as possible opportunities for residents to feel in control of their lives. Here we maintain that one of the administrator's major tasks is to create and enforce as many as possible opportunities for staff to feel in control of their work. Not an easy task for either group. The forces on institutionalization appear to naturally move toward removing control from the residents. Similarly, the forces of regulations and the accompanying need for conformity in the workplace naturally move toward removing control over work from the staff members. In a study of staff self-perceived influence on decision making (498 staff in 51 nursing homes), nurse assistant involvement in shift reports, frequency of unit staff meetings, and administrators' decision-making autonomy from the governing board were found associated with increased levels of nurse's aide involvement in decision making (Kruzick, 1995, p. 207; Maddox & Sussman, 2001, p. 549).

One administrator gives nurses' aides 50 cents an hour for each employee they get and *keep* at the facility. When the administrator asked an aide how she was doing, she replied, "My company's fine." She had 6 employees in her "company" and was earning $3.00 more per hour now. Creative incentives are endless.

Respect for the Creative Potential of Each Employee— Maintaining Passion

The "business" of every nursing facility is providing resident care. In *A Passion for Excellence,* Peters and Austin (1985a) insist that there are only two ways to create and sustain superior patient care: first, by taking exceptional care of patients by providing superior services and quality of care; and second, by constantly innovating.

According to them, this is not accomplished by the genius of the administrator or by mystical strategic moves. Excellence in patient care comes from "a bedrock of listening, trust, and respect for the dignity and the creative potential of each person in the organization" (Peters & Austin, 1985a, p. 20).

High patient care depends on whether the administrator has been able to enable the employees—the housekeepers, kitchen staff, laundry workers, maintenance persons, accountant, and secretary, as well as the nursing staff—to "buy" into the facility.

Stow the Fire Hoses

Most individuals and organizations tend to resist change. It has been observed that the only persons who really welcome change are patients with wet diapers and busy cashiers. There is a tendency to "fire hose" employee's suggestions or ideas for new ways to accomplish the facility's goals. "It's not within the budget," "it'll never work," "we've already tried that," "yeah, but, things are fine the way they are," and "we don't do it that way around here," are common responses to new suggestions.

According to Kriegel (1991), conventional wisdom holds that everything happens in cycles. The belief is that things will cycle back—back to normal, back to the good old days. Such criticizing of new ideas leads to sticking with the tried and true approach. Kriegel argues that the new reality is that change will be followed with change, that the waves will not flatten out. Rather, waves will continue to get bigger and come at the facility faster.

Membership on a Team

We have mentioned the team concept several times and will return to it in the discussion of resident care planning.

Industries have repeatedly discovered that small groups produce higher quality, more personalized service, and more innovations than do larger entities (Johns & Saks, 2001, pp. 533–535). American companies, such as General Motors, Hewlett-Packard, and Emerson Electric now typically limit the size of the plant they will build to between 200 and 500 employees. The Japanese organize their largest industrial plants into small teams of 10 to 40 workers. Ask each worker, "What do you need to do a better job?"

A Natural Head Start

The nursing home enjoys a natural advantage over these companies. Federal regulations have demanded a small-team approach. Those who drew up the federal requirements already knew what industry is beginning to realize: Employees perform better when they are part of a team (Noe et al., 2000, p. 26).

Team membership is a valuable tool in efforts to retain employees, because it helps meet the employee's need for social involvement, communication with other employees, and meaningful personal involvement in the real work of the facility.

As a matter of practical reality, the work of a nursing facility cannot be successfully accomplished without the departments functioning as a single team. Achieving and maintaining this necessary teamwork is one of the nursing facility's constant challenges.

Trying Easy

Ever more intense regulatory efforts and continuous squeezing of the funds made available to nursing facilities can lead to a faster is better mentality, what Kriegel refers to as the Gotta's (1991, p. 53), for example, "I gotta make medication rounds quickly, finish all the paperwork, cut costs, get the patient ready for that meal, get the trays out fast . . ."

A Lesson From Chaplain

Kriegel cites the old Charlie Chaplain film *Modern Times,* in which he is happily decorating cakes on the assembly line, adding a rose here, a fancy frosting there. Then the assembly lines speeds up and in his haste the icing gets sprayed everywhere, and the cakes begin falling off the end of the assembly line, falling onto a growing mound on the floor. The more recent equivalent is, in Japan, known as *karoshi,* or death from overwork. Many Japanese workers have been driven to work in perpetual overdrive leaving the worker frustrated, nervous, and irritated—a true Type A lifestyle requirement.

The pressures from low reimbursement levels to give more service with fewer employees in the nursing facility can lead to reduced quality and service. Creativity and innovation are losers to speed. The turnover rate among directors of nursing and the nursing assistants are testimony to this. Caudill and Patrick (1992) developed a 56-item questionnaire for nursing assistants completed by 996 of them. Weekly and permanent resident assignments were favored over rotating responsibilities. Aides responsible for larger number of residents left more often (Caudill & Patrick, 1992, pp. 29–32). Kriegel (1991) relates his experiences with athletes trying out for the Olympic team. After recording their times the first round he told them to run at nine-tenths their capacity, not flat out. Each ran faster the second time. An Arkansas study of long-term care nurse administrators by Vaughn-Wrobel and Tygart (1993) confirmed that most nurse administrators are ill-prepared by prior administrative training for their positions.

Turnover

Turnover rates are as high as 60% The nurse administrator position normally requires a 110% or greater effort from persons without adequate prior training. Conventional wisdom, Kriegel (1991) notes, tells us to move at 110% to get the necessary work done. The administrator can assist employees to give a passionate 90% rather than pressuring for 110% efforts. A passionate 90% is more effective than a panicked 110% effort. From an "easy" passionate 90% the employee gets job satisfaction; from the "harder" 110% effort the employee gets job dissatisfaction. Patients who hear the proverbial "we're working short today" know that the necessary 110% effort will lead to lower quality and care that shift (Johns & Saks, 2001, pp. 119–120; Noe et al., 2000, p. 358; Robbins & Coulter, 2007, p. 389).

Ninjas of Joy

Work ought to be fun. Several West Coast Silicon Valley firms, have led the way toward the concept that work ought to be fun. Dress is California informal, life is laid back, having fun is an important value. Aristotle observed that pleasure in the job puts perfection in the work (Kriegel, 1991, p. 258). If nurses who love nursing can be hired, if nursing assistants who love taking care of older people can be hired, if maintenance persons who love to tinker and repair and maintain can be hired, the facility will be a pleasant place to spend one's hours.

The Importance of Having Fun

It is perhaps more important to have fun in a nursing facility than in most work settings. As one writer observed, coal miners used to take birds into the shafts as early warnings of danger. Laughter and good humor are the canaries of the work shift—when laughter dies its an early warning that life is slipping from the facility (Kriegel, 1991, p. 260). Ben and Jerry's, the ice cream manufacturer, has appointed "joy gangs" whose responsibilities are to put more joy into the facility. These gangs must figure out activities and events that encourage the employees and residents to loosen up and have fun with each other.

Not necessarily an easy task in the nursing home environment, therefore all the more important.

Turnover is high, and burnout is high among nursing facility staff. Kriegel (1991) observes that conventional wisdom says play to win. Kriegel says "*play, to win*" (p. 256). There is a saying that getting there is more than half the fun. Actually, winning must take place not at the end of the game, but every day on the way. Work must be fun each day if employees and residents are to experience quality living. He who laughs, lasts. This is true both of employees and residents.

Meeting the Employee's Need for Economic Security

For the purposes of this discussion of ten activities available to employers seeking to retain staff, by the term *security* we mean the finance-related benefit package provided for the employees. Often employee behaviors are rewarded through incentive plans (any rewards that motivate employees), which are designed to achieve facility goals (Argenti, 1994, p. 218).

A Simplified Model

One way to view what employees need from the facility is the following:

What	Knowledge of what the organization needs
How	Skills to do what the organization needs
Will	The desire to do what the organization needs
Equipment	The tools to get the job done to professional standards
Time	Enough staff to permit the desired behaviors

2.9 Evaluating Employees

Job Performance Evaluation: A Line Manager Function

Job performance evaluation is a task assigned only to line managers. Such responsibility distinguishes staff from line management functions: Staff, having no line authority, should not be assigned line responsibility for human resources matters—hiring, evaluating, promotion, reprimanding, suspending, or discharging employees—because to do so violates the concept of each employee reporting to but one manager.

Purpose of Job Performance Evaluation

W. Edwards Deming's (1982) third deadly sin is:

> Evaluation by performance, merit rating, or annual review of performance.

These, Deming, asserted, destroy teamwork and nurture rivalry. Performance ratings build fear, leave people despondent, bitter, beaten, and encourage mobility of management.

Having acknowledged this, what is a department manager to do? How is the facility to judge the performance of its employees over time? There are those such as Deming who would argue that being the member of a productive team affords the facility managers sufficient evaluation and control over an employee's performance. Perhaps so.

There may be problems with doing away with annual or other reviews of employee performance. The frequent change of staff, including department managers in the average nursing facility, means that the organization's "memory" can be short. For an employee seeking to "build a career" at a facility, if there are no records, their progress over an extended period is more subject to the impressions of department managers who may pass through (Noe et al., 2000, p. 303).

As a practical matter, all of us are judged by ourselves and our coworkers as we go about our daily work. The organization needs some method of creating a track record, both to reward the good employee and to identify employees who function at the margin of competence and for whom considerable documentation must be in place when the time comes for dismissal.

A basic purpose of the job performance evaluation is to focus the energies of the employee on the performance level expected of them (Johns & Saks, 2001, pp. 40–43). Whereas on-the-job and inservice training are part of the directing role of department heads, job performance evaluation is a function of comparing and controlling personnel performance quality. The goal of the performance evaluation is, of course, to nurture the performance needed for the success of the facility, and, so far as practical, to reward good work (Noe et al., 2000, p. 305).

The Equal Employment Opportunity Commission (EEOC), and more recently, the Americans with Disabilities Act (ADA) have done much to stimulate employers to keep accurate evaluation records of employees' work. Court hearings have also contributed to the desirability of carefully documenting worker performance.

Performance Evaluation: Three Basic Objectives

Three basic objectives of performance evaluations are: (a) to give employees feedback about their work performance, (b) to provide a basis (plan) for directing future employee efforts toward organizational goals, and (c) to provide a basis on which managers will decide on promotions, compensation, and future job assignments (Johns & Saks, 2001, pp. 40–43; Noe et al., 2000, p. 306; Robbins & Coulter, 2007, p. 337).

The performance evaluation can force communication to occur that might not otherwise occur concerning the manager's feelings about the employee's work. Setting up a performance evaluation system may simply be a needed formalizing of the department managers impressions of the daily work of the employee. Most industries use the performance evaluation. A study by the Bureau of National Affairs revealed that among the industries studied, 84% had regular procedures for evaluating office personnel and 58% for evaluating line workers (1975, pp. 1–3). The majority of evaluations were given on an annual basis.

On balance, the absence of any written system for evaluation of long-term performance exposes the individual more nearly to the "whim" of managers who head the employee's department.

Outline of the Performance Evaluation Process

First, the manager defines the functions, tasks, demands, and expectations of the job and translates them into performance criteria (Johns & Saks, 2001, p. 90; Noe et al., 2000, p. 306; Robbins & Coulter, 2007, p. 338). To implement this, forms and procedures, including standardized methods of rating employees to be used by supervisors in conducting evaluations, must be developed.

Approximately 2 weeks before an evaluation date, the manager completes the form, sending a copy to the employee, together with notification of time and place of the evaluation. This gives the employee time to prepare for the meeting.

At the evaluation the manager reviews the completed form and may modify sections, if appropriate. Performance goals for the next time period are reviewed, modified if employee and manager concur, and, if possible, mutually agreed upon.

At the end of the session both employee and manager sign the evaluation. Provision is normally made for any addendum the employee may wish to write or for the employee to indicate disagreement with the findings. In the event of such a difference of opinion, appeal procedures are normally available.

As Deming has been eager to point out, the performance evaluation process is not without its faults.

The Performance Evaluation Process: Problems Encountered

Whatever the importance to the facility, and however rational the evaluation process may seem, resistance to its effective utilization often arises, making the program difficult to implement (Johns & Saks, 2001, pp. 89–91).

Often evaluations are given at the time the employee hopes for an annual raise, focusing primary attention on past performance rather than future performance goals. The managers are not normally rewarded when they take time to give thorough evaluations. Most managers are uncomfortable with face-to-face judgmental roles. Employees are highly sensitive to negative evaluations, leading managers to avoid conflict. Employees desire that the appraising manager meet at least three criteria. The appraiser should have had adequate opportunity to observe the employee's work (Johns & Saks, 2001, p. 413). Employees want the appraiser to thoroughly understand the employee's job and have clearly stated standards by which to judge the employee's efforts (Smith, 1984, p. 51). The manager ought to judge the work from an informed viewpoint. Nurse's aides, for example, want someone trained as a nurse, who presumably understands the nature of their job, to write their evaluation.

Performance evaluations sometimes fail. One major nursing home corporation has identified as contributing causes: (1) lack of previously agreed-upon objectives, (2) poor skill of the manager, (3) lack of a defined evaluation process, and (4) managerial behavior that does not contribute to the self-esteem/self-image of the employee. Employees, the corporation points out, do not normally outperform their self-image: If their self-image is high, high performance can be anticipated, and the converse can be expected if their self-esteem is low. Performance evaluation, they point out, should not be the first time people hear about things. A major goal is to be a coach, not a critic. A point to remember: Evaluate performance, not the person. One can be candid and specific about performance without attacking the person.

Methods of Rating Employees

Rating Scales

Rating scales are consistently used. They list a number of characteristics, traits, and requirements of the employee's position on a line or scale. The evaluator checks off the degree to which the employee is believed to meet a train or requirement. For example, a scale recording degree of initiative might appear thus:

Initiative

Lacks initiative   Meets requirements   Highly resourceful

Work Quality

Needs to improve   Meets standards   Exceeds standards

Global Ratings

Often the manager will be asked to provide a global rating for the employee. This normally is regarded as a summary score based on the components of the evaluation. Generally, each employer establishes a numeric or alphabetic scale for the facility.

For example, 1 might represent the highest and 5 the lowest rating. Inevitably, the scale comes to resemble the grading system everyone has known in elementary and secondary school: Whatever the symbols used, the person comes to understand that they are an A, B, C, or D performer—or an F, in which case a termination notice might be pending. However much or little the manager may write or discuss with the employee, the employee's real concern is, "Am I a "1" performer, and if not, why not?" because the employee knows that the "1" performers get first chance at whatever rewards the system has to give, be it promotions, bonuses, salary increases, or high status.

Errors Made by Managers Using Rating Scales

Rating scales, too, have their problems. At least three types of errors occur.

The Leniency Error

To avoid conflict, some supervisors give consistently high ratings. The lenient supervisor's ratings are difficult to accurately compare with those of a stricter and more demanding supervisor.

The Error of Central Tendency

Other supervisors consistently give only moderate scores to employees regardless of whether their performance is poor or outstanding (Johns & Saks, 2001, p. 72).

The Halo Effect

The halo effect occurs when a supervisor who values one particular type of job behavior, punctuality, for example, permits the presence or absence of this one trait to color several or most other traits ratings. A habitually late employee might be excellent in resident care, but be rated low in most categories because the supervisor is irritated by the persistent tardiness (Robbins & Coulter, 2007, pp. 408, 198).

Rating by Essay

The use of essays or paragraphs describing employee progress is less frequent than rating scales. It is especially difficult to compare employees when the essay method permits supervisors simply to write whatever evaluative comments occur to them. A brief essay at the end of a rating scale can be valuable, however.

Possible Outcomes From Evaluations

Evaluations are primarily intended to give feedback to the employee about performance to date and projected activities. Some of the possible results can be transfer, promotion, or demotion, or, in the case of the reductions in force, the basis for discharge.

Transfer

A transfer is the placement of an employee to another position that is approximately equivalent to the present position. A nurse, for example, may find that working on the medically complex hall is beyond their current level of technical skills and ask for a lateral transfer to a lighter care hall.

Promotion

A promotion is placement of an employee at a higher level within the facility or group of facilities (promotion to a job at the corporate level). There are at least two recognized bases for promotions: merit and seniority. Seniority is concerned with length of service and tends to be automatic. The merit system relies on performance evaluations of supervisors for placement of a worker at a higher level. Under the seniority system a nurse who serves the required number of months or years at Level 1 is automatically promoted to Level 2. Under the merit system a nurse may or may not be promoted from Level 1 to Level 2, depending on evaluation decisions of the supervisor.

Demotion

Demotion is the change of assignment of an employee to a lower level in the organization, usually with less pay, fewer responsibilities, and reduced status. Demotions are often accomplished by the use of transfers (Noe et al., 2000, p. 333). A formerly more productive employee may be transferred to another position, with pay and status remaining intact. Another alternative to demotion is promotion to a position with little responsibility or power.

Layoff

Layoffs are normally temporary dismissals and are potentially demoralizing to the remaining employees as well as to those laid off. Unambiguous layoff policies can reduce anxiety among the remaining employees. However, such policies also tie the hands of management, who might, for example, seek to retain a recent but especially valued employee. Layoffs are carefully scrutinized by employees for fairness and equability in their implementation.

Discharge

When companies downsize, some basis for deciding who is dismissed is exercised. Discharging those employees with the lowest evaluation ratings first is a frequently used approach.

Cop Versus Coach

One of the reasons Deming advises against performance evaluation reviews is that it places the manager more nearly in the role of policeperson than of coach. The performance evaluation usually focuses on "areas for improvement," the negative side of the employee's work. The focus is on what the employee is not doing right, rather than on strengths. The department manager is the employee's coach. The coach's job is to bring out the best in the individual. When managers cite employees' weaknesses in the performance evaluation the employee feels more busted than trusted. It is the employee's strengths, not weaknesses that will carry the employee through to success. As Kriegel (1991) observes one can get by improving upon weaknesses, one can become great by building on strengths.

Evaluation Do's and Don'ts Learned by One Corporation

A major national nursing home chain suggests the following useful ideas about evaluations:

- Evaluation information should be given only to those who have a definite reason and legal right.
- Evaluations should be conducted in private.
- It is unfair to an employee not to be frank with him or her in an evaluation interview and discuss areas of needed improvement.
- The evaluation form should accurately reflect the employee's performance.
- Effective evaluation interviews that produce results take time.
- Evaluations should be made only on those things that are relevant to the job.
- A supervisor will find it difficult to follow up on an "I'll try harder!" solution from the employee.
- If policy permits, the employee has a moral and ethical right to see his or her evaluation form.
- Overrating all employees is a mistake in the long run.
- Recent events, both positive or negative, can unduly bias a performance evaluation interview.

2.10 Paying Employees

The nursing home is labor intensive. In most facilities wages and benefits make up more than half of the operating costs. About 65% of nursing home expenditures are personnel costs. Estimates are that benefits made up 39% of employee compensation. A 1997 survey revealed that employee compensation nationally was 55% of all industries and 62% of nursing industry costs (Noe et al., 2000, p. 388).

Careful management of wages and benefits is one of the major sources of cost control available to the nursing home administrator.

Money Is Liquid Value

Benefits

Economic theory holds that employees prefer a dollar in cash over a dollar's worth of any specific commodity, because the cash can be used to purchase the commodity or something else, that is, cash is less restrictive. Nevertheless, benefits as a percentage of wages and salaries has increased from 17% in 1955 to 42% by 1997 (Noe et al., 2000, p. 451; Robbins & Coulter, 2007, p. 474). Government programs requiring certain benefits, such as Social Security benefits, have partly caused this shift. Favorable tax treatment of certain benefits, for example, tax deferred 401k plan contributions, have also contributed to this trend (Noe et al., 2000, p. 452).

The wages paid the employees normally determine their standard of living (Johns & Saks, 2001, pp. 164–170). Wages also affect their status in both the facility and in the community. Wages are perceived as a statement by the facility about the relative worth of the skills of each employee.

The most liquid benefit a facility can give to its employees is the paycheck. Health insurance, sick leave, and the like, are important, but the benefit most highly valued by the employee is the dollar value of the paycheck, which provides maximum control over the product of the employee's work effort.

For the typical nursing home employee the wage rate is salient, and even a difference of a few cents per hour can spell satisfaction or dissatisfaction with wages for an individual making comparisons with a similarly qualified coworker.

Theories of Compensation

Compensation is generally considered the reward given employees in exchange for their work effort. How willing an employee may be to work hard and assist the facility toward its goals can depend on how justly the employee feels their wages and benefits fit their work effort (Noe et al., 2000, p. 389).

Equity Theory

According to equity theory, employees seek an exchange in which their wages and benefits are equal to their work effort, especially when compared to wages and benefits paid to similarly situated coworkers (Johns & Saks, 2001, p. 147; Robbins & Coulter, 2007, p. 465). If the individual feels equitably paid, less tension may exist. If however, they suspect that others with similar skills and investment of effort receive more, a tension exists that most employees will seek to resolve.

Typical worker responses to perceived inequities are to ask for a pay raise, reduce their effort, file a grievance, or, in some cases, seek employment elsewhere. Alternatively, the employee may encourage those perceived as similarly situated, but benefiting more, not to work so hard. Reactions to perceived inequities can take many forms.

Wage Polices

Developing and administering compensation policies are important administrative duties. Policies should cover such areas as the following (Johns & Saks, 2001, pp. 166–167; Noe et al., 2000, p. 390; Robbins & Coulter, 2007, p. 475):

- The rate of pay, set below, at, or above the prevailing community practice;
- The discretion supervisors can exercise in differentiating an individual's pay from the set scale;
- The amount of spread between pay rates for employees with seniority and pay rates for new employees; and
- The periods between raises and the weight given to seniority and merit in determining a new pay rate.

Hourly Wages or Salaries?

Most facilities distinguish between hourly employees (wage earners) and persona paid stated salaries periodically. Wage earner or hourly employees generally are required to punch in and out on a time clock and are paid only for hours worked as verified on the time card. Salaried workers, in contrast, are paid a set wage regardless of the hours worked, which may or may not be required to be recorded on a time clock. Usually, department managers in the nursing facility are paid set salary. However, some department managers, for example, the head of dietary who encounters numerous occasions for long days, may negotiate to work on an hourly basis.

How Much to Pay: The Wage Mix

Determining wage rates and benefits is a complex task affected by a number of factors called the wage mix (Noe et al., 2000, pp. 392, 424):

- the labor market
- prevailing wage rates
- cost of living increases
- ability to pay
- collective bargaining
- individual bargaining
- value of the job

The Labor Market

Once governmental requirements for minimum wage rates are met, and sometimes the influence of unions also taken into account, supply and demand dramatically affect the wage rate. During the early decades of the 20th century physicians were able to restrict their numbers and keep them lower than the demand; this resulted in favorable influences on their incomes, which now average well over $150,000 per year. Similarly, the nurse shortage of the early 1990s resulted in dramatic increases in the wages earned by nurses in the facility. In many cases the director of nurses' salary increased beyond that of the administrator. For many administrators this had the benefit of pushing their own wage upward to enable it to continue to be above that of the director of nurses.

Prevailing Wage Rates

According to a government study, more than half of businesses surveyed indicated that the prevailing wage scale in their communities for comparable jobs was the most influential factor in determining wages actually paid (Noe et al., 2000, p. 392).

This tends to be true for nursing facilities, which generally are viewed as paying somewhat lower salaries to employee categories such as nurses than do local hospitals. In general, the local hospital's wage rate sets the prevailing wage rate against which the other health care providers set their own pay scales.

Wage surveys for the community or region are taken by many organizations. They may be carried out by a single facility, or through agreements with others to share this information. In most communities nursing facilities share wage information with each other and other health providers.

Cost of Living Increases

During periods of inflation, cost of living adjustment may be made in wage rates. The purpose of cost of living increases is to assist workers to maintain their purchasing power. These increases, often embodied in escalator clauses of labor contracts, provide for wage adjustments based on some index, usually the Consumer Price Index (CPI). The CPI is a government-defined measure of the cost of living compared to a base point, usually of a few years earlier, which is designated as 100. Any increase or decrease in the cost of living is then expressed as a percentage of the base figure of 100.

Collective Bargaining

Where employees are unionized, nursing homes are subject to union influences, regardless of wage rates paid.

Individual Bargaining

Individuals with especially desirable skills may be able to negotiate a higher wage than others in similar positions. When a highly qualified maintenance director or director of nurses is sought, the facility may bargain with such a person and offer them a premium.

Key Job Comparisons

In the nursing facility the wages paid to the nurses tend to become the benchmark against which the earnings of other staff members are compared and established (Noe et al., 2000, p. 393).

Wage Classes and Rates

To approach equity and achieve some flexibility for supervisors evaluating employees, wage classes or grades and wage rates are normally established. All jobs within that class are paid at the same rate or within the same rate range. A rate range is the variation permitted within a class or grade (Noe et al., 2000, p. 392).

Merit Pay

Use of merit pay is a complex matter. Usually a merit increase grid is developed for each merit pay position. The size and frequency of pay increases are tied to (1) the individual's performance rating, and (2) the position of that individual's pay in the merit increase grid. Merit pay often increases individual competition among staff thus reducing willingness to perform as a team. A fair and accurate performance system satisfactory to most employees is difficult to develop and administer, thus leading to increased levels of employee dissatisfaction, and perhaps, turnover (Noe et al., 2000, p. 429). Group incentives are useful, but also have limitations inasmuch as they may pit groups against each other. This is undesirable in the intimate atmosphere of the nursing home setting where all departments (groups) must cooperate with each other (work as a team) if quality of care is to be delivered (Noe et al., 2000, p. 436).

2.11 Disciplining Employees

The following are some of the more common staff disciplinary problems faced by nursing facilities:

- excessive or unexcused absences or tardiness
- leaving the facility or work area without permission
- violation of rules about smoking, intoxication, narcotics, gambling, fighting, firearms
- failure to follow safety procedures, especially the Bloodborne Pathogens Act requirements
- failure to accept direction
- failure to report accidents
- failure to take resident safety and welfare into account
- verbal, physical, or other abuse of residents
- theft, punching another employee's time card, falsifying records
- insubordinate behavior or abusive language
- failure to report their own condition of illness
- solicitation or acceptance of gratuities from residents, or families, or significant others
- immoral, indecent, or disorderly conduct

Need for Rules and Their Consequences

Each facility should carefully state and consistently enforce policies regarding disciplinary actions (easier said than done!). The employees must be made fully aware, before any infraction occurs, of both the facility's rules and the disciplinary action that will be its consequence. Although policies and rules may have been clearly formulated, these policy statements remain confusing unless they are continually reinforced by positive (motivating) and negative (disciplining) actions. Unless the facility can document that it had a "just cause" for firing an employee there is a significant chance that the employee will be able to collect unemployment benefits.

Grievance Procedures

Grievance procedures are an important safety valve for policies regarding disciplinary actions. Employees need to know that there are equitable procedures through which their reactions and views can be expressed when they feel they have been dealt with unfairly.

Progressive Discipline

For most offenses, progressive discipline—beginning with verbal warnings, followed by written warnings for any subsequent violations—makes the most sense. Progressive discipline may prevent repetition of the offending behavior after only a verbal warning, thus bringing about an early solution to the problem.

Employees who are dismissed have the right to present their case to the employment security commission, and many do. It is necessary for the employer to keep a well-documented record of having made every reasonable effort to persuade the employee to conform to facility policy before dismissal. Normally, administration must be able to demonstrate that disciplinary actions taken were based on rational judgments about the offending behavior, not on personal vindictiveness or excessive emotional reactions of supervisors to employee behavior.

Each facility needs to define clearly its own policies governing suspension and discharge procedures. Normally, several managers, including the administrator, participate in a decision to suspend or discharge an employee.

One major nursing facility chain recommends the following be assured:

- That the requirement reasonably relates to the operation of the facility and that the requirement has been properly communicated.
- That management has investigated the matter fairly, objectively, and in a timely manner.
- That the requirements and penalties are and have been administered fairly and objectively, without any form of discrimination.
- That the situation is dealt with and a penalty determined in a manner consistent with past practice for similar situations.
- That the penalty is appropriate to the seriousness of the infraction.
- That misconduct (e.g., patient abuse, theft, and substance abuse) is reported to the appropriate agency for investigation according to state or federal regulations.
- That where discharge is the penalty, employees have warning or knowledge of the probable consequences of their actions.

Discharging Employees

The process of terminating employees, especially executives, can be eased through helping that person find alternative employment. This is called disemployment, outplacement, or dehiring (Noe et al., 2000, p. 361; Robbins & Coulter, 2007, p. 392). The managers themselves may assist the employee to find another position or hire an employment firm to do so. This is sometimes known as outplacement counseling or transferring problems (Noe et al., 2000, p. 361).

REFERENCES

Allen, J. E. (2006). *Nursing home federal requirements and guidelines to surveyors and survey protocols.* New York: Springer Publishing Company.

Argenti, P. A. (1994). *The portable MBA desk reference.* New York: Wiley.

Argyris, C. (1972). A few words in advance. In A. J. Marrow (Ed.), *The failure of success.* New York: AMACOM.

Bureau of National Affairs. (1975). *Employee performance: Evaluation and control.* Washington, DC: Author (Personnel Policies Forum Survey No. 108).

Caudill, M. E., & Patrick, M. (1992). Turnover among nursing assistants: Why they leave and why they stay. *Journal of Long Term Care Administration, 19,* pp. 29–32.

Chruden, H. J., & Sherman, A. W., Jr. (1980). *Personnel management* (6th ed.). Cincinnati: South-Western Publishing.

Deming, W. E. (1982). *The Deming Management Method.* New York: Putnam.

Department of Health and Human Services. (2005). Centers for Disease Control and Prevention, National Center for Health Statistics. Hyattsville, MD: Author.

Department of Health and Human Services. (2006a). Centers for Medicare and Medicaid Services, Oscar Form 672: F78–F142.

Department of Health and Human Services. (2006b). Centers for Medicare and Medicaid Services, Oscar Report, 18S.

Dunnette, M. D., & Kirchner, W. K. (1965). *Psychology applied to industry.* New York: Appleton-Century-Crofts.

Equal Employment Opportunity Commission, Civil Service Commission, Department of Labor, & Department of Justice. (1987). Uniform guidelines on employee selection procedures. *Federal Register, 43*(166), pp. 38,290–38,315.

Givnta, J. (1984). For good job training, you need a good beginning. *Supervisory Management, 29*(6), pp. 19–21.

Gordon, G. K., & Stryker, R. (1983). *Creative long term care administration.* Springfield, IL: Charles C Thomas.

Grant, D. A., & Kemme, J. (1993). How to conduct security checks on prospective employees. *Nursing Homes, 30,* pp. 12–14.

Harrington, C. H., Carrillo, M. S., Thollaug, S. C., Summers, P. R., & Wellin, V. (2000). *Nursing facilities, staffing, residents, and facility deficiencies, 1993 through*

1999. San Francisco: University of California at San Francisco, Department of Social & Behavioral Sciences.

Hitt, M. A., Ireland, R. D., & Hoskisson, R. E. (2001). *Strategic management: Competitiveness and globalization* (4th ed.). Cincinnati, OH: South-Western College Publishing.

Ivancevich, J. M., Szjlagyi, A., & Wallace, M. (1977). *Organizational behavior and performance.* Santa Monica, CA: Goodyear Publishing.

Johns, G., & Saks, A. (2001). *Organizational behavior* (5th ed.). Toronto: Addison Wesley Longman.

Kriegel, R. J. (1991). *If it ain't broke ... break it.* New York: Time Warner.

Kruzick, J. M. (1995). Empowering organizational contexts: Patterns and predictors of perceived decision-making influence among staff in nursing homes. *The Gerontologist, 35*(2), pp. 207–216.

McGregor, D. M. (1960). *The human side of enterprise.* New York: McGraw-Hill.

Maddox, G. L., & Sussman, S. W. (2001). *The encyclopedia of aging* (3rd ed.). New York: Springer Publishing Company.

Miller, D. B. (Ed.) (1982). *Long term care administrator's desk manual.* Greenvale, NY: Panel Publishers.

Noe, R. A., Hollenbeck, J. R., Gerhart, B., and Wright, P. M. (2000). *Human resource management: Gaining a competitive advantage* (3rd ed.). Boston: McGraw-Hill Companies, Inc.

Patchner, M. A., & Patchner, L. S. (1993). Essential staffing for nursing home care: The permanent assignment model. *Nursing Homes,* pp. 39–40.

Peters, T., & Austin, J. (1985a). *A passion for excellence: The leadership difference.* New York: Random House.

Riter, R. N. (1993). Some practical advice for the new nursing home administrator. *Journal of Long Term Care Administration, 21,* pp. 40–41.

Robbins, S. P, & Coulter, M. (2007). *Management* (9th Ed.). New York: Pearson / Prentice Hall.

Rogers, W. W. (1980). *General administration in the nursing home* (3rd ed.). Boston: CBI Publishing.

Rotondi, T., Jr. (1976). Behavior modification on the job. *Supervisory Management, 21*(2), pp. 22–28.

Ruhl, M. J., & Atkinson, K. (1986). Interactive video training: One step beyond. *Personnel Administrator, 51*(5), pp. 360–363.

Scott, S. (1983). Finding the right person. *Personnel Journal, 62*(11), pp. 894–902.

Seasons Seminars. (2004). *National Sample Survey of Registered Nurses.* Retrieved from www.seasons-seminars.com.

Smith, K. E. (1984). Performance appraisal: A positive management tool. *College Review, 1*(2), 43–62.

Thomas, W. H. (1996) *Life worth living: The Eden alternative in action.* Acton, MA: Vander Wyk & Burnham.

Vaughn-Wrobel, B. C., & Tygart, M. W. (1993). Management education needs of nurse administrators in long term care. *Journal of Gerontological Nursing,* pp. 33–38.

Vroom, V. H. (1964). *Work and motivation.* New York: John Wiley and Sons.

PART III

Finance/Business

3.1 The Administrator's Role as Financial Manager

An administrator's duties encompass nearly every aspect of managing the facility, from assisting in the recruitment of professional medical staff to assuring the efficient operation of the laundry department. Not surprisingly, the administrator is also finally responsible for the income and expenses of the facility. It is, in reality, the administrator who is the one person held accountable for the entire financial operation of the facility.

Selecting and Evaluating Financial Personnel

Although we will explore their individual functions in more detail later, let us say here that the *bookkeeper* primarily records the daily cash transactions of the facility, keeping track of all money going out or coming in. The *accountant* uses the information compiled by the bookkeeper to generate reports on the financial standing of the facility. The bookkeepers and accountants record the financial transactions, but the administrator is chief financial officer of the facility, not the bookkeepers, accountants, or even the business manager or the one who holds the title of chief financial officer (CFO).

The administrator must ensure that the business office process runs smoothly—that the bookkeeper is qualified for the job and has access to the information needed for recording all the facility's financial transactions. Thus, the administrator must have some knowledge of bookkeeping in order to know whether this important task is carried out as it should be.

The administrator may also have to select an accountant, either as an employee or as a consultant for the facility. If the administrator manages one of a chain of nursing homes, the accountant will probably be an employee of the corporate office. The administrator should therefore have some understanding of accounting to be able to assess the accountant's performance.

Increasingly, the administrator must understand and monitor the manner in which the Minimum Data Set (MDS) is being completed to assure that the facility receives the highest reasonable and accurate Resource Utilization Group (RUG) score for each resident served.

The administrator must be able to interpret the financial reports developed by the accountant and the corporate office. The administrator's primary role as financial manager is to use the financial information to make informed decisions about the facility. The administrator needs to know how these reports, especially the Medicare / Medicaid reimbursement requests, are prepared.

"Corporate" Purposes; Facility Ownership Patterns

Corporate offices often use individual facilities for various purposes, for example, to balance the cash flow and tax affairs of the corporation through the network of facilities rather than by actual individual facility performance. A single facility may be carried on the books as having a high debt load while another, similarly situated, may be considered as having a low debt load. The administrator must grasp the nuances of these matters to be able to compare their figures after debt service and taxes with those of a sister facility carried at a different debt load. They may vary, yet the level of success of staff performance may be comparable.

Nursing facility ownership patterns have been somewhat stable for a number of years. During the 1993, 1999, and 2006 period the percent of for-profit facilities remained about 66%, nonprofits about 27% to 28%, with government-owned facilities showing a steady decline from 6.9% in 1993 to 6.1% in 2006 (see Figure 3.1). Ownership patterns vary widely across states. Alaska and Wyoming have a high percentage of government-owned facilities. Alaska; Washington, DC; Minnesota; North Dakota; Pennsylvania; and South Dakota have a high percentage of nonprofit facilities. Arkansas, Oklahoma, and Texas have the highest percentage of proprietary facilities.

Maintaining Enough Income

In addition to bookkeeping and accounting, we will also take a close look at costs. There are many different types of costs, and we will explore how viewing costs in different ways can provide the administrator with information not included in the financial reports prepared by the accountants.

As the facility's ultimate financial manager, the administrator must assure the availability of funds for conducting business: to purchase supplies and pay salaries and to meet the regular payments on any borrowed funds. Without these purchases and payments, the facility cannot operate. When money is

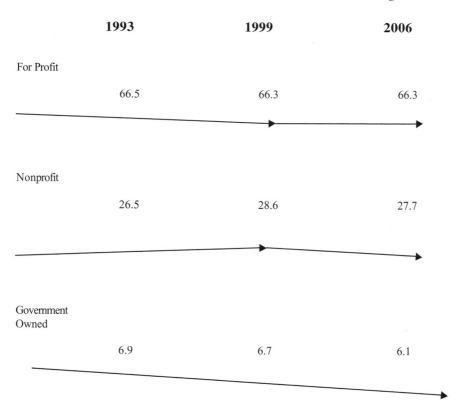

FIGURE 3.1 Trends in percent distribution of U.S. nursing facilities by ownership, 1993, 1999, and 2006.
Source: DHHS, 2006, F12.

not available to meet expenses, the facility cannot continue to operate for very long and may be obliged to close its doors.

Facility income is derived from the data entered into the MDS and sent periodically to the federal government. MDS forms can be obtained from a variety of sources such as Briggs Corporation or Med-Pass, Inc., which mark the quality indicators items in blue ink and the reimbursement level determination items in red ink. If the MDS is not accurately filled out the facility may be losing significant amounts of income by under reporting the amount of care being given each resident as measured by classifying resident reimbursement rates under over 40 RUGs. The more resources used, the higher the RUG score. The higher the RUG score the higher the reimbursement rate for each resident.

The Centers for Medicare and Medicaid Services (CMS) carefully monitor the level of care deemed appropriate for each resident each days. If the resident is left at a higher RUG score (level of reimbursement) for a week longer than CMS deems it appropriate while doing the annual survey the facility may be asked to reimburse Medicare for the excess dollars received.

Setting Rates

How does the administrator (or corporation) guarantee that the facility will receive sufficient funds? The administrator needs to know how to set rates for the services offered and how to produce the number of residents who will require these services. Appropriate rates for resident care services must reflect their true full costs, so the administrator must be able to measure these costs.

Besides being available in sufficient amount, funds must be received on a timely basis. The good financial manager understands the billings and collections procedures that keep money owed to the facility coming in regularly enough to meet financial obligations.

Planning and Budgeting

Financial management is important to planning and budgeting. To make a financial plan, or budget, the administrator must be able to predict both the costs of running the facility and the money it can expect to earn in the coming year(s). Knowledge of the facility's past financial performance and insight into the reason for earlier budget shortfalls or successes are essential for preparing a realistic and useful budget. The administrator who is not familiar with the cost and earnings of all the departments cannot expect to guide the organization on a reliable path in the future.

Responsibility to Others

Finally, by virtue of their position as director, the administrator is responsible for the effective operation of the nursing facility—to its residents and their significant others, to the employees, to the owner(s) or stockholders, and to the governing body of the facility. When signs of ineffective financial management become apparent, it is to the administrator that each of these parties turns for explanation.

Because nearly every decision made will have financial implications, an understanding of financial management is incumbent on the administrator, the person ultimately responsible for the performance of the facility, even in chain-operated homes.

However good the relationship of the manager with staff or however capable they may be in other aspects of administration, if finances are poorly or improperly handled, the administrator is likely to be judged ineffectual by the board of the facility owners.

Maximizing cash flow into the facility is part of the administrator's financial goal. This goal may be achieved by assuring that the facility receives maximum reimbursement from payers such as Medicare, Medicaid, and private insurance companies. Section G of the MDS, which measures the activities of daily living (ADLs) for example, heavily impacts a resident's revenue (RUG) categorization. Assistance in ADLs is normally provided by nursing assistants, one of the lower cost employees. The heaviest care scenario can be set as the amount of resources used. For example, a resident may need one person to help them transfer from bed to toilet on the day shift, but require two persons to assist them in the evening. This resident may be classified as a two-person assist for transfer for reimbursement purposes.

Being reimbursed for the most appropriate level of rehabilitation care can be another case in point. If, for example, the point at which the resident is reimbursed at a higher level of care is 280 minutes of care and staff is providing 270 minutes of care week after week, an opportunity to be appropriately reimbursed at a higher level may be being missed. Staff care about what the administrator cares about. If the administrator is paying careful attention to the minutes of reimbursable rehabilitative care being received and appropriateness of the RUG category levels of reimbursements for number of minutes served, the staff may also.

If the resident is not accurately assessed by the MDS coordinator the facility may lose many thousands of dollars of revenue annually. If, however, the MDS coordinator or administrator claims heavier care levels (hence more reimbursement dollars) than actually permitted the facility may be fined and required to pay back "extra" monies received. This is a complex assignment, because Medicare contracts with several intermediaries (usually large health insurance companies) to manage Medicare reimbursements, and these intermediaries interpretations vary over time and from intermediary to intermediary. For reasons such as these the financial accounts have established what are known as the Generally Accepted Accounting Principles (the GAAPs).

3.2 Generally Accepted Accounting Principles—The GAAPs

The accounting system defines the manner in which financial records must be kept, and it is used by nearly every type of organization, including nursing homes. Financial records refers primarily to the books and financial statements of the facility. Books are a set of records that list, in a prescribed manner, each monetary transaction (all money earned or spent) of the facility.

Maintaining the books constitutes bookkeeping. The books are used to prepare the financial statement. The financial statements are simply a summary of all the transactions recorded in the books, and they reflect the soundness of the organization's financial status.

The books and financial statements are prepared according to a series of rules known as the Generally Accepted Accounting Principles (GAAPs). These are consistent standards of accounting that allow the financial records to be understood by the various parties who have an interest in the financial position of the facility and also permit the financial statements of different homes or other organizations to be more easily compared. A discussion of selected GAAPs follows.

Entity Concept

Entity is a basic concept of accounting, under which the nursing facility is regarded as a whole, entirely separate from the affairs of the owners, managers, or other employees. This means that if the owner, for instance, withdraws from or adds to the funds of the facility, this transfer must be recorded in the books to reflect the effect on its finances.

Ongoing Concern Concept

Another basis rule of accounting is the consistency concept. This concept requires that the accounting reports for a facility be prepared in the same

230

way from year to year, in order to compare accurately the reports between two or more different time periods. This does not require that the organization prepare reports in a manner that is not suitable to the needs of management, but suggests that the method of reporting be carefully selected and that changes occur infrequently, if at all. Clearly, financial statements that are prepared in a different format every year will make comparisons difficult.

Concept of Full Disclosure

Related to consistency is the concept of full disclosure, which means that all financial information, that is, all money spent, earned, invested, or owed by the facility, must be shown in the financial records to represent accurately its financial standing. The concept of full disclosure has important legal implications, because failure to disclose all financial information may affect the amount of taxes the facility owes or the level of reimbursement it should receive from Medicare, Medicare, and other third-party payers.

Time Period Concept

Also known as the accounting period, the time period is the interval covered by the financial reports, usually 1 year. The accounting period should be consistent from one year to the next; that is, the fiscal year (the 12-month period designated for financial record keeping) should begin on the same date every year. Accounting records are frequently prepared more often than once a year, usually monthly, to provide management with current information. These shorter time periods should also remain consistent. Typically, monthly financial reports are prepared and distributed to the management, while quarterly (every 3 months) and annual reports are prepared and distributed to both managers and ownership.

Objective Evidence Concept

The objective evidence concept requires accounting records to be prepared with documentable records that are kept by the facility. Every transaction should be accompanied by a documented record, that is, by a piece of "paper" that confirms it. These "pieces of paper" (or equivalent electronic information) are the objective evidence of the transaction; they include receipts for bills that have been paid, bills (or invoices) for money owed by the facility, bank statements indicating interest earned periodically, or case receipts for money received by the facility each day or designated period. These are called the *source documents* of the transactions. Objective evidence is necessary so that estimates need not be used.

Instead of estimating the cost of supplies purchased during a month, for instance, all invoices are filed in an orderly fashion and used as objective source documents in determining the cost of supplies for the month. Estimates should be used as infrequently as possible, as this introduces an element of error and inconsistency in the accounting reports. When estimates are necessary, the process used in arriving at the estimated figure should be noted in the financial statement.

3.3 Two Approaches to Accounting: Cash Accounting and Accrual Accounting

There are two systems of accounting: cash and accrual. The difference between the two is primarily the time period in which expenses and revenues are recorded in the books. Revenues, the money coming into the facility, can be recorded for the period when, for example, the money from resident care is earned or when the cash payment is actually received by the facility.

Expenses, which will be defined in more depth later, are the money spent by the facility, and can also be recorded in two ways. An expense can be recorded when payment is made for items purchased. In accounting terminology, money paid out is called an expenditure. An expense can also be recorded when the items purchased are actually used up by the facility.

The difference in the time of recording is the difference between the two systems of accounting and results in two very different ways of preparing the financial records.

Cash Accounting Approach

In cash accounting, expenses are recorded when the cash is actually disbursed, and revenues are recorded when the money from, for example, resident services is received by the facility. Thus, the cash system of accounting simply records expenditures and receipts (the actual flow of cash out of and into the facility) as they occur. Organizations using the cash system of accounting, therefore, do not include in their accounting records noncash expenses, such as depreciation, because depreciation, the cost of wear and tear on equipment, for example, is a cost of providing services to residents that does not involve a cash expenditure.

Cash accounting also does not recognize those expenses that are prepaid, such as insurance paid up for months or years ahead. If the premium for a 3-year insurance policy is paid in the first year that the facility is covered by the policy, an insurance expense would be recorded in the month it is paid and would be listed only as an insurance expenditure for that 1-month time period. The fact that it was a prepaid expense and would last over several accounting periods is not acknowledged. Also, money that is owed to the facility for services already provided would not be recorded as accounts receivable, but would be counted as revenue only after the facility received payment. The chief advantage of cash accounting is simplicity; it is similar to one's personal checking account.

Cash accounting, however, has several disadvantages. One is that expenses and revenues for a single time period are not attributed to that same period. For example, medical supplies might be paid for in August but actually used up over the next 4 months. The cost of providing medical services in September would not include the cost of the medical supplies, as that expense would have been recorded in August. Thus, the total cost and revenues, and therefore the real profit or loss for those months, could not be accurately measured.

As already mentioned, the cash accounting system does not recognize the very real cost of depreciation of the facility's building, or plant, major equipment, or other capital items. It also does not recognize money that is owed to creditors by the facility (known as accounts payable, a deferred expense) or money that is owed to the facility by residents for services provided (accounts receivable, a deferred revenue).

Lastly, because the only means of recording expenses and revenues is when cash changes hands, the accounting records are subject to mismanagement by those involved in the accounting process. For these reasons, the cash system is infrequently used. Perhaps 99% of all nursing facilities use the accrual accounting approach.

Accrual Accounting Approach

Under the accrual system of accounting, revenues are recorded when they are earned and expenses when they are incurred, regardless of the time the cash transactions take place. The previous definition of expense can now be more precisely stated as a cost that is used up, or "expensed."

Using the example of the medical supplies, the cost of the supplies purchased in August is expensed over the next several months. The accounting records for September would show a medical supplies expense equal to the cost of the supplies used in September, and so on. This should help the reader understand why understanding the accounting and record-keeping procedures discussed in the next sections is necessary. The accrual system requires that every expense incurred by the nursing facility be attributed to the period, usually the month, in which it is incurred and all revenues to the month in which services are rendered.

This complexity is the main disadvantage of the accrual basis of accounting, but it has numerous advantages. Most important, it allows the facility to measure the revenues earned after expenses have been paid, or losses incurred, by matching revenues and expenses for each time period. It also includes depreciation, accounts payable, accounts receivable, and prepaid expenses in the accounting records, providing a more accurate picture of the facility's actual financial position. It is less subject to tampering, as expenses and revenues are usually backed by several forms of objective evidence. The following discussion of accounting and record keeping will be based on accrual accounting.

3.4 The Two Main Steps in the Accounting Process: Recording Transactions and Preparing Financial Statements

Recording Transactions in Journals and the General Ledger

The accounting process involves two main steps: keeping the books and preparing the financial statement. *Bookkeeping* is a system of recording all revenues and expenses, and matching those revenues to expenses during the same time period. This process is necessary for the preparation of the *financial statements,* which are a summary of the nursing facility's financial well-being within a time period.

The accounting process is fairly universal and will be described here in chronological order, from the chart of accounts to the preparation of the financial statements.

Chart of Accounts

The chart of accounts is simply a list of every account in the facility. The accounts are organized into six main groups:

- assets—things owned by the facility
- liabilities—things owed by the facility, or its obligations
- capital—money invested in the facility, also known as the facility's net worth
- revenues—earnings from operations or other sources
- expenses—costs of salaries, supplies, and so forth, that have been used up, usually through the provision of services
- fund account—any funds that have been established for restricted or unrestricted uses

As can be seen from the sample Chart of Accounts in Table 3.1, each account has a number. The first digit indicates the categories into which the account falls; the second digit usually is a subcategory. For example, registered nurse (RN) salaries are an expense (category 5) in the nursing department and have an account number 5201.

Note that the salary expense account number for every other department ends with 1 also. This system of classifying accounts is useful, as it identifies every account of the facility and thus is a means of control; expenses, for example, are automatically applied to a specific source so that random or unauthorized expenses cannot accumulate unnoticed. The numbered system also saves time by recording a number rather than a long title on many documents. It is especially convenient for a computerized bookkeeping system.

The Journals

Any transaction that takes place will affect some account. The journals are the first place that transactions are recorded; they are the books of original entry. Each facility will have its own system, but generally there are six journals:

- Cash Receipts Journal—records all cash received for services provided, for example, sales refreshment machines
- Billings Journal—lists all bills sent for services rendered
- Accounts Payable Journal (purchase journal)—records all purchases made that will be paid within the next few months
- Cash Disbursements Journal—records all payments made for services and supplies used for resident care and for all other operations of the facility
- Payroll Journal—summarizes all payroll checks distributed during the pay period
- General Journal—a record of nonrepetitive entries

The journals are characterized by another concept of accounting: double-entry bookkeeping. For each transaction, two entries are made in the appropriate journal, a debit and a credit.

A *debit* in accounting simply means the left side of the journal account; credit refers to the right side. When all debits and credits are totaled at the end of each month, they should be equal. Thus, for every debit entered, one or more credits are entered that equal the debit, and vice versa. Table 3.2 indicates which transactions are recorded as debits and which as credits.

TABLE 3.1.   Chart of Accounts, Old Well Home

Assets		Liabilities	
	Current Assets		Current liabilities
1101	Cash-petty	2102	Accounts Payable—supplies
1103	Cash-payroll account	2104	Notes Payable—short term
1106	Cash-operating fund	2107	Mortgage Payable—short term
1112	Investments-money market fund	2109	Debts Payable—current
1114	Investments-C of D	2111	Emp. Benefits Payable
1117	Investments—depreciation fund	2113	Emp. Health Ins. Payable
1122	Accounts Receivable—Medicare	2115	Salaries Payable
1123	Accounts Receivable—Medicaid	2201	Taxes
1124	Accounts Receivable—Private	2204	Taxes Payable—state
1126	Accounts Receivable—other	2205	Taxes Payable—municipal
1131	Interest Receivable	2207	Taxes Payable—federal
1163	Unexpired Liability Insurance	2221	Interest Payable
	Noncurrent Assets		Noncurrent Liabilities
1302	Land	2303	Notes Payable—long term
1305	Land improvements	2313	Mortgage Payable—long term
1402	Building—Main	2323	Bonds Payable
1414	Building—Welsh Hall	2401	Pensions Payable
1426	Building—garage/storage		
1430	Building Improvements		Capital
1502	Furniture—Main	3001	Owner's Equity
1504	Furniture—Welsh Hall	3101	Net Income (Loss)
1512	Equipment—Main		
			Revenue
1514	Equipment—Welsh Hall		Nursing Care
1516	Equipment—office	4001	Medicare
1518	Equipment—kitchen	4003	Medicaid
1519	Equipment—laundry	4005	Private
1521	Equipment—transportation		
1524	Equipment—land maintenance		Ancillary
		4212	Physical Therapy
	Contra Assets, Accum. Depr.	4214	Occupational Therapy
1602	Accum. Depr.—main bldg.	4216	Social Services
1604	Accum. Depr.—Welsh Hall	4218	Speech Therapy—contract

(Continued)

TABLE 3.1.   (Continued)

Assets		Liabilities	
1606	Accum. Depr.—garage/storage		
1636	Accum. Depr.—bldg. Improvements		Uncompensated Care
1642	Accum. Depr.—furn., main	4311	Contract. Discount-Medicare
1644	Accum. Depr.—furn., Welsh	4313	Contract. Discount-Medicaid
1651	Accum. Depr.—equip., main	4315	Contract. Discount-Other
1654	Accum. Depr.—equip., Welsh	4332	Donated Care
1666	Accum. Depr.—office equip.	4341	Bad Debts
1668	Accum. Depr.—kitchen	4351	Patient Refunds
1669	Accum. Depr.—laundry		
1671	Accum. Depr.—transportation		
1674	Accum. Depr.—land maintenance		
1680	Accum. Depr.—bldg. Improvements		

Expenses			
	Administration	5411	Payroll tax
5001	Salaries—administration	5432	Supplies
5002	Salaries—clerical	5442	Repairs
5003	Consultation fees	5461	Contract services
5006	Health Insurance		Housekeeping
5011	Payroll tax	5501	Salaries
5013	Taxes—income	5506	Health Insurance
5015	Taxes—property	5511	Payroll tax
5022	Insurance—liability	5532	Supplies
5026	Pension fund	5542	Repairs
5032	Supplies		
5034	Telephone		Rehabilitation
5035	Travel		Physical Therapy
5037	Postage	5601	Salaries
5039	Licenses and Dues	5606	Health Insurance
5042	Repairs	5611	Payroll tax
		5632	Supplies
	Plant Operation	5642	Repairs
5101	Salaries		
5106	Health Insurance		Occupational Therapy:
5111	Payroll tax	5661	Salaries
5122	Utility—electricity	5666	Health Insurance

(Continued)

TABLE 3.1.   Chart of Accounts, Old Well Home (Continued)

	Expenses		
5124	Utility—gas	5671	Payroll tax
5126	Utility—water	5682	Supplies
5128	Utility—sewage	5692	Repairs
5132	Supplies		Social Services
5142	Repairs	5701	Salaries
	Nursing	5706	Health Insurance
5201	Salaries—registered nurses	5711	Payroll tax
5202	Salaries—licensed practical	5732	Supplies
5203	Salaries—aides	5742	Repairs
5206	Health Insurance		Activity
5211	Payroll tax	5801	Salaries—beautician
5222	Pharmacy	5802	Salaries—crafts
5224	Laboratory	5806	Health Insurance
5232	Supplies	5811	Payroll tax
5237	Uniform	5832	Supplies—beauty
5242	Repairs	5833	Supplies—crafts
	Dietary	5835	Transportation
5301	Salary—dietician	5837	Special Events
5302	Salary—food service	5842	Repairs
5306	Health Insurance		Capital Expenses
5311	Payroll tax	5904	Interest—mortgage
5332	Supplies	5907	Interest—long-term debt
5342	Repairs	5914	Debt Service—mortgage
	Laundry	5917	Debt Service—long-term debt
5401	Salaries	5934	Depreciation—plant
5406	Health Insurance	5936	Depreciation—equipment

Journal entries are set in the shape of a T and thus are often called T-accounts. Data from the journal entries are the source documents, the objective evidence referred to at the beginning of this section.

To illustrate the process of journalizing, the example of the Billings Journal is used. When a bill is sent to a resident or to that person's payer, the bill represents revenues earned by the facility that it expects to receive. This

TABLE 3.2.   Transactions Recorded as Debits and Credits

Debit	Credit
(+) Increase in assets	(-) Decrease in assets
(+) Decrease in liability	(-) Increase in liability
(-) Decrease in capital	(+) Increase in capital
(-) Decrease in revenues	(+) Increase in revenues
(-) Increase in expenses	(+) Decrease in expenses

account receivable is an asset, because it is cash to which the facility is entitled. Thus, a bill to Ms. Jones for $1,000 would be recorded in the debit column as an increase in assets. On the credit side, $1,000 would be recorded as in increase in revenue. This journal entry is illustrated in Figure 3.2. The source document for this entry would be a copy of the invoice sent to Ms. Jones.

When the billings to all service recipients for the month are entered in the journal in this manner, the sum of debits should equal the sum of credits at the end of the month. Notice that the Billings Journal is used only for the billing of a service; the service recipient's payment of the bill will be recorded in the Cash Receipts Journal. The complete transaction would be recorded as follows.

Billings Journal

Debit _____	Credit _____
3/02	Acc/Rec $1,000.00 (account receivable)
3/02	Revenue $1,000.00

OLD WELL HOME
Billings Journal

			Debits	Credits
3/02	Acc't Receivable – Jones, F.		1 0 0 0 00	
3/02	Revenue			1 0 0 0 00
3/02	Acc't Receivable – Ross, M.L.		2 0 0 00	
3/02	Revenue			2 0 0 00

FIGURE 3.2 Old Well Home billings journal.

Cash Receipts Journal

Debit _____   Credit _____
4/22   Cash $1,000.00 (account receivable)
4/22   Acc/Rec $1,000.00

The credit in the Cash Receipts Journal would not be due to an increase in revenue, but to a decrease in accounts receivable. As mentioned, under the accrual system of accounting, revenue is recognized when the services are provided, rather than when the cash is received.

Role of the General Journal

The *General Journal* records transactions that do not properly fit into any of the other journals. Note that the first five journals all record cash transactions; the General Journal is used to make adjustments in the books to conform to the accrual system of accounting.

As with medical supplies, the supplies purchased in August will be only partially consumed in that month, but the Cash Disbursements Journal would record the cash expenditure for the supplies purchased in August. Under the accrual method of accounting, only the costs of supplies used in August would be included in the August financial reports, so the total cost of providing services can be compared with the revenues earned in the same period. Therefore, an entry must be made in the General Ledger to adjust the medical supplies expenditure in the Cash Disbursements Journal to the cost of medical supplies used up in August. This is known as an *adjusting entry*.

If an expenditure of $300 for medical supplies is made in August, and the inventory records compiled at the end of August revealed that $75 remained in inventory, the adjusting entry in the General Journal would be as follows.

General Journal

Debit _____   Credit _____
8/29   Med Supp $225.00 (an increase in expenses)
8/29   Inventory $225.00 (decrease in expense)
8/29   Inventory $75.00 (increase in asset)
8/29   Med Supp $75.00 (decrease in expenses)

In addition to adjustments for inventory, entries for depreciation and pre-paid expenses are also recorded in the General Journal to reflect the cost of using the plant or equipment over the time period, as well as the amount of prepaid expenses used up.

Finally, the General Journal can be used to correct errors made in the other journals. The General Journal accounts are usually repeated from month to month and therefore should be standardized to the extent possible. This prevents omission of unapparent, but very real costs.

The General Ledger

At the end of each month, when all adjusting entries have been made in the journal accounts, the financial information in all journals is *posted* (written or entered in) to the General Ledger.

The *General Ledger* can be thought of as a summary of all debits and credits contained in the journals for the time period. It usually has a page for each account in the Chart of Accounts.

The purpose of the ledger is twofold. First, it keeps a continuous balance of the amount in any account for each month. It also enables a "trial balance" to be done. Before the financial statements can be prepared, the total of all debit columns in all journals must equal the total amount from all of the credit columns. By accumulating all journal entries in one book, the ledger, debits and credits can be easily added up and compared. When total debits equal total credits, the books are said to "balance," and thus a trial balance has been calculated. If total debits do not equal total credits, then there is an error in one or more of the journal entries.

Under the double-entry concept of accounting, each debit recorded in a journal must be matched by a credit of an equal amount. The trial balance, therefore, indicates whether or not an error has been made in recording transactions.

With so many accounts, there is ample opportunity for error. Thus, accuracy in preparing the journal and ledger entries will save a great deal of time spent in a search for possible mistakes. The relationship between the journals and General Ledger is shown in Figure 3.3 and Figure 3.4.

The General Ledger should be arranged in the order that the accounts will appear in the financial statements. Once the trial balance and gain/loss statements are prepared, the ledger is closed. This process will be discussed in the following description of the financial statements.

Preparing the Financial Statements: The Income Statement and the Balance Sheet

The financial statements are the summary of all transactions made during a particular time period and their effect on the finances of the facility. The GAAPs require that the financial statements include four reports.

1. Income statement, or profit/loss statement
2. Balance sheet, or statement of financial position
3. Statement of changes in financial position
4. Notes to the financial statements

The income statement and balance sheet are prepared directly from the General Ledger (Figure 3.4) and will be described in later sections. The statement

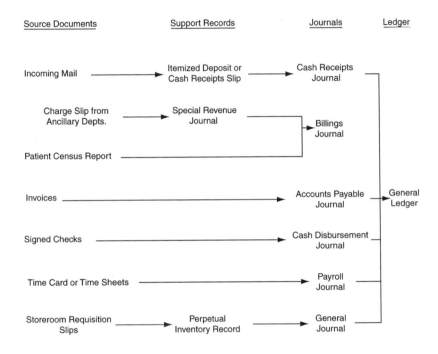

FIGURE 3.3 Source documents, support records, journal, and ledger. Adapted from Catholic Hospital Association, p. 14.

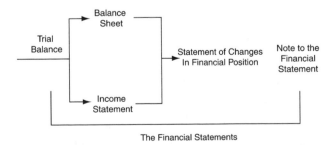

FIGURE 3.4 The financial statement.

of changes in financial position and the notes to the financial statements are prepared from the income statement and balance sheet, and they will be discussed in less detail.

Profit and Loss: The Income Statement

The income statement shows whether revenues were sufficient to cover expenses, whether the facility made or lost money during the time period.

In accounting, income does not refer to the funds coming into the facility, but to revenues minus expenses, or the profit or loss experienced by the facility (or income compared to expenses in not-for-profit operations). While net income indicates that the facility made money, or had some revenues in excess of expenses, a net loss indicates the facility lost money in the time period covered by the income statement. A net loss, or any negative figure on the financial statements, is usually shown in parentheses.

The income statement in Table 3.3 shows a net income of $833 for the month of July and $35,625 for the year until then. Revenues are listed first on the income statement, usually starting with the largest source of revenues. From the General Ledger, all of the revenues earned from providing room and board and other services are calculated as routine services, separated by the level of care or type of service.

When all revenues earned from providing services, or operating revenues, from the General Ledger have been computed, any deductions from revenue are subtracted from the gross operating revenues. Deductions from operating revenues might include money owed to the facility that cannot be collected (known as bed debts or charity care), or they might be due to contractual discounts.

In the process of setting rates at which they will reimburse the facility for care, Medicare, Medicaid, or other third-party payers sometimes pay the nursing facility somewhat less than the facility's full charges. This discount from the regular price of providing care is known as a contractual discount. This discounted rate is the price at which the facility has agreed to provide care when it admits the insured resident. Contractual discounts are therefore deducted from operating revenues instead of included as an expense. Today, most hospitals are forced by competition to offer contractual discounts to large groups such as HMOs. Nursing facilities are similarly affected by competition and the desire to admit residents from such large third-party payers.

This also works in reverse. The nursing facility can negotiate discount rates from providers thus paying less than the face amount of bills received by the facility. It may be possible, for example, for physicians to permit the facility

TABLE 3.3. Old Well Home Income Statement

Revenues	July 'XI	Year to date	Vertical Analysis Percentages (YTD)
Operating revenues			
Nursing	357,603	2,207,814	
Total nursing	357,603	2,207,814	
Ancillary			
Physical therapy	9,974	61,839	
Occupational therapy	9,890	59,340	
Social services	2,866	16,909	
Total ancillary	22,730	138,088	
Gross operating revenues	380,333	2,345,902	
Less deductions	45,640	281,508	
Net operating revenue	334,693	2,064,394	
Nonoperating revenue			
Miscellaneous			
Meals	430	2,494	
Concession	1,358	8,691	
Beauty shop	790	4,819	
Total miscellaneous	2,578	16,004	
Interest	2,640	15,312	
Nonoperating revenue	5,218	31,316	
Total revenues	339,911	2,095,710	
Expenses			
Operating expenses			
Salaries			
Nursing	135,192	833,151	68%
Dietary	15,582	93,492	8%
Administration	9,551	54,441	49%
Laundry	3,409	20,454	2%
Housekeeping	13,435	81,282	7%
Maintenance	5,287	32,145	3%
Physical therapy	9,652	.60,808	5%
Occupational therapy	3,450	20,735	2%

(Continued)

TABLE 3.3.   (Continued)

Revenues	July 'XI	Year to date	Vertical Analysis Percentages (YTD)	
Social serv	2,146	13,305	1%	
Total salaries	197,705	1,209,812	100%	59.0%
Supplies	31,393	189,928		9.2%
Activity	2,065	12,390		0.6%
Capital equipment	200	1,600		0.1%
Utilities	8,764	52,584		2.6%
Telephone	163	1,043		0.1%
Insurance	4,000	24,018		1.2%
Taxes (real estate)	3,313	19,878		1.0%
Capital costs				
Interest	27,816	166,896	30%	8.1%
Mortgage payment	24,029	144,174	26%	7.0%
Depreciation	39,627	237,762	43%	11.5%
Total capital costs	91,472	548,832	100%	
Total expenses	339,078	2,060,085		100%
Net income (loss)	833	35,625		
Income tax (@ 45%)	375	16,031		
Profit after tax	458	19,594		

to pay them what Medicare would pay them, not the dollar amount the physician's office bills.

Total deductions are subtracted from the gross operating revenue to get the new operating revenue. Net operating revenues for the Old Well Home for July are $334,693 (Table 3.3). Nonoperating revenues, income from sources other than direct resident care, are listed next. In July, the Old Well Home earned $900 in interest from funds invested in a local bank and $4,318 from a certificate of deposit. Miscellaneous sources of revenue are also included directly from the appropriate page in the General Ledger. Miscellaneous revenues for Old Well Home are from guests' meals, the beauty shop, or concession income.

Expenses are listed next, starting with the largest item, which is usually salaries. All salaries are listed by department. The salary expense generally includes any employee benefits and payroll taxes paid by the facility.

Supplies, which are separated by department in the ledger according to the Chart of Accounts, are combined into one expense item in Old Well's income statement. A capital expense of $200 was incurred in July by the purchase of equipment.

Capital equipment is an asset that will be used by the facility to provide services for more than 1 year and will not be sold in the course of operations. In addition to equipment, capital items also include such assets as the building, beds, and furniture. If we were to look at the General Ledger under the Chart of Accounts number for capital equipment expenses, we would discover that the $200 was used to purchase office equipment for Old Well.

Further down on the income statement there is an expense called capital costs. A capital cost is an expense related to the use of capital items. At some earlier time the Old Well Home had borrowed money for new dining and lounge furniture and money to purchase the building, both at an annual interest rate of 14%. For the month of July the total interest expense was $27,816. Interest expenses, then, are one cost of using capital.

A mortgage payment expense of $24,029 for July is a second source of capital costs. Another cost of using capital is depreciation; the cost of wear and tear on old Well's depreciable assets was estimated to be $39,627 for 1 month. (See section on depreciation for estimation of this expense.)

To compute the net income, or profit or loss, the total expenses are subtracted from total revenues. This gives the net income before taxes. Subtracting percentage for income tax shows that Old Well's profit after taxes is $458. Although depreciation is a real cost of providing services, it does not represent an actual cash outflow, and depreciation may be added to the after-tax profit to give the actual cash standing of the facility.

The income statement, then, shows the operating performance of the facility for a period of time, and it is usually prepared on a monthly and annual basis.

Closing the Books

Because revenues and expenses must be measured for finite periods of time, these accounts must be brought to a sum of zero so that they can be recorded over again for a new time period. Bringing the expense and revenue accounts to zero defines "closing the books."

To Close the General Ledger:

1. For all revenue and expense accounts with a credit balance, add a debit equal to the credit to bring the account to zero.

2. For all revenue and expense accounts with a debit balance, add a credit equal to the debit to bring the account to zero.

According to the double-entry accounting, compensation must be made for these new debits and credits in some other account.

1. Add up all the newly added debits.
2. Add up all the newly added credits.
3. Subtract the debits from the credits.
4. Enter the difference in the retained earning account, as follows:
   - If the difference is a profit, enter it as a credit.
   - If the difference is a loss, enter it as a debit.

Thus, all revenue and expense accounts have been brought to zero, and the books are balanced and ready for a new time period.

Statement of Financial Condition: The Balance Sheet

Unlike the income statement, which summarized operating performance over a period of time, the balance sheet records the financial position of the nursing facility at one point in time. Whereas the income statement shows the ending balance of the revenue and expense accounts, the balance sheet summarizes the assets, liabilities, and capital accounts of the facility. This document is called a balance sheet because the asset accounts must balance with the liability and capital accounts. This relationship can be expressed as an equation, called the accounting equation:

$$Assets = Liabilities + Capital$$

The balance sheet for the Old Well Home for the year is shown in Table 3.4. Assets are listed on the left in order of liquidity.

Current assets refers to those possessions of the facility that will be or theoretically can be, turned into cash within 12 months. Prepaid insurance is considered an asset because the coverage is something owned by the facility. The income statement records the proportion of the prepaid insurance that was used in the month of July ($4,003), and the balance sheet shows the amount of insurance that remains.

Noncurrent assets, of course, refers to those assets that will not be liquidated within the year; they usually include plant (the building), property, and equipment. These are also called fixed assets and are recorded at their cost at the time of purchase, rather than their current market value.

TABLE 3.4.   Old Well Home Balance Sheet

Assets	July 31, 'XI	July 31, 'XO
Current assets		
Cash	60,700	2,834
Accounts receivable		
(Less Bad Debts of $9,032)	53,517	61,397
Securities	225,275	10,500
Inventory	62,006	54,880
Prepaid insurance	2,400	3,600
Total current assets	403,898	133,211
Noncurrent assets		
Equipment	1,983,000	1,981,200
Plant	5,767,004	5,767,004
Less Accumulated Depreciation	2,772,192	2,362,300
Plant and Equipment	4,977,812	5,385,904
Property	2,650,000	2,650,000
Total fixed assets	7,627,812	8,035,904
Total assets	8,031,710	8,169,115
Liabilities		
Current liabilities		
Accounts payable	2,852	24,606
Notes payable	33,625	355,271
Benefits payable	24,843	630,388
Current portion of		
long-term debt:		
Mortgage	230,680	192,233
Long-term debt	75,000	75,000
Total current liabilities	367,000	1,277,498
Noncurrent liabilities		
Mortgage payable	3,460,202	3,690,883
Debts payable	675,000	750,000
Total noncurrent liabilities	4,135,202	4,440,883
Total liabilities	4,502,202	5,718,381
Net worth		
Retained earnings		
Year to date	35,625	27,507
Total	370,956	335,331
owner's equity	3,122,927	2,087,897
Total net worth	3,529,508	2,450,735
Total liabilities and capital	8,031,710	8,169,115

The *historic cost* concept is another basic tenet of accounting and relates to the ongoing concern concept: Because capital assets will not be liquidated any time soon, their current market value is of little relevance. The value of these assets to the facility, however, must include the depreciation on plant and equipment over the years, and so this accumulated depreciation is subtracted from the historic cost of the depreciable assets. Although land usually appreciates in value over time, it does not do so simply through the operations of the facility and is therefore recorded at historic cost, with no depreciation from its value.

Depreciation, therefore, is an expense associated with the use of an asset, so depreciation is included both as an expense on the income statement and a contra asset (literally, "against an asset") on the balance sheet. Note that employees are not included as an asset. This is because assets are those things owned by the facility; an organization cannot own its employees.

Liabilities are the obligations of the facility. Current liabilities are those obligations that must be met within the next 12 months, such as bills from suppliers of foodstuffs and medical or office supplies and short-term bank loans.

On this particular date (Table 3.4), Old Well owes its suppliers $2,852. If this debt were paid tomorrow and a balance sheet made up for that day, Old Well would have no accounts payable on its balance sheet. Notes payable refers to loans that must be repaid within 12 months. Old Well owes $33,625 to a local bank for interest on its borrowed funds, as well as a portion of a long-term debt due within the year. The noncurrent liabilities sections shows which debts these are. Old Well has a payment due on its debt for new furniture, and a portion of its mortgage payment is due also.

Capital accounts, or new worth, are recorded below the liabilities. This section is also called owners' equity, shareholder's equity, fund balance, or retained earnings, depending on the origin of the funds that make up this section. It includes funds that the owners have put into the facility, whether the owners be one person, a partnership (two or more unincorporated owners), a corporation, or a charitable organization. Net worth also usually includes retained earnings, or the net income that has been put back into the facility over the years.

If the facility incurs a net loss, this amount is subtracted from the net worth. The Old Well net worth includes the retained earnings of the year to date and the retained earnings from its earlier years of operation. It also shows that the owners have invested $3,122,927 in the facility over the years. If this amount was from stockholders, it would be called shareholders' equity; if from a charitable organization, it would be a fund balance.

The most important thing to remember about the net worth is that it is not a pool of cash. The funds recorded as net worth are monies that have been put into the facility at some time; it is merely a record of these funds, not cash available for operations or investment.

To summarize, the balance sheet shows the financial position of the facility for only one point in time. Its relation with the income statement is the retained earnings, which usually include the net income in the net worth.

Thus, the basic accounting equation can be expanded to

$$\text{Assets} = (\text{Liabilities} + \text{Owner's Equity}) + (\text{Revenues} - \text{Expenses})$$

Two Additional Financial Statements

Statement of Changes in Financial Position

Also simply called the statement of changes, this financial report shows the major transactions that occurred over the period covered by two balance sheets, or the way that working capital was used during that period. Working capital simply refers to the current assets and current liabilities from the balance sheet. The amount of working capital available is:

$$\text{Current Assets} - \text{Current Liabilities}$$

The statement of changes shows the transactions that caused the amount of working capital to change over a time period. It is therefore a very useful document for those interested in knowing how the facility acquires and uses its funds.

Sources of Funds

Sources of funds are generally an excess of revenues over expenses of operations, interest income, an contributions to the facility (or owners' equity). Noncash items, such as depreciation or money designated for repayment of debts, are added as a source of funds because this is still cash (a current asset) owned by the facility.

Uses of funds would include nonoperating expense such as repayment of a portion of a debt or additions to property. The uses of funds are subtracted from the sources of funds to give the change in working capital over the time period. This difference should equal the change in working capital calculated from the balance sheets at the beginning and end of the time period covered.

Notes to Financial Statements

The notes to financial statements are included to explain the accountant's interpretation or calculation of figures, or variation in the books due to a change in their organization, which may not be readily understood by those reviewing the financial statements. The financial statements are not considered complete without each of these notes.

Staff Functions in the Accounting Process

The number of staff persons in the business office and their degree of specialization will vary with the size, complexity, and ownership of the facility. In general, however, those responsible for the accounting functions will be the bookkeeper, the accountant or comptroller, and the administrator.

The bookkeeper maintains the journals and ledger and performs the trial balance. An accountant or comptroller may also check the trial balance, but their primary task is the preparation of the financial statement.

For all practical purposes, it is legally mandatory that a nursing facility have its books officially audited, that is, audited by a person who is a certified public accountant (CPA). It is almost impossible to do business without having the facility's books audited by a CPA, who, in effect, serves as the public's representative.

Administrators of a chain-owned facility will generally send the data from the books to a regional or corporate office, where the financial statements, as well as a variety of other schedules, will be compiled and returned.

3.5 Putting Financial Statements to Work: Working Capital, Ratio Analysis, and Vertical Analysis

The net income is an important and readily identifiable item of interest on the financial statements. What other information can be gleaned from these reports? There are several the administrator can use. Three tools are discussed in this section.

Working Capital

Current assets minus current liabilities equals the working capital available. This can also be considered the funds available to the facility.

Suppose the administrator of the Old Well facility wants to learn if enough funds are available to purchase $60,000 worth of capital equipment for the nursing department. Where can this information be found?

The net income for the month of July—and the entire year—has been reinvested in the facility, as indicated by the net worth section of the balance sheet; these funds may or may not still be available. Although the net worth shows the funds that have been invested in the facility, it is not a pool of cash. Recall that the net worth is merely a record of the funds that have been invested in the facility over time and that most of the funds shown here are therefore not available for spending or investing.

The administrator might also check the cash accounts of the Old Well to see if the cash for purchasing the items is available. But this is not suitable either, for if the Old Well owes $367,000 to various creditors, as indicated by the current liabilities section on the balance sheet, any available cash may be needed to meet these obligations.

In order to get an idea of the funds available to purchase the needed equipment, the administrator must look at the amount of working capital available. Current assets remaining after current liabilities have been subtracted yields the amount of money that the administrator has at their discretion.

The administrator finds that there is only $36,898 in working capital available to purchase equipment for the nursing department and that the facility probably should not purchase new equipment at this time. Since current assets include relatively nonliquid accounts, such as inventory and prepaid insurance, the working capital may be calculated by excluding these accounts from the total current assets.

Ratio Analysis

Another common approach to analyzing financial statements is to perform a ratio analysis. Financial managers generally express the information in financial statements as a series of ratios.

There are an infinite number of ratios that may be derived from financial statements, but the discussion here will be confined to several of the more common measures of financial performance.

Usefulness of Ratios

Ratios are useful in several ways. First, financial ratios are no more than fractions using the numbers in the financial statement and are therefore fairly simple to calculate quickly and easily.

Ratio analysis allows the administrator to identify trends in many measures of financial performance of the facility by comparing the same ratio for several periods. Ratio analysis of the financial statements can also be used to compare the financial performance of several facilities. It is one of the most useful tools the administrator has.

As previously mentioned, the amount of working capital available is calculated by subtracting current liabilities from current assets. A positive amount of working capital indicates that the facility is able to meet its current obligations with its current assets.

If all resident revenues were collected before or immediately after they were earned, the facility would have no need of excess working capital. But because third-party payers, such as Medicare and Medicaid, pay nursing facilities for services sometimes well after services were rendered, the facility must maintain a certain level of working capital to meet expenses during the "lag time" before the payments are received. (If part of a chain or group of facilities, the same problem is faced by the corporate managers who have the same gaps between services rendered and payments received, but on their larger scale.) Even nursing facilities that have predominantly privately paying residents must plan for collections of resident bills to extend over a period of weeks to months. How much working capital should the facility maintain to cover its lag time? One way to get an idea of an appropriate amount is to perform a current, or acid-test ratio.

Current Ratio

Current Ratio = Current Assets / Current Liabilities

The Old Well Home has $403,898 in current assets and $367,000 in current liabilities, so:

$$\$403,898 / \$367,000 = 1.1$$

A current ratio greater than 1 shows that the Old Well is able to meet its current obligations, with a surplus of working capital. Does this mean that a current ratio of 2.5 is even better? Not necessarily; a high current ratio may show that the facility has too much money tied up in current assets and that it may make better use of some of these funds by investing them in an interest-bearing bank account or its equivalent.

Interpreting Ratios

Interpretation of an appropriate current ratio exemplifies a point of caution with the use of any ratio. One ratio itself reveals very little about the performance of the facility. Ratios must be compared either over time or with the rest of the industry. A current ratio of 1.1 may be fine if the ratio for the Old Well in the past has been as follows:

Year 1	Year 2	Year 3	Year 4
.80	.85	.90	1.0

A ratio of 1.1 could also indicate a decline in working capital if past ratios have been much higher than 1.1. Industry comparisons are also important. If the average current ratio for the nursing facility industry, preferably in the same region, is 1.0, then the Old Well may be managing their working capital well. If, however, the industry average is .9, then Old Well might rethink the amount of funds it is keeping available. Thus, interpretation of all ratios is relative to both past performance and industry averages. The administrator of the Old Well will find out what the appropriate current ratio is and adjust their own working capital to maintain that ratio.

The Quick Ratio

Another commonly used ratio is the quick ratio. This ratio is similar to the current ratio, but is a more rigorous and representative measure of current assets, as only cash and accounts receivable, and sometimes marketable securities are used to cover current liabilities.

Quick Ratio = (Cash + Acc. Rec. + Mkt'ble Sec) / Current Liabilities

The quick ratio reveals that Old Well is not quite able to cover its current obligations with its most available assets, but is quite close to the industry average.

Average Collection Period Ratio

The average collection period ratio is another useful ratio, showing the average lag time of accounts receivable. Although the administrator of the nursing facility will have relatively little influence in expediting the collection of funds paid by third parties such as Medicare and Medicaid, the facility should attempt to collect privately paid monies from patients as soon as possible in order to decrease working capital needs. This is therefore an important ratio.

Average Collection Period = 365 x Acc. Red. / Net Operating Revenues
365 x $53,517 / $334,693 = 58 days

Because most insurers reimburse the nursing facility sometimes up to 3 to 5 months after billing, an average collection period of 58 days may be appropriate for a facility with a majority of publicly paid for residents. The length of time between billing Medicaid and receiving payment varies radically among the states, some paying immediately, some deliberately delaying payment for months in order to manage the state's own cash flow. A number of states now require that all Medicaid billing be submitted electronically.

Accounts Payable Average Payment Period Ratio

A related ratio is the accounts payable average payment period, which shows the average number of days used to pay creditors. Too many days in the payable period may develop into a poor credit relationship with suppliers, and too few days may indicate that funds should be invested for a longer time before creditors are paid.

Average payment period = 365 x Accounts Payable / Supplies Expense
365 x $2,852 / $31,393 = 33 days

Because payment for bills is generally sought by the 30th day at the latest, Old Well seems to be performing well in its efforts to make timely payments to suppliers. If the average payment period were much shorter, Old Well might consider waiting for 30 days to pay some of its creditors and investing these funds in an interest-earning account. If a discount is offered for payment within 10 days or some short specified period, early payment of accounts payable might be more cost-effective.

For both accounts payable and accounts receivable considerations, the opportunity cost (loss of use otherwise available for these funds) must be considered. In times of low interest rates, when the use of money is low, the opportunity cost is less than in times of high interest rates, that is, when using money is more costly.

Net Operating Margin Ratio

The net operating margin is the proportion of revenues earned to the amount of expenses used to earn those revenues. A low operating margin may indicate that rates for services should be raised or expenses reduced.

The Old Well's negative operating margin shows that operating revenues do not cover operating expenses and that the administrator should consider increasing charges for services, if the market will allow it, or reducing operating costs in order to increase the facility's operating margin. Another approach to this ratio is operating income as a percentage of revenues. This ratio is best compared with industry averages for an indication of performance.

Debt-to-Equity Ratio

The debt-to-equity ratio is a measure of the long-run liquidity of the facility, or the ability of the facility to meet its long-term debts. A "small" proportion of debt to equity indicates that the facility could incur more long-term debt, other things being equal, if needed; whereas a high debt-to-equity ratio (when compared to the industry) probably shows that the facility may have more debt than may be advisable, all other things being equal. This ratio is of particular interest to would-be creditors.

$$\text{Debt} / \text{Equity} = \text{Long-Term Debt} / \text{Total Equity}$$
$$\$4,135,202 / \$3,529,508 = 1.17$$

These are some of the more commonly used ratios. There are, of course, many other parameters of financial performance that will be of interest to the administrator.

Other Formulas of Value to the Nursing Home Administrator

$$\text{Average Length of Stay} = \frac{\text{total patient days in the year}}{\text{Number of admissions in the year}}$$

$$\text{Percent of Occupancy} = \frac{\text{Average daily census}}{\text{Number of beds}}$$

$$\text{FTE (full time equivalent)} = \frac{\text{total number of hours worked or budgeted}}{40 \text{ (an FTE is a position that only works 5 days/week)}}$$

FTEs x 1.4 = number of line staff positions; if you want to know how many nursing assistant positions, for example, you can have 7 days/week

$$\text{Costs per patient day} = \frac{\text{costs in month}}{\text{Total patient days in month}}$$

$$\text{Hours per patient day} = \frac{\text{number of hours worked}}{\text{Number of patients}}$$

$$\text{Turnover rate in percent} = \frac{\text{number employees terminated x 100}}{\text{Number of total FTEs (Can be monthly or annually by department)}}$$

Vertical Analysis

A third method of analyzing the financial statements is to perform a vertical analysis. A vertical analysis converts each item on the income statement, balance sheet, or other financial report to a percentage of some total item on the same document.

A vertical analysis of the Old Well income statement, using the year-to-date values, is shown in Table 3.5. Like the ratios given previously, these ratios are useful when compared over time, or with other facilities. For example, an unusually high ratio of supplies to total expenses in July may indicate that supplies are being wasted or pilfered, provided there has not been a change in the type of services that would warrant a greater use of supplies. On the other hand, although their percentage for July may be higher than for any month that year, if supplies as a proportion of total expenses are consistently higher in July than any other month, then the administrator knows that this is a pattern that may or may not be a matter of concern.

The administrator can accumulate valuable information from the financial statements by performing both ratio and vertical analyses. By comparing these

TABLE 3.5.   Old Well Home Income Statement: Vertical Analysis

	July 'XI	Year to date	Vertical analyses	
Revenues				
Operating revenues				
Nursing				
Skilled				
Intermediate				
Total nursing	357,603	2,207,814	100%	94%
Ancillary				
Physical therapy	9,974	61,839	45%	
Occupational therapy	9,890	59,340	43%	
Social services	2,866	16,909	12%	
Total ancillary	22,730	138,088.	100%	6%
Gross operating revenues	380,333	2,345,902	100%	
Less deductions	45,640	281,508	12%	
Net operating revenue	334,693	2,064,394	88%	
Nonoperating revenue				
Miscellaneous				
Meals	430	2,494	16%	
Concession	1,358	8,691	54%	
Beauty shop	790	4,819	30%	
Total misc.	2,578	16,004	100%	51%
Interest	2,640	15,312	49%	
Nonoperating revenue	5,218	31,316	100%	
Total revenues	339,911	2,095,710		
Expenses				
Operating expenses				
Salaries				
Nursing	135,192	833,151	68%	
Dietary	15,582	93,492	8%	
Administration	9,551	54,441	4%	
Laundry	3,409	20,454	2%	
Housekeeping	13,435	81,282	7%	
Maintenance	5,287	32,145	3%	

(Continued)

TABLE 3.5. (continued)

	July 'XI	Year to date	Vertical analyses	
Physical therapy	9,652	60,808	5%	
Occupational therapy	3,450	20,735	2%	
Social serv	2,146	13,305	1%	
Total salaries	197,705	1,209,812	100%	59.0%
Supplies	31,393	189,928	9.2%	
Activity	2,065	12,390	0.6%	
Capital equipment	200	1,600	0.1%	
Utilities	8,764	52,594	2.6%	
Telephone	163	1,043	0.1%	
Insurance	4,000	24,018	1.2%	
Taxes (real estate)	3,313	19,878	1.0%	
Capital costs				
Interest	27,816	166,896	30%	8.0%
Mortgage payment	24,029	144,174	26%	7.0%
Depreciation	39,627	237,762	43%	11.5%
Total capital costs	91,472	548,832	100%	
Total expenses	339,078	2,060,085	100%	
Net income (loss)	833	35,625		
Income tax (@ 45%)	375	16,031		
Profit after tax	458	19,594		

ratios over time and with other facilities, trends and patterns in the operation of the facility can be identified, which is perhaps one of the most important functions of financial statement analysis. Awareness of such patterns enables the administrator to pinpoint problem areas in the facility and make more knowledgeable financial decisions.

3.6 Additional Accounting Procedures That Help the Administrator Maintain Control Over the Facility

Although accounting processes are similar in every institution, the procedures for managing finances will vary from facility to facility, and so will the best methods of control.

In financial management, control refers to the development and maintenance of systematic ways to identify problems when they occur to permit the administrator to intervene appropriately. To maintain control, the administrator and the staff normally develop policies for all office procedures. Identification of possible financial problems as soon as they arise enables the staff to deal with them effectively through the use of recognized policies.

There are several tools available to assist the administrator in controlling financial operations. Procedures should be arranged so that no single person has complete responsibility for any area of the facility's finances. A system of checks and balances can be established so that part of one person's task is completed or reviewed by another. Furthermore, each employee can be required to take vacation time so that no one has uninterrupted control of certain office tasks. It is important to have procedures in place that reduce temptation to a minimum. Even the best procedures set up by the most sophisticated corporations have not been able to prevent an occasional embezzlement of funds at facilities. Eternal vigilance is necessary in such money matters.

Accounts Receivable: Billing for Services Rendered by the Facility

The facility cannot receive moneys for services rendered until the resident has been billed for them. Delays in billing create an opportunity cost: the loss of use or availability of funds when cash owed to the facility is not yet in its possession.

Financial Review of Applicants

Some states require that admissions be on a first-come, first-served basis for any applicant for whom the facility is capable of providing appropriate care. Other states allow the facility to make admissions decisions based, in part, on financial considerations.

At the time of admission the payment source should be established. If the client is not paying with their own funds, written agreement to pay must be obtained from the person who controls the resident's funds. In addition, present and potential Medicare and Medicaid needs should be determined. These agencies will normally pay for care only after an authorization number has been established for a recipient. A significant number of persons who enter the facility as Medicare or private paying persons quickly spend down their savings. The social worker must anticipate which persons will become Medicaid eligible and begin the application process several weeks in advance of actual eligibility in order to achieve a steady payment stream for care rendered.

Just as the facility must remove temptations from its employees to embezzle facility funds, so also must the facility constantly seek to minimize temptations for resident's money managers to withhold moneys legitimately due the facility. Experience has taught that social security and similar checks that have been pledged to pay for the resident's care are best sent directly to the facility rather than to a family member who may feel more pressing financial needs than payment of the facility charges.

Resident Ledger Card

When the resident's source of payment has been confirmed, a Resident Ledger card is made up for each person admitted, listing the name, room number, source of payment, and daily (or routine) service charges. The charges and the billing and collections procedures must be explained to each resident or sponsor.

Preparation of Invoices

In every case, charge slips for each service not bundled into the daily rate must be collected from each service center on a periodic basis (daily or weekly). Because these charges are distinct from routine room-related services, a Special Revenues Journal(s) may be created to record them.

Routine Charges

Once the ancillary charges for the billing period have been determined, they are added to the resident's routine charges. The routine charge is the charge for "room and board" services, which usually include basic nursing care, room, and meals. Facilities will package their charges variously, depending on a number of considerations. Some offer a broad continuum of services from which residents may choose.

Daily Census Form

$$\text{Average Daily Census (ADC)} = \frac{\text{total patient days}}{\text{days in the month}}$$

The routine charge may be determined on a daily, weekly, or monthly basis and is calculated with the aid of the Daily Census Form. This is a summary of the facility's occupancy that lists daily admissions, discharges, and transfers by level of care, if more than one is offered by the facility. The Daily Census Form is normally prepared by the nursing unit (often called the "midnight census") and is submitted to the business office.

Patient Census Report

A patient census report is drawn up by the bookkeeper (usually for the month) by compiling the information from the Patient Census Forms (Figure 3.5).

The Patient Census Report is in turn used to calculate the total routine charge for each resident or service recipientt (e.g., outpatient physical therapy charges). Routine and ancillary services are finally calculated for each resident and service recipient and entered on each resident's or service recipient's Accounts Receivable Ledger card (Accounts Receivable, Invoice Supplement; see Figure 3.6) and in the Billings Journal.

To expedite the billing process, the Billings Journal should be divided by payer type (private pay, Medicare, Medicaid, Veterans Administration [VA], hospital reserve bed contract, HMO, PPO, IPO, Worker Compensation Fund, or similar third-party payer). (The VA, in addition to building new long-term care facilities of its own, is subcontracting with private nursing homes for care, usually shorter termed, of the now-aging and exploding aged veteran population.) The number of nursing home stays being paid for by the VA increased from 47,000 in 1970 to 93,000 in 2003 (Department of Health and Human Services [DHHS], 2005, p. 402). The number of veterans being cared for in VA-owned facilities compared with contracts with individual nursing facilities

PATIENT CENSUS REPORT

OLD WELL HOME

| MONTH/YEAR | AREA |
| 06/x1 | Skilled |

ROOM AND BED	ROOM RATE	PATIENT NAME LAST	INITIAL	PATIENT NO.	1	2	3	4	5	6	7	8	9	10	11	12	13	14	15	16	17	18	19	20	21	22	23	24	25	26	27	28	29	30	31
117	70	Jones			x	x	x	x	x	x	x	x	x	x	x	x	x	x	x	x	x	x	x	x	x	x	x	x	x	x	x	x	x	x	
118	70	Rose			x	x	x	x	x	x	x	x	x	x	x	x	x	x	x	x	x	x	x	x											

DAY OF MONTH

TOTALS				
Private	Agency	Medicaid	Medicare	Other
240.00		2100.00		
100.00		1400.00		

TOTALS
Billings
2340.00
1500.00

FIGURE 3.5 Patient census report.

LEDGER CARD   ADDITIONAL CURRENT ENTRIES – COMPLETE SECTION A AND B

ACCOUNTS RECEIVABLE
INVOICE SUPPLEMENT

ADJUSTMENTS TO PRIOR MONTHS – COMPLETE SECTION A AND C

S	FACILITY NO.	FACILITY NAME									
E		OLD WELL HOME		YRMO x100	NUMBER /	PATIENT NAME Rose, M. L.					
C	PATIENT NUMBER	INVOICE NUMBER 3012-700-01				INVOICE DATE 6/29/X1					
A											

STATUS CODES
1 = PRIVATE
2 = AGENCY
3 = MEDICARE
4 = VETERAN
5 = OTHER

AREA
C = CERTIFIED
S = SKILLED
I = INTERMEDIATE
R = RESIDENTIAL

LEVEL
UNCLASSIFIED
SKILLED
2 – 6 INTERMEDIATE
7 = RESIDENTIAL
9 = HOLDOVER

TRAN CODE	DATE MO/DAY	OPEN ITEM	DESCRIPTION	PRIVATE	AGENCY	MEDICARE	VETERAN	OTHER	STATUS	NON-COLLECT
	/									
	/									
	/									

TOTAL

TRAN CODE	DATE MO/DAY	ROOM-BED	NO DAYS	RATE	AREA	LEVEL	PRIVATE	AGENCY	MEDICARE	VETERAN	OTHER	STATUS	NON-COLLECT
	6/29	118	30	70.00	S	S	275.00		2100.00				
	/												
	/												

TOTAL   275.00   2100.00

TRAN CODE	DESCRIPTION	OPEN ITEM	NO. OF DAYS	RATE	AREA	LEVEL	PRIVATE	AGENCY	MEDICARE	VETERAN	OTHER	STATUS	NON-COLLECT
	PHYSICAL THERAPY								240.00				

TOTAL   240.00

EXPLANATION OF ADJUSTMENTS

ADJUSTMENTS
SECTION C

TRAN CODE	TRAN CODE	OPEN ITEM	NO. OF DAYS	RATE	AREA	LEVEL	PRIVATE	AGENCY	MEDICARE	VETERAN	OTHER	STATUS	NON-COLLECT
65													
65													
65													
65													
65													
65													
65													
65													
65													
65													
65													
65													
65													

TOTAL

FIGURE 3.6 Ledger card.

is not available. The billing process and services covered vary with each payer. Each bill should itemize any ancillary charges (when permitted by the payer) to expedite the processing of invoices by third-party payers. Increasingly, billing may be done by electronic submission using computers and modems. Some state Medicaid programs require electronic submission. This normally means that the facility receives payment on a more timely basis.

Billing Medicare, Medicaid, Other Third Parties, and Private Payers

Billing is an increasingly complex process because of the increasing variety of payment agreements nursing facilities are negotiating with third parties. Medicaid patients care costs are normally billed and paid for monthly, usually with one composite bill for all Medicaid residents submitted to the state or its designated payer. Medicare bills, on the other hand, are normally submitted for each individual resident and sent to a fiscal intermediary. Medicare (and Medicaid) payers sometimes pay promptly; yet, sometimes they send for clarification on bills, the purpose of which is to delay the final payment to the facility in order to ease cash flow problems being experienced by the third-party payers. It is a complicated game in some states.

More and more third-party payers are negotiating contracts with nursing facilities that also vary in method of payment. Often a third-party payer, a health maintenance organization, for example, will negotiate a separate payment schedule for each member they send to a nursing facility. Other third-party payers may negotiate a flat rate for all members it refers to a particular nursing facility, regardless of acuity level. For some residents the monthly fee negotiated by their third-party payer will be all inclusive, others will be on an itemized service use basis. It is in these circumstances that both the facility administration and the third-party payer administration are jockeying for a position that, whatever the payment arrangement, covers their actual costs.

Electronic Health Records Systems

The health care industry is being pushed toward completely electronic records. The federal goal is to have all health care records in electronic form by the year 2014. The first electronic medical record products for the national system were approved in July, 2006. Increasingly staff in the facility will use laptop computers and handheld devices to track resident data, give medication, and chart resident information.

A number of firms are now developing electronic record systems that track decubitus ulcers (pressure sores), check prescriptions against residents' known drug allergies and whether a given medication is covered by the resident's Medicare prescription plan . . . the tracking possibilities are endless. Such systems also provide the administrator with an "audit trail" that allows errors to be identified and corrected on a real time basis.

Intense pressures on third-party payers to hold down costs are being passed on to the nursing facility.

Accounting for Deductions From Revenue

Besides contractual discounts, charity care and bad debts are also sources of deductions from revenue. Charity care is provided to a resident when the service is not reimbursable and cannot be paid for privately. Bad debts, on the other hand, are resident accounts that are past due, but are still subject to collection.

Contractual discounts are often the largest source of deductions from revenue in nursing facilities. Because most deductions cannot be confirmed until payment has been received, they are accounted for in the Billings Journal when known rather than estimated. The payment from public insurers will be accompanied by a Medical Assistance Remittance and Status Report. This report lists the resident's name and claim number, the service dates, the description of services rendered, the total amount billed to the program, and the allowed and nonallowed charges, with an explanation code stating why the service was not reimbursed. The T account for deductions from revenue would be:

Billings Journal

Debits	Credits
2/27	Cont. Disc. $450.00
2/27	Acc. Rec. $450.00

Submitting and Resubmitting Claims

The amount of the deduction is also included on the resident's Accounts Receivable Ledger Card. If the deduction is invalid, the fiscal intermediary should be contacted for an explanation of the deduction. The claim can then be resubmitted accompanied by the information needed to justify the request for payment. Medicare intermediaries are constantly issuing bulletins defining and redefining what covered charges include and exclude. Understanding Medicare billing, especially Medicare Part B billing, is one of the more complex, yet important tasks of the facility staff. In an era of razor thin net operating margins, appropriate billing can have a significant impact on the result. So can inappropriate billing, however.

Medicare has many rules, one of which is that facility bills will be paid as expeditiously as possible so long as the amount of "inappropriately" billed services do not exceed 5% of all the facility's Medicare billings. What Medicare deems appropriate and inappropriate is a moving target requiring constant business office attention. Once this 5% threshold is violated, each bill submitted by the facility for a future time period is scrutinized and payment slowed. Some facilities have found that the best way to assure that Medicare billings are appropriate is to have weekly "Medicare Meetings" attended by nursing (usually the director of nurses and other relevant nurses), the business office manager, the director of rehabilitative therapies, the admissions/social worker director, and the administrator. At these meetings each Medicare resident is reviewed for appropriateness of Medicare specific care being given and an assessment made of future days of appropriate Medicare coverage that can be anticipated during the 100-day limit for each spell of illness experienced by this person.

Medicare Part D

Medicare Part D benefits facility cash flow inasmuch as some drugs are covered for the first time under Medicare Part D.

Medicare Cost Reconciliation Settlement

When Medicare pays a facility for providing care to patients/residents, the amount of reimbursement is based on the cost of that care. However, instead of calculating the actual cost of providing care for each Medicare beneficiary in each facility, Medicare makes an estimate of how much the care for residents in each facility should have cost and then pays the facility periodically, based on that estimate. If this estimated amount of reimbursement received during the year is less than the cost of providing the care, Medicare will make up the difference at the end of the year by paying the facility a Medicare Cost Reconciliation settlement, or requiring any overpayment be returned. Any funds due from Medicare are recorded in the Cash Receipts Journal as follows:

Cash Receipts Journal

Debits _____	Credits _____
11/23	Due from Medicare $375.00
11/23	Cont. Disc. $375.00

Sometimes services that are not allowable by their insurer (e.g., occupational therapy or some types of dental care) will be provided to patients who cannot pay for them. These services are considered charity care and are "written off" as essentially nonbillable. A special account should exist in the Chart of Accounts for this type of care, separate from other types of uncollectibles. Each facility needs policies to govern the circumstances and extent of charity care that will be given.

Collecting Money Owed to the Facility

An appropriate collections policy will depend on the facility's past experience with its payers. For bills delinquent by 1 month, a letter may be sent as a reminder. A telephone call to the payer (logged into a written record) may be made after an appropriate interval. The collections policy must indicate if and under what circumstances a collections agency or other procedure will be used.

Account Write-Off Recommendation

Problem collections are most effectively handled with an attitude of diplomacy and firmness, and an effort should be made to accommodate the payer if there is a valid reason for delinquent payment. If a patient's accounts are eventually determined to be uncollectible, some type of Account Write-Off Recommendation form (Figure 3.7) is filled out, with one copy retained in the resident's file and another going to the accountant, so that the total of uncollectible accounts can be recorded in financial statements.

Nursing facilities, like hospitals and other health care providers, are victims of the cost shifting phenomena in the United States. Because of public relations and other considerations, it is exceedingly difficult for facilities to discharge residents whose bills are uncollectible, but who have no place else to go.

Handling Cash

Cash is easily mismanaged. It is easily concealed. The typical facility will keep only a small amount of cash on the premises, often not more than $500, as most transactions will take place through business office accounts.

Cash Handling Procedures

All cash must be handled by at least two employees, both of whom are bonded. One person should be responsible for receiving the cash, for example, opening

Facility _____ # _____ Date _____

Patient Name _____ # _____ P__ A__ M__ VA__ Other __ Balance $_____

Admission Date _____ Discharge Date _____ Expired: Yes ☐ No ☐

Readmission Date _____ Discharge Date _____

Readmission Date _____ Discharge Date _____

Name and address of responsible party _____

_____

Home phone _____ Business phone _____

Date and amount of last payment _____

Brief History of account: (attach copy of form H-0611) _____

_____

_____

_____

Should account be assigned to a collection agency? Yes ☐ No ☐

Facility opinion by _____ Date _____

*Regional concurrence by _____ Date _____

**Corporate concurrence by _____ Date _____

If Medicare—Include all intermediary correspondence.

Is coinsurance involved? Yes ☐ No ☐   If yes, please provide dates and amounts: _____

_____

_____

_____

_____ /_____
Administrator   Date

_____ /_____
Regional Controller   Date

_____ /_____
District Director/Director of Operations   Date

*For all accounts over $250.00
**For all accounts over $500.00.

FIGURE 3.7 Recommendations for write-off of uncollectible account.

the mail or taking a check in person. This should not be the same person who is responsible for making bank deposits. Checks should be stamped "For Deposit Only" in the name of the facility immediately upon receipt and a daily remittance list prepared for all cash received. One copy of this list should be retained by this employee, and another should go to the person making the bank deposits.

Cash receipt slips should then be prepared, with one copy going to the payer and another to the accountant or the accountant's file. The bookkeeper should record the cash received in the Cash Receipts Journal and also on the patient's own sheet in the Patient Accounts Receivable Ledger (Figure 3.8).

Cash should be deposited in the bank daily to prevent it from being mislaid and to earn the maximum amount of interest on available funds. At the end of each month entries in the Cash Receipts Journal are posted into the General Ledger and these figures checked against the cash receipts entries in the Patient Accounts Receivable Ledger.

Accounts Payable: The Facility's Bills

Accounts payable are moneys owed to creditors for purchases made by the facility. A nursing home's creditors usually furnish foodstuffs, linens, medical supplies, pharmaceuticals, laboratory tests, and office, housekeeping, and maintenance supplies, for example. A file should be set up for each regular vendor or supplier, as well as a Miscellaneous Vendor file for all unusual or incidental purchases.

When a purchase order is made out and sent to the supplier, a copy of the purchase order should be placed in the appropriate file. When the order is received, all supplies should be delivered to a storeroom with the exception of food stuffs. A receiving slip will accompany the shipment; this should be checked against the items as they are being received and against the purchase order to make sure all items purchased were delivered (and, incidentally, that supplies that were *not ordered* are not delivered and signed for). Any back-ordered items on the receiving slip should be noted. The approved receiving slip is then placed with the purchase order in the vendor file.

Invoices from creditors are usually sent to the facility at the beginning of each month. The receiving slip and purchase order should be checked against the invoice to confirm that the unit price is the same as when the shipment was ordered and that all supplies charged in the bill were actually received.

All invoices should be approved by the administrator according to most owner policies, but practically speaking the administrator designates appropriate individuals to share in this task. These invoices are then recorded in the Accounts Payable Journal by department. For example, medical supplies and pharmaceuticals may be attributed to nursing, foodstuffs to dietary, linens to housekeeping, and so on. Invoices are placed in an invoice file.

At the end of the month the accounts in the Payables Journal are added up, and this sum should equal the total of all invoices in the invoice file. Bills are usually payable within 30 days. Creditors should be paid on the latest

FACILITY NO. _____   PAGE _____ or _____

DATE OF DEPOSIT 09/12/19X1   FACILITY NAME Old Well Home

PATIENT'S NAME LAST NAME INITIAL	C A S H	MISCEL- LANEOUS	PRIVATE	AGENCY	MEDICARE	VETERAN	OTHER	POSTED TO INVOICE NO.
Jones, F.A.					2375 00			3012- 756-01
TOTALS FOR EA. COLUMN	Ⓐ							
		ACCOUNT	1211	1212	1213	1210	1217	

MISCELLANEOUS RECEIPTS SUMMARY				REDEPOSITED ITEMS RECEIVED FROM	AMOUNT
ITEM	ACCOUNT	AMOUNT			
EMPLOYEE MEALS - FOOD SALES	4820				
VENDING MACHINE INCOME	4860				
TOTAL A MUST EQUAL TOTAL B		Ⓑ			

TOTAL OF
THIS DEPOSIT $_____
                          ACCOUNT 1130

FIGURE 3.8 Accounts receivable record.

possible date, unless a discount is offered for early payment. This does not mean that accounts payable should be chronically delinquent while available funds remain in the bank; it is important to maintain a good credit relationship with suppliers. Suppliers, often middlepersons, are dependent on reasonably prompt payment of invoices for their own business operations.

At the beginning of the month the invoices in the invoice file should be used to pay all bills due in that month. Checks should be signed by two designated employees, and all payments should be recorded in the Cash Disbursements Journal at the time checks are written. Invoices should be marked "Paid" and placed in the vendor file, along with the receipt of payment statement when it is received. These source documents are retained until the end of the year for the accountant's records.

Inventory: Controlling Supplies and Equipment

A system of inventory control is needed to measure the amount and type of supplies used by each department. Under accrual accounting one must be able to measure all expenses incurred in order to match them with the revenues earned in a time period. Consistent records of the cost of supplies consumed enable comparisons to be made over time between departments or services. These records are also valuable in the budgeting process.

A system of inventory control discourages waste and pilferage of supplies and provides a means of keeping supplies at optimal levels. Overstock, especially of time-dated supplies, has an opportunity cost: the cost of moneys unnecessarily tied up in inventory and a possible cost of obsolescence. Excess inventory also increases the opportunity for pilferage. On the other hand, frequent shortages of needed supplies can impinge on the quality of care and result in frustration among staff or require that costly rush orders be used to meet supply needs. Late last century a management approach to this continuing problem called "just in time" inventory was initiated. One well known example was the Harley Motor Cycle Company, which moved to just in time inventory with notable success. Today, their management views just in time inventory as much a liability as an asset. (The real problem at the Harley plants, it turned out, was not the timing of the arrival of inventory, but the quality and appropriateness of the inventory whenever it arrived.)

Ideally, the focal point of inventory control is a locked central storeroom (Figure 3.9). All supplies should be delivered to a central storeroom as soon as they are received. A limited number of employees should have access to central storerooms, usually one employee on each shift, though access to supplies must be balanced so that supplies may be obtained when needed but are not subject to unwarranted use. Smaller facilities may find a central storeroom impractical, in which case decentralized storerooms can become the responsibility of personnel in the individual department.

Perpetual Inventory

A perpetual inventory system is recommended to maintain a precise count of inventory on hand, that is, an accurate count of supplies used and those remaining in the storeroom. At the beginning of each fiscal year, probably more often, all inventory in central stores (or the decentralized storerooms) should be physically confirmed. This is the Beginning Inventory for the time period.

Additions to inventory are noted from the receiving slips included in each shipment of supplies. The Beginning Inventory and the Inventory Received by the storerooms make up the Total Available Inventory. When supplies are removed from a storeroom, a requisition slip identifying the supplies and date issued, by department, must be filled out. Supplies issued by storerooms may be taken as the supplies actually used in providing services. This, of course, does not account for those supplies remaining in each department or subloca-tion that have not yet been used.

For this reason, department heads should be encouraged to keep initial levels of supplies in their departments. Requisition slips should be initialed by a department head or other designated person. Requisition slips not only provide a check on the unjustified removal of supplies from the storeroom(s), but are the objective measure of the supplies consumed during a particular period.

The receiving slips and requisition slips are the source documents for keeping the perpetual inventory record (Table 3.6). At the end of each year, or other time

FIGURE 3.9 Perpetual inventory record.

period, the inventory in the storerooms should be counted and compared with the ending inventory from the perpetual inventory record. If the physical count of the storerooms and the inventory record do not match, this may indicate pilferage, misuse of requisition slips, or inaccuracies in the record-keeping system.

It is advisable for the business office to maintain a list of all inventory items used by the facility, the number of items in one unit, and the current price per unit. This log acts as a reference for determining the cost of the inventory used by each department and for establishing the total volume of supplies remaining in the storeroom(s).

LIFO / FIFO

To account for the effects of inflation or deflation on the price of inventory, the GAAP recognizes two methods of inventory costing—last in, first out (LIFO) and first in, first out (FIFO). The LIFO method assumes that inventory added last to stores is used first, thus making (in the case of inflation) the value of the goods remaining in inventory lower than that of the goods used to provide services. The FIFO method assumes the opposite, that the older and less expensive supplies (in the case of deflation) are used for services, and the higher priced goods remain in inventory longer. The difference in the effect of these two methods is shown in Table 3.7. Either method of inventory cost

TABLE 3.6.   Old Well Home Perpetual Inventory Record

Item #400 Syringes, disposable	# Units	Cost/unit	Cost
July			
Beginning inventory	4	$7.00	$28.00
Goods received	5	$7.00	$35.00
Total goods available	9	$7.00	$63.00
Ending inventory	3	$7.00	$21.00
Goods used	6	$7.00	$42.00
August			
Beginning inventory	3	$7.00	$21.00
Goods received	6	$7.00	$42.00
Total goods available	9	$7.00	$63.00
Ending inventory	4	$7.00	$28.00
Goods used	5	$7.00	$35.00

may be adopted, but the one selected should be used consistently and should be mentioned in the notes to financial statements.

Payroll

Payroll is another source of cash outflow. It is the largest expense in the nursing facility, accounting for over 50% of total costs in most cases. It also makes up about 85% of the facility's controllable costs. A controllable cost is one over which the administrator has influence. Because it is the primary expense of the facility, accurate accounting records are essential.

Payroll Journal

The Payroll Journal lists all paychecks disbursed in the time period, by department. At the end of the pay period the hours worked are entered in the Payroll Journal, as derived from the time cards or sheets and the salaried employee's

TABLE 3.7.   Inventory

Item #400 Syringes, disposable	# Units	Cost/unit	Cost			
August						
Beginning inventory	3	$7.00	$21.00			
Goods received	6	$7.00	$42.00			
Total goods available	9	$7.00	$63.00			
Ending inventory	4	$7.00	$28.00			
Goods used	5	$7.00	$35.00			
September		Last in, first out			First in, first out	
Beginning inventory	4	$7.00	$28.00	4	$7.00	$28.00
Goods received	5	$8.00	$40.00	5	$8.00	$40.00
Total goods available	9	4 @7.00 5 @8.00	$68.00	9 OR	4 @7.00 5 @8.00	68.00
Ending inventory	5	4 @7.00 1 @8.00	$36.00	5	$8.00	$40.00
Goods used	4	$8.00	$32.00	4	$7.00	$28.00

staffing plan. Overtime hours are compensated at a higher rate and are listed in a column separate from the regular rate. Gross pay is then calculated by multiplying hours worked by the hourly rate:

$$\text{(pay rate x reg. hrs.)} + \text{(Overtime rate x Overtime hours)} = \text{gross pay}$$

Payroll Deductions

Payroll deductions must be subtracted from gross pay to arrive at the employee's net pay. They include federal, state, and sometimes municipal taxes, as well as various other deductions that must be made.

The amount of federal, state, and local tax deducted is a percentage based on the employee's income. The percentages are supplied by the various government agencies. The Federal Insurance Contribution Act (FICA) deduction is the employee's contribution to the Social Security fund.

A certain proportion of the employee's paycheck is withheld, matched by the employer, and remitted on a quarterly basis to the Internal Revenue Service (IRS), which collects taxes for the federal government. Because this payroll tax is part of the cost of providing services, it must be attributed to the time period in which the employee was earning the wages. The cumulative amount of payroll tax is entered in the Payables Journal for each month as a credit to the taxes payable and a debit to cash.

Other deductions from the employee's pay may include meals and uniform expense. If the employee health plan requires some contribution by them, this would also be noted in the Payroll Journal as a deduction. Deductions for each employee are calculated and subtracted from gross pay to give the net pay. A separate column should exist for bonuses or other adjustments to net pay. At the end of each month, salary totals for each department are posted to the General Ledger. A page from a typical Payroll Journal is shown in Figure 3.10.

The employees who divide their time between two or more departments should be listed in the department where the majority of hours are spent, with a portion of their earnings and taxes allocated to the second department. Some reimbursement programs, such as Medicare, may require record keeping for the hours each day spent by an employee attributable to each Medicare resident.

Separate Payroll Bank Account

The facility should maintain a separate bank account solely for payroll. The person preparing the payroll does not write their own paycheck. All paychecks should have two signatures or be approved by the administrator before being

FIGURE 3.10 Page from payroll journal.

disbursed. The paycheck number and the date of issue are recorded in the Payroll Journal to identify checks that are misplaced or to stop payment on checks that are not cashed within a reasonable period of time. Checks are best distributed to each employee in person.

Preparation and maintenance of the payroll is largely a bookkeeping function, although larger homes may have a separate department devoted to this task. In recent years a number of electronic payroll services have been offered by banks and other financial service groups. A telephone call to the bank or data transmission by a telephone line-operated or computer modem accomplishes transmission of information to the financial service or corporate office, which in turn delivers the checks to the facility at a specified time. The modem is an electronic device that can transmit computer data over telephone lines from the facility computer to the bank computer.

Protecting the Residents' Funds

Legal Responsibilities

Nursing facilities are frequently asked by residents to safeguard their assets. Any agreement to take responsibility for these assets must be conformed through a legal contract signed by both the facility and the resident or the sponsor. This contract establishes a trust relationship between the resident and the facility, and sound procedures for managing these assets must be adhered to so that the relationship is not violated. Administrators vary in what they will protect for residents. Some may keep jewelry and similar items in safekeeping. In general, experience suggests that cash be the primary or only resident asset the facility will take responsibility to safeguard. Valuables other than cash are best managed by a legal representative of the resident.

Separate Accounting

As a check on patient cash, a separate book should be kept to record the information, shown in Figure 3.11. A copy of a receipt signed by the patient or sponsor is kept in an envelope accompanying this book.

Use of Interest Bearing Accounts

Patient funds deposited with the facility are to be managed in accordance with §483.10(c) of the federal requirements.

		Page _____ of _____			
Facility Old Well Home _____		# _____	Month ending 06/30/X1		

Patient Name	Beginning Balance	Deposits	Disbursements	Ending Balance
Jones, F.A.	$210.00	$90.00	$25.00	$275.00

FIGURE 3.11 Patient trust funds trial balance.

Note

Matters such as inventory and payroll should not occupy too much of the administrator's time. However, it is important that all of these details be properly managed by the staff, and experience seems to show that when the administrator understands the fine points of financing and occasionally reviews these matters knowledgeably with them, the staff tend to pay attention to details also. The result is that the administrator is thus freed to deal with broader policy while procedures such as payroll and managing resident accounts function smoothly.

3.7 The Concept of Depreciation

Depreciation has been mentioned to some extent already. Capital assets are those used to provide services during more than one time period; in the course of operations they lose value as a result of use, wear and tear, or obsolescence.

To account for this loss of value to capital assets in the accrual system of accounting, the cost of the asset is spread over the time period that it is used. This must be done because the total cost of acquiring the asset could not properly be attributed to the month in which it was purchased, when it is actually an expense of providing services for several years to come.

Identifying Depreciable Assets

Assets that can be capitalized or depreciated differ from other assets of the facility in that they are used in operations for more than one time period and will not be converted into cash within the year. Many facilities set a minimum value for depreciable assets, usually about $500. A calculator, for example, may be used in the business office for many years, but its acquisition cost may be so low that the depreciation expense over its useful life would be negligible. The asset must be tangible and by definition must be owned by the facility. Thus, leased equipment cannot normally be depreciated. (Some leases, in which the lessor agrees not to take depreciation, can under some circumstances be depreciated.)

All new assets meeting these criteria are considered depreciable assets. Any alterations of the present fixed asset that affect either its value or its useful life, such as renovation, are depreciable expenses. Repair of damages or regular maintenance of the asset cannot be considered part of the depreciable expense.

Determining Depreciation Expense

There are several methods of calculating depreciation expense, but all methods are based on the historical cost of the asset, its useful life (sometimes preset by tax or other regulations), and its salvage value, if any.

Historical Cost

The historical cost of the asset is the cost of acquiring the asset that is depreciated over several time periods. In addition to the purchase price, the cost of taxes, shipping delivery, installation, and so forth can be included along with any other one-time costs associated with acquiring the asset.

Useful Life

The useful life of the asset is the number of years the item can be expected to be used by the facility. This must be an estimation. However, the IRS has useful life estimates for most assets that are mandated in reporting taxes or, in most instances, in calculating depreciation reports for Medicare, Medicaid, and some other third-party payers.

Salvage Value

A capital asset may have some value at the end of its useful life. A van, which normally has an IRS determined useful life of 5 years, might be such an asset.

Straight Line Depreciation

There are several methods for figuring the depreciation expense, once the historical cost, useful life, and salvage value are determined. Straight-line depreciation is a depreciation method in which the historical cost of an asset is spread evenly over its useful life so that the depreciation expense is the same in every time period that it functions.

Historical Cost / Useful Life = Annual Depreciation Expense

If the Old Well purchases new physical therapy equipment worth $20,000 with an estimated useful life of 5 years, the annual depreciation expense for the equipment would be:

$20,000 / 5 = $4,000 per year depreciation

After the first year the value of the physical therapy equipment on the books would be:

$20,000 − $4,000 = $16,000

Hence, the $16,000 is called the book value of this asset.
Straight-line depreciation has the advantage of simplicity.

Accelerated Depreciation

This method attributes most of the depreciation expense to the first years of the asset's life, thus enabling the facility to write it off more quickly, thereby gaining a tax advantage through earlier tax recognition of the investment. Among the several types of accelerated depreciation are the sum-of-the-years digits and double declining balance.

Purposes of Depreciation

We have already mentioned that depreciation must be calculated to adhere to the accrual system of accounting. To ignore the very real cost of depreciation is to underestimate the expense of providing services and to overestimate the value of the assets of the facility. For this reason, depreciation is included on the Income Statement as an operating expense and is subtracted from the historical cost of fixed assets on the balance sheet to reflect its impact on the financial position of the home.

Asset Replacement

Probably the most important reason for recognizing depreciation is for asset replacement. Because the asset will eventually have to be replaced, the present asset should be expensed over its useful life to accumulate the funds needed for its replacement. Chances are, however, that an asset purchased 10 years earlier will be more expensive than the original. This is not always the case. Some assets remain about the same for replacement while others actually may decrease in replacement costs. Computers, for example, have become less and less expensive to provide the same computing capacities because of advances in technology and competition among computer makers (Johns & Saks, 2001, p. 512).

Few facilities actually "fund" depreciation, that is put cash in an interest bearing account reserved for replacing equipment. Such a fund would appear in the Capital or New Worth section of the balance sheet as "Funded Depreciation."

Entering Depreciation Into the Accounting Records

A portion of the depreciation expense may easily be attributed to each time period by dividing the annual depreciation expense by the number of accounting periods in the year. Because depreciation is entered in the General Journal at the end of each month, the Old Well's new physical therapy equipment depreciation expense after the first month of purchase under straight-line depreciation would be as follows:

General Journal

	Debit _____	Credit _____
1/29 Depreciation expense	$333.33	
1/29 Reserve for depreciation		$333.33

Categorization of Fixed Assets

The Chart of Accounts should have an account for each type of fixed asset owned by the facility. These assets can be categorized generally as:

- land and improvements,
- buildings,
- fixed equipment,
- major movable equipment, and
- minor movable equipment,

or in more specific categories that are more useful to the facility.

In addition, depreciation schedules should be maintained for each category of assets (Table 3.8) and for each type of depreciation, if accelerated and straight-line are both used.

If two differing schedules are used to depreciate the same assets—one for reimbursement and one for other purposes—there will be a difference in depreciation expense for each asset every year. Because the total amount of depreciation taken for each asset should be the same (total depreciation will equal the historical cost less salvage value), this difference between the two depreciation expenses is a timing difference. Depreciation in this case may be regarded as a charge that must be deferred to another time period or as revenue that is accrued if depreciation will be recognized in a later accounting period.

TABLE 3.8. Old Well Home Depreciation Schedule

Item	Cost	Date Purchased	Life	Method Depreciated	Year	Depreciation, per year Annual	Cumulative
Plant: main	$5,767,004.00	6/19X0	30	Strt. line	X0	$192,233.47	$192,233.47
Hall welsh					X1	192,233.47	384,466.94
Hall & Garage					X2	192,233.47	576,700.41
					X3	192,233.47	768,933.88
					Etc.		
Kitchen	$398,600.00	6/19X0	15	Strt. line	X0	$26,573.33	$26,573.33
Equipment					X1	26,573.33	53,146.66
					X2	26,573.33	79,719.99
					X3	26,573.33	106,293.32
					Etc.		

3.8 Using "Costs" in Managerial Decisions

Efficiency

Efficiency may be defined as input over output, or the amount of input used for a certain level of output. Costs, as a component of input, are generally easier to control than revenues or other measures of output. Revenues are subject to limitation by competition from providers of similar services and government regulation through insurance and medical assistance programs. Knowledge of costs and the ability to control and reduce them permit liquidity of limited funds, making them available for other uses.

3.8.1 TWO TYPES OF COSTS: VARIABLE AND FIXED

Variable Costs

All costs can be regarded as variable, fixed, or semivariable. Variable costs are those that fluctuate directly and proportionately with changes in volume. That is, if volume is increased or decreased by a certain percentage, variable costs will rise or fall, respectively, by the same percentage. The cost of disposable medical supplies in the nursing department will vary directly with the number of similar care type and level patients served. The cost of food in dietary or the cost of postage for resident billing will also vary with resident volume.

Fixed Costs

Fixed costs, on the other hand, do not relate to changes in volume. The cost of the director of nursing's salary will not change with fluctuations in the number of residents. This does not mean that the director's salary cannot change at all, but it will result from an administrative decision rather than responding to patient volume, because federal regulations require that there be a full-time director of nursing. Clearly, if volume varies enough, many "fixed" costs will not remain the same. If resident volume increases substantially, a new administrative position in the nursing department may have to be created to accommodate the additional patient load. Fixed costs, then, are said to be fixed only over a relevant range of volume.

3.8.2 AN ADDITIONAL TYPE: SEMIVARIABLE COSTS

Semivariable costs do not fit neatly into either a variable or fixed category, as they vary disproportionately with volume. Examples of semivariable costs might be total nurse's aide's salaries, which depend more on resident volume and resident level of care needs than does the director of nursing's salary, which does not fluctuate directly with these variables.

Utility costs that are based on ranges of usage rather than actual usage may also be considered semivariable costs. It is helpful to think of semivariable costs as having a much narrower relevant range than fixed costs. Semivariable costs are often broken down into fixed and variable components for use in calculations, and so our discussion here will be limited to fixed and variable costs for the sake of simplicity.

Total Variable Costs

While total variable costs (TVC) change with volume, variable costs per unit do not. If disposable syringes are $1 each, the cost per syringe per patient will be $1, whether 100 or 150 patients receive injections using syringes purchased at one cost in one batch. Total fixed costs (TFC), however, do vary per unit with changes in volume. If the director of nursing's salary is $44,000 (exclusive of benefits, etc.) and they oversee the care of 100 residents, the director's salary cost per resident would be $440 (exclusive of benefits, etc.). If that same director of nurses oversees 150 residents, the cost drops to $293 per resident. Familiarity with the costs of the facility maximizes the administrator's ability to control its finances.

The behavior of variable and fixed costs is summarized in Table 3.9. As can be seen, fixed costs decrease with an increase in volume. Because the nursing facility generally has a high proportion of fixed costs, maintaining a high volume of service is of paramount concern to their administrators.

A closer study of the concept of fixed and variable costs reveals how it can be used to aid in decision making. Because all costs can be considered fixed or variable (even semivariable costs),

Total Fixed Costs + Total Variable Costs = Total Costs

TABLE 3.9.   Behavior of Fixed and Variable Costs

Patients	Director of nursing		Disposable medical supplies	
	(TFC)	FC/Unit	TVC	VC/Unit
100	$44000.00	440	100	$1.00
125	$44000.00	352	125	$1.00
150	$44000.00	293	150	$1.00
	(No change)	(Change)	(Change)	(No change)

Because total variable costs are a function of the variable cost per unit and the number of units, the above equation can be expanded to

Total fixed costs + (variable cost per unit x volume units) = total costs

$$\text{Total fixed costs} + \left(\frac{\text{variable costs}}{\text{units}} \text{ x volume units} \right) = \text{total costs}$$

$$\text{Break-even Volume in Units} = \frac{\text{Fixed Cost}}{\text{Rate}} - \text{Variable Cost}$$

Thus, if three of these values are known, the remaining value can be calculated.

The administrator of Old Well wants to find the average variable cost of medical supplies used per resident during the month. The General Ledger shows that the total costs of the nursing department for 1 month are $12,000. The administrator has determined that fixed cost accounts in that department amount to $9,000 and that medical supplies are its only variable cost. The patient Census Report for the month shows that there have been 3,000 resident days or an average of 100 residents over 30 days. To calculate the variable cost per patient in the nursing department:

$$\frac{(\text{Total Costs} - \text{Total Fixed Costs})}{\text{Volume units}} = \frac{\text{Variable Costs}}{\text{Units}}$$

($12,000 – $9,000) / 100 residents = $30 per resident

Thus, the variable cost of providing nursing services in this particular month was $30 per resident.

Volume of Service Units

These equations can be used to determine the volume of service units required to break even. Because total costs (TC) equal total revenues (TR) at the break-even point, total revenue (TR) can be substituted for total costs (TC) in the above equations to give the costs or volume needed to bread even.

If the total costs of the physical therapy department are $6,500 per month, the total fixed costs are $5,200, and the variable cost per patient visit to physical therapy is $8, how many patient visits are needed per month to break even in this department?

```
Total Costs   = Total Revenue
              = $6,500 = $5,200 + ($8 x Volume Unit)
Volume units ($6,500 – $5,200) / $8
Volume units = 162.5 visits per month
```

We have assumed that the physical therapists are employees of the facility and that their salaries comprise a significant portion of the fixed costs of the department. If physical therapy is provided on a contractual basis, the therapists' salaries would become a variable cost if they were paid for each visit.

3.8.3 ADDITIONAL TYPES OF COSTS

Indirect Costs and Direct Costs

Costs may also be categorized as direct and indirect. In order to discuss them, however, we must first define revenue and cost centers.

Revenue Centers

Revenue centers are units of the facility, usually departments, that generate revenue, usually through resident care. Revenue centers in the nursing facility will normally be nursing, possible physical therapy, occupational therapy, pharmacy, laboratory, and medical support. It may also be any other department or center earning revenue, such as a cafeteria that serves a large number of guest meals or a profitable day care program. If pharmaceuticals or medical supplies are included as part of the routine care and are not separately charged, they would not be revenue centers.

As facilities add service areas such as assisted-living wings, home health, and hospice care, these become additional revenue centers. If the facility earns a significant amount of revenue from interest on investments, interest may also be considered a revenue center.

Cost Centers

Cost centers are units of the facility identified with certain costs. Revenue centers are almost always cost centers because the revenue-earning departments also have costs directly associated with them. Interest as a revenue center has little or no costs associated with it. All other departments, such as administration, maintenance, housekeeping, and usually dietary and laundry, are cost centers. Depreciation, interest, insurance, telephone, utility, and transportation expenses may also be considered cost centers. These are all identifiable costs of the facility, and the concept of cost centers will become clearer as we proceed.

Direct Costs

Direct costs are those directly attributable to a revenue center or directly providing resident care. In the nursing facility direct costs are often called resident care costs. Direct costs of the nursing department would include all nursing salaries, payroll taxes, benefits, medical supplies, expenses associated with capital equipment used only in the department, and any other costs associated directly with this department.

Indirect Costs

Indirect costs are those that cannot be directly associated with a revenue-producing center, yet support the functions of the resident care centers (or other care centers, such as an adult day care center). Indirect costs of the nursing department would be administration, payroll, utility, housekeeping, maintenance, dietary, laundry, plant depreciation, tax, and interest expenses that keep these departments running. For this reason, indirect costs are also known as support service costs.

Support Service Costs

These indirect costs must be allocated to all the revenue-producing departments that are also cost centers in order to be included in the charge for services in each revenue center and to reflect the total cost of providing that service. To find the total costs of the revenue-producing department, the support costs must be spread over all revenue-producing departments in some systematic way. This process is known as cost finding, as it yields the total costs of the resident care centers (and other centers such as adult day care).

The concept of cost finding is illustrated schematically in Figure 3.12. The total costs of both the support and service (or revenue-earning centers) are shown. To find the total cost of providing resident services A and B, some portion of the support centers must be allocated to the revenue centers. Support Center No. 1 divides its support equally between service centers A and B, so 50% of Support Center No. 1's costs are attributed to each Resident Service Center.

Support Center No. 2 provides more services to patient Center B, and this is reflected in the proportion of Support Center No. 2's costs that go to Service Center B. When the costs of both support centers are allocated, the total cost of providing services A and B are known.

Values of Cost Finding

Cost finding yields a representative picture of the entire expense of providing each service. This information is used in deciding whether a particular service should be discontinued or supported. For example, unless all direct and indirect costs of providing a service, such as adult day care, are calculated, it is difficult to determine the cost-effectiveness of offering such a service. Cost allocation is a subjective process in that there is an almost

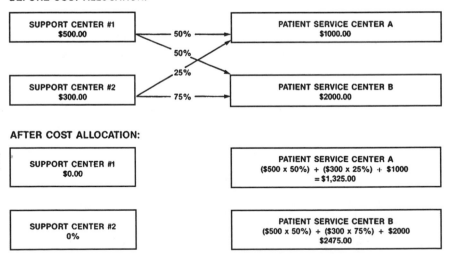

FIGURE 3.12 Cost allocation between two support and revenue centers.

infinite number of ways to perform cost allocation properly. Numerous facilities offered adult day care a few years back, but when they stopped to determine the full actual costs of earning the daily charges for day care, they discovered that most of the programs were cost-ineffective (Maddox & Sussman, 2001, p. 130).

Allocating Indirect Costs

There are several methods for allocating indirect costs, among them the step-down and reciprocal methods. Providers who are reimbursed on a cost basis must usually use the step-down method unless another method is approved. We will discuss the step-down method in some detail here and briefly explain the reciprocal method at the end of this section.

The step-down method derives its name from the shape of the completed worksheet and involves the systematic allocation of all cost centers over all other cost centers that use the "services" of the cost-center expenses being allocated. Support costs are spread not only over revenue centers, but also over other support cost centers.

Once a support cost is divided among the other cost centers, no more costs can be allocated to that department. Therefore, the order in which support costs are allocated affects the final cost of the revenue centers. As a rule, cost centers that are used by most of the other cost centers are allocated first.

The basis of allocation also affects the outcome of the cost-finding process. In allocating housekeeping costs to the departments that use housekeeping services, the basis for allocation might be the number of employees in the department, the square footage of the departments, or some other criteria. Likewise, administrative costs might be allocated on the basis of number of employees, total salary of employees, volume of services provided, or total revenues earned in each department. These alternatives are examples only; clearly, the basis for allocation varies.

Third-party reimbursement will indicate the basis for allocation that should be used for residents for whom they reimburse, but in any case the method the facility uses should remain consistent to enable comparison of the resulting costs in different time periods.

The Step-Down Process

Cost allocation is best illustrated through a step-by-step example of the step-down process. The one provided in Table 3.10 is necessarily simplified; cost allocations for most health care organizations are usually performed by

TABLE 3.10.   Old Well Home Step-Down Worksheets: Preliminary Worksheet

Cost Centers	Capital (sq. ft.)	Plant (sq. ft.)	Admin. (1) (-FTE)- (1)	Main. (1) (sq. ft.)	Laundry (lbs. dry)	House- keep (sq. ft.)	Dietary (meals)	Soc. Serv. (visits)	P.T. (visits)	O.T. (visits)	NURS- ING	TOTAL
Sup- port & revenue centers												
Adminis- tration	3.0%	3.0%										
Mainte- nance (2)	1.5%	1.5%	0.5%									
Laundry	9.0%	9.0%	3.0%	9.4%								
House- keeping	8.0%	8.0%	7.4%	8.4%	5.0%							
Dietary	10.0%	10.0%	7.3%	10.5%	15.0%	12.8%						

(Continued)

TABLE 3.10. Old Well Home Step-Down Worksheets: Preliminary Worksheet (Continued)

Cost Centers	Capital (sq. ft.)	Plant (sq. ft.)	Admin. (1) (-FTE)-(1)	Main. (1) (sq. ft.)	Laundry (lbs. dry)	House-keep (sq. ft.)	Dietary (meals)	Soc. Serv. (visits)	P.T. (visits)	O.T. (visits)	NURS-ING	TOTAL
Social services	0.5%	0.5%	0.1%	0.5%		0.6%						
Physical therapy	7.0%	7.0%	2.5%	7.3%	2.5%	8.9%						
Occupational therapy	2.0%	2.0%	0.4%	2.1%	2.5%	2.6%						
Nursing	59.0%	59.0%	78.8%	61.7%	75.0%	75.2%						
TOTAL	100.0%	100.0%	100.0%	99.8%	100.0%	100.0%	100.0%	100.0%	100.0%	100.0%	100.0%	100.0%

1. FTE = Full Time Equivalent Employees.
2. Total Maintenance costs include all utility costs.

computer because of the volume and complexities involved in larger, more departmentalized, or multiprogram facilities.

Other Methods of Cost Finding

Two other approaches to cost finding are the reciprocal and cost-apportionment methods. The reciprocal is similar to the step-down method, except that it recognizes reciprocal services provided between cost centers, such as administration and maintenance. Because of the calculations involved and the extent of these services in most organizations, reciprocal allocation is performed by computer.

Rate Setting

One of the primary uses of the cost-finding process is to develop a basis for setting rates for the services provided by the revenue centers. Once the costs of the revenue centers are known, the average cost per unit of service can be calculated by dividing the total cost of the revenue center by the expected service volume.

First, the unit of service must be determined. In the physical therapy department a unit of service is normally calculated as a 15-minute segment for which charges are made.

The average cost per unit of service offers a basis for rate setting, because rates should approximate the cost of providing the service. But other factors, such as demand for services, competitive rates, expected inflation rates, contractual discounts, and frequency of uncollectibles must be considered in achieving realistic rates.

3.9 Budgets and Budgeting

Considerations in Budgeting

The budgeting process in the nursing facility is a period of planning. The physical budget is more than a record of anticipated expenses for the next fiscal year. It represents a careful examination of internal and external changes that management believes will affect the operation of the facility and the strategy to deal with these changes for some time to come. Thus, the budget is a reflection of the administrator's short- and long-term goals for the facility. Most organizations also have a 3–5 year budget plan following the next fiscal year as a guide to long-range planning.

The budget is a tool to be used throughout the year, rather than a document that, once completed, is filed away to remain only in the memory of the budget participants. The budget can be changed as conditions change. It provides a meaningful comparison between actual and projected expenditures and revenues.

Most facility administrators use the budget in a monthly review with department managers on how the year is unfolding and what changes need to be undertaken.

3.9.1 TWO METHODS OF BUDGET PREPARATION

Budgeting is done in any number of ways, and each individual facility or multifacility operation will develop its own particular style. In general, two methods of budget preparation are used: the top-down and the participatory method.

Top-Down Approach to Budgeting

With the top-down approach, the administrator (or corporate) alone prepares the annual budget with little or no guidance from department heads. This method is most suitable for smaller facilities with few departments, where the administrator is familiar with all the costs of the facility. Top-down is also often the approach used by chains, in which case the local administrator is given a "suggested" budget with the corporation's goals already built into it. The top-down method is quick, but it has the disadvantages of possibly stifling innovation or of imposing an unpopular or unrealistic budget on department head or chain facility administrators.

The Participatory Approach

The participatory method of budgeting requires input from staff members on several levels of the organization. The administrator provides guidelines for the preparation of departmental budgets, prepared by the department heads and other key personnel. These budgets are then reviewed by the administrator, adjusted as necessary, and combined into one organizational budget.

Participatory budgeting is more appropriate for larger facilities. Although it is time-consuming, it furnishes an opportunity for communication between the administrator and department heads and results in input into the budget from those who are most knowledgeable about the daily operation of the individual departments.

Participatory budgeting will be used to describe the budgeting process in this section, as it is considerably more involved than the top-down approach. However, the process described is equally applicable to the latter.

Participatory budgeting augments the role each participant plays in the operations of the facility. Department heads and others become more aware not only of the costs of their areas and the resources available to the facility, but also of the needs of the other departments. Budgeting also brings greater recognition of their own roles to the participating staff, and although the budget process is often time-consuming and frustrating, the staff is rewarded by the knowledge that their experience and ideas are valued.

Finally, the budget communicates information about the facility to external parties who have an interest in its status, such as the board of directors or stockholders, third-party payers, planning agencies, accreditation teams, rate review commissions, and unions. The administrator must often be able to justify proposed expenses and revenues to them.

3.9.2 FIVE STEPS IN THE BUDGETING PROCESS

There are any number of ways to prepare the budget, whether by the administrator alone or with the input of key personnel. The optimal method will depend on, among other considerations, the size of the facility, whether it is freestanding or a unit in a small or large chain, and the administrator's time constraints.

In designing the budgeting process the administrator first decides what information is desired and how detailed it must be and then maps out the logistics of the activity. The administrator determines who the participants will be. In the case of top-down budgeting, the administrator and perhaps other administrative personnel, such as the bookkeeper, comptroller, or business manager, will be involved. Participatory budgeting usually includes the administrator, the accountant or the comptroller, bookkeeper, human resources director, and department heads and their assistants. The budget timetable must also be defined. At least 2 to 5 months before the beginning of the next fiscal year should be allowed for the entire process.

Step 1: Assessing the Environment

The initial step in the budgeting process is the assessment of the external and internal environments (Hitt, Ireland, & Hoskisson, 2001, pp. 54–55). The budget cannot be prepared in a vacuum. The political, economic, and social environments outside the nursing facility walls are not static. Although the administrator does not have control over these aspects of the external environment, ignorance of the trends affecting the nursing facility industry, and failure to anticipate their effects on the operations of the facility, leave the administrator less able to deal effectively with changes (Hitt et al., 2001, pp. 52–55). Such trends may occur as one or more of the following:

- increased or decreased competition
- new types of competition, for example, local hospital opening long-term care beds or increasing capacity to treat at home by local home health agencies or emergence of additional hospice care agencies
- altered reimbursement policies
- amended licensing laws
- revised quality review regulations
- swings in the economy
- inflation, deflation, or stagnation
- changes in prevailing wage rates
- reduction or enlargement of the potential service population
- changes in availability of key personnel
- changes in disease patterns among residents
- changing system pressures from hospital discharge patterns due to Diagnostic Related Group (DRG) pressures
- changing third-party payer situation, with new patterns of providing and paying for care emerging

- increasing acuity level among the resident population
- other

Some, if not most, of these fluctuations in the external environment may affect the plans and operations of the facility.

Step 2: Programming

After the external environments and their anticipated effects on the facility have been evaluated, the facility's objectives for the coming year are determined. This process is sometimes known as programming; in effect, it results in a program for the facility to follow. Through this "programming" the administrator can alter internal operations over which they have control to respond to the external (and internal) influences on the facility.

How might an administrator use programming to cope with external events? In periods of rising inflation the cost of living goes up. This usually results in a demand for higher wages. If the administrator is aware of this trend, an objective might be to index the salaries, that is, raise them by a certain percentage to approximate the increased costs of living by a certain time during the following year. An increase in salary expense can then be included in the budget, thereby preventing a situation in which funds are not set aside for this purpose. Such an oversight could result in recruiting problems, high staff turnover, or a strain on operating funds when a salary increase is finally provided.

Similarly, if a competitor is opening a facility quite close by, a contingency fund could be set aside in the following year's budget to raise salaries to meet the new competitor's salary scale, should this become necessary (Hitt et al., 2001, pp. 81–86).

Other considerations for programming are changes in (a) service volume, (b) services offered, (c) payer mix, (d) human resources needs, and (e) capital needs. The cumulative effect of expected external and internal events should determine the objectives of the facility for the next year(s), which in turn form the basis of assumptions made in the budgeting process.

The completed budgeting process should result in four types of budgets: the operating budget, the cash budget, the capital budget, and the pro forma financial statements.

Step 3: Developing The Operating Budget

The operating budget has two parts: the expense budget and the revenue budget.

The Expense Budget

The expense budget, the type with which we are most familiar, lists the antici-pated expenses of the facility for the coming year and is prepared largely by the department heads. The budget timetable should indicate when the final departmental expense budgets are due.

The heads of all service units should indicate the expected resident service volume, while support departments (such as dietary) should be able to estimate the number of meals that will be served. Budgeting offers an opportunity for communication among departments. After all, dietary must learn the expected resident volume in the different areas of the facility to be able to calculate the number of meals to be served and types of diets likely to be prescribed.

Additionally, department heads should review staff positions and note any recommended changes in the staffing pattern. In larger facilities recommen-dations for salary changes may be the responsibility of the personnel director and may be based on competitive salaries in the community or union agree-ments if employees are so organized.

Department heads should also check equipment in their departments for repair or replacement needs. Included in this assessment would be estimates of the costs of repair or replacement, supported by professional estimates, manufacturer price sheets, and the like. If equipment needs are extensive, it may be worthwhile for department heads to develop a plant and equipment budget for their departments, which will facilitate preparation of the capital budget.

The cost of supplies and other expenses are often a significant portion of depart-mental costs. Any change in the volume of supplies needed and the cost per unit should be noted on the budget. Catch-all or miscellaneous categories should be kept to a minimum, as there can be little control over unidentified costs.

Anticipated expenses should be broken down by months or another cus-tomary accounting period used in the facility. Monthly expense budgets also facilitate preparation of the cash budget.

Determining Expenses

In determining expenses several strategies can be used. One tactic is to increase all of the current year's expenses by a certain percentage. Although this method is quick, it defeats the purpose of budgeting and the effort involved in envi-ronmental assessment and programming.

It is more productive for the department head to identify monthly and yearly trends in costs and utilization to help reduce expenses. For example, occupancy of the nursing unit might be consistently below average during the winter holidays, but regularly above average in late January and February. Identification of such trends is useful in budgeting for monthly costs on volume levels. It is also often helpful to identify the source of variances in the current year's budget and allow for them in the preparation of the new budget.

In setting up the expense budget a checklist can be used to make sure all expense items in departments are included. A good source for this checklist is the Chart of Accounts, which should list all expense accounts by department.

All budget participants ought to know how and by whom the final budget levels are decided. Finally, the organizational expense budget is separated by months, and the individual department budgets retained for comparison of actual with budgeted performance in each department throughout the year.

The Revenue Budget

The second section of the operating budget is the revenue budget, which projects the monthly income for the next fiscal year. The revenue budget need not be prepared on a departmental basis; fewer departments are involved in determining revenues than in determining expenses, and nonoperating revenues are generally under the control of the administrator. Also, service revenues are based on the prices charged for services, which are determined by administrative decision. Hence, the revenue budget is usually prepared at the administrative level.

Operating Revenue Estimates

To estimate operating revenues, all revenue centers are listed, with the number of residents appearing by type of payer. Total resident service revenues are calculated by multiplying the expected service volume in each revenue center by the charge per unit of service. As mentioned in the section on cost finding, rates for services may be determined in several ways. For publicly insured persons, the allowable rate per unit of service may be somewhat less than charges; the reimbursable rate should be used in projecting revenues for these persons.

For privately paying residents, charges can be based on the cost plus profit for providing the service, using the results of the cost-finding process and break-even analysis. Rates may also be based on competitive charges for similar services in the community or on the price that the market will bear.

Nonoperating Revenues

Nonoperating revenues, such as interest income, borrowed funds, and charitable donations, are dependent on any number of factors but are relatively predictable on a monthly basis. These revenues are added to the monthly operating revenues to arrive at the total expected revenues.

Total revenues can then be compared with total budgeted expenses. If revenues seem inadequate to meet expenses, the administrator can check the validity of the predicted service volumes. If service levels seem reasonable, the administrator can seek to increase patient service volume, reduce budget expenses, or raise rates.

Using the Operating Budget: Variance Analysis

As a managerial tool, the operating budget is used throughout the fiscal year to measure performance by a technique called variance analysis, which is a comparison of actual versus budgeted monetary and volume values at the end of each month.

Actual expenses that deviate significantly from the budgeted amounts can be investigated to identify the source of the variance. Such variances may be anything from an inadvertent miscalculation of costs or patient volume to serious mismanagement by a particular department. Typical sources of overage are items such as more pool labor being used than anticipated, or a number of employees working unanticipated or unauthorized overtime. Once the source of variances is known, the budget can be adjusted accordingly or the cause of the variance can be dealt with. Budget variance analysis provides the administrator with an important means of control over the finances of the facility.

Step 4: The Cash Budget

The next step in the budgeting process is preparation of the cash budget. As its name implies, it is prepared on the cash basis of accounting, although it is based on the revenues and expenses from the operating budget. Note that the operating budget is prepared on the accrual basis of accounting: Projected revenues are based on the income earned in the time period, not on the amount of cash received for services during the month.

The cash budget is an estimate of the cash inflows and outflows for the next 12 months, enabling the administrator to identify months with possible cash shortages and overages. This information can be used to defer nonurgent expenditures to a month with high cash inflows or retain overages in one month to cover anticipated cash shortages in the next. A cash budget is useful for anticipating effects of such events as three pay periods occurring in one month, or anticipated large Medicare payments at known intervals. Facilities having corporate ownership may have little need of a cash budget inasmuch as the corporate funds can cover any temporary shortages in cash flow needs of the facility. Some administrators rely on the cash budget for daily operations and sometimes prepare weekly or even daily cash budgets a month in advance.

Determining Cash Inflows and Outflows

To develop the cash budget, cash inflows and outflows must be determined. Because the facility has less control over cash inflows, especially those received from third-party payers, projecting them is somewhat complicated. First, all payer sources must be identified. These will usually be private payers, Medicare, Medicaid, insurance companies, HMOs or IPOs or similar organizations, the Veterans Administration, and all other known or anticipated sources of income for services expected to be rendered. The lag time between the billing of services and receipt of payment is determined. Most private payers do so within 30 days of billing, but time lags for Medicare and Medicaid may vary considerably. This can be used to measure the percentage of revenues that will be received from each payer in each month.

When cash inflows from resident services are known, monthly cash receipts from nonoperating sources are computed to give total cash receipts for each month.

Cash outflows are somewhat easier to estimate, because most cash disbursements, such as salaries and supplies, are made at prespecified intervals. Using the expense budget and the facility's experience with suppliers and other creditors, the amount of cash disbursements can be determined for each month. An insurance policy that is paid on a triennial basis may be due in February, for example.

As with the operating budget, the cash budget is updated as conditions or needs change throughout the year, whatever the reason. The cash budget can be a useful planning tool.

Step 5: The Capital Budget

The capital budget is a summarization of all anticipated capital (items with a life of more than 12 months) expenditures in the budget year. Although many capital purchases and projects may be needed, all might not be readily affordable in the course of a single year. The capital budget is the result of the decision concerning capital projects that will be undertaken, and, most important, how they will be financed. If a competitor is to open a large, all-new facility nearby, for example, a contingency capital item might be funds for renovations of a portion of the facility to compete should census drop precipitously.

Pro Forma Financial Statements

The budget process concludes with the development of the pro forma financial statements. The pro forma statements are the preliminary financial statements based on budgeted amounts. The pro forma income statement, for instance, is derived from the operating budget and shows the net income (or loss) expected under the budgeted expenses and revenues.

The budgeting process can be costly in terms of time for the administrator and all other budget participants. However, it involves a thorough investigation of the facility's finances through such tools as cost finding, break-even analysis, rate setting, programming, and cash flow analysis. Through these processes, budgeting familiarizes the administrator with the costs of running the facility and maximizes their ability to manage successfully.

3.10 Finance

We now turn to examine the broader business and financial context within which the nursing facility manages its affairs.

In this section we will

- glance briefly at the sources of law and the court systems
- review a number of legal terms
- discuss the issue of risk management for a nursing facility
- examine a number of business and financial concepts and terms, insurance terms, and terms associated with wills and estates

3.10.1 SOURCES OF LAW

The daily business of the nursing facility is conducted within the context of the U.S. legal system.

Constitution

The Constitution is the written agreement establishing the fundamental law of the United States of America, setting forth the conditions, mutual obligations, and rights of the federal and state governments and laying basic principles of government. The Bill of Rights guaranteed specific individual rights.

Statutes

Statutes are the law under which we live. In the United States they are the acts passed by the federal and state legislatures (Noe, Hollenbeck, Gerhart, & Wright, 2000, p. 74). Lesser governmental bodies, such as county commissions, adopt ordinances; administrative agencies function by means of regulations.

Common Law

Common law is the accumulation of opinion handed down by judges. It is an outgrowth of court decisions over hundreds of years. Our common law originated in England, where judges followed unwritten principles of "common sense" in addition to statutory laws. Common law principles change over time with the changing values and needs of society.

Regulations

To implement statutes (laws) passed by legislative bodies, the executive branch of government (the president and the various federal agencies the president oversees), through these administrative agencies, writes regulations (Noe et al., 2000, p. 75). These regulations are the official interpretations of the intent of each statute. As a consequence, regulations become, in effect, part of the law. One may challenge a regulation on the grounds that the "official interpretation" is unconstitutional or inconsistent with the legislative intent of the statute the regulation implements.

The federal requirements for nursing facilities are an example of regulations. These were written by the executive branch of the federal government during the process of spelling out the details of how the legislation will be interpreted and implemented. The federal requirements for nursing facilities were written by the employees of the Health Care Finance Administration, which administers Medicare and Medicaid. The federal requirements published in the Federal Register as, for example, the OBRA regulations (the Nursing Home Reform Amendments of 1987) have the effect of law when federal inspectors visit a nursing facility and issue deficiencies based on both the written regulations and a set of "interpretive guidelines." These interpretive guidelines, although not law or regulation per se, are very real; they are the "guidelines" used by federal certification inspectors to record deficiencies and levy fines.

These requirements (not the interpretive guidelines), along with other federal administrative agency regulations, are published in the *Code of Federal Regulations* (often refereed to as C.F.R).

The President of the United States has the prerogative of issuing executive orders under various statutes. Executive orders also have the effect of law. President Johnson, for example, issued Executive Order 11246 requiring all federal contractors to use affirmative action guidelines designed to hire and promote women and minorities within their organizations (Noe et al., 2000, p. 75).

Code

A code is a compilation of statutes and regulations. The statutes, together with the regulations written by the administrative assigned to implement each statute, are systematically collected and placed into codes of law. The U.S. Code (USC) is an example.

3.10.2 THE COURT SYSTEMS

Federal Courts

The U.S. Constitution authorizes the creation of the Supreme Court and any additional courts Congress chooses to establish. Currently, entry into the federal court system is at the level of federal district courts (general courts of original jurisdiction). Jurisdiction is the power to hear and decide a case. Situated between these and the federal Supreme Court are 12 courts of appeal, which together cover the 50 states and hear cases in the event a party is dissatisfied with the judgment of the federal district court based on what the dissatisfied party views as an error (Noe et al., 2000, p. 75).

The federal government also operates other courts, such as a Court of Claims, the Court of Customs and Patent Appeals, the Tax Court, and federal bankruptcy courts.

State Courts

The court systems vary from state to state. The lowest level of the state system is the magistrate court, which deals with misdemeanor cases, traffic violations, and small claims (about $1,000 or under). Above the magistrate courts are the state circuit courts, or district courts, where more serious cases are tried.

Circuit or district courts have original jurisdiction over both civil and criminal cases. Most states have state courts of appeal, which normally do not have original jurisdiction and therefore limit themselves to appeals from lower courts in the state. Finally, each state has a state supreme court. This is the court of final appeal in all matters except those that involve a federal issue appealable to the U.S. Supreme Court.

3.10.3 LEGAL TERMINOLOGY

Accuse—To directly charge a person with committing an offense that is recognized as being against a law. The accused person becomes the defendant and must answer the complaint or accusation through the legal process.

Acquit—To set a person or corporation free of accusation(s). Acquittal is a decision (verdict) of not guilty and is rendered either by a jury or a judge (in nonjury trials). Under the principle of double jeopardy, a person or corporation cannot be tried again for the same accusation after a verdict of not guilty.

Actionable—Conduct giving rise to a cause for legal action. For example, actionable negligence occurs only when a person unreasonably fails to perform a legal duty, resulting in damage or injury to another person. If there is no resulting damage, there may not be actionable negligence even though the person made a mistake.

Adjudication—Decision or disposition of a case by the announcement of a judgment or decision by the court or other body.

Admission—The acknowledgment of certain facts by a party in a civil or criminal case. An admission does not necessarily constitute a confession of guilt. For example, the defendant may admit that they were driving the automobile but deny running the red light. The term "confession" is generally restricted to an acknowledgment of guilt.

Affidavit—A written statement given under oath before an officer having authority to administer oaths. A notary public is such a public officer and is authorized to signify by their signature that they witnessed the execution (signing) of certain documents, such as affidavits, deeds, and wills.

Aggrieved party—One whose legal rights have been invaded or who has suffered a loss or injury. *Aggrieved party* is frequently used in connection with proceedings by administrative agencies. For example, a person contesting the revocation of their professional license in an administrative proceeding is an aggrieved party.

Amicus curiae—Literally, a friend (amicus) of the court (curiae). An amicus curiae brief is a written document that provides the court with information that might otherwise escape attention. A long-term care ombudsman might, for example, appear in a court case on behalf of a resident. The "friend of the court" has no absolute right to appear in the proceeding, so must obtain the court's permission prior to intervening.

Appeal—The request by a party to a lawsuit for a higher court to review a lower court's decision when they believe the lower court committed an error.

Appearance—The coming into court of a person on being summoned to do so. Appearance without receiving a summons is a voluntary appearance. Appearance in court after papers have been served is an involuntary appearance.

Arbitrator—An impartial person chosen by the parties to an argument to decide the issue between them. Arbitration is used to avoid unnecessary and costly court actions.

Arraignment—An early step in a criminal proceeding at which the defendant is formally charged with an offense.

Assault—See Torts.

Battery—See Torts.

Burden of proof—Also known as burden of persuasion, it's the obligation of the person bringing an action to prove facts in a dispute. In criminal cases the state must prove its case beyond a reasonable doubt. In civil cases the burden of proof is met by a "preponderance" of the evidence, that is, at least 51%.

Civil law—Pertains to a crime; any act the government has deemed to be injurious to the public and actionable in a criminal proceeding. The criminal acts may be felonies (serious crimes such as murder, arson, rape, or armed robbery) or misdemeanors (less serious crimes such as minor traffic violations). A criminal violation may result in either a jail sentence, a fine or both. To picture the interaction of civil and criminal law, assume an employee intentionally runs over a resident in the facility parking lot. The employee may be sued by the resident for money damages in a civil action suit and may also be brought to trial on criminal charges by the district attorney for the same act. (The nursing facility probably will be sued civilly by the resident too, particularly if the employee has very little money.)

Consent, informed—Consent given after full information regarding the matter has been provided to the person consenting. In the nursing facility context, patients must understand the nature and risks of certain treatments before the facility can claim exemption from responsibility for resulting complications. A diabetic resident may, for example, volunteer to participate in an experimental diet program. Unless the resident fully understands the risks involved, the facility may be held liable for subsequent complications. The facility should require the resident to sign a properly prepared consent form. Consent to one treatment or procedure is not necessarily consent to another treatment or procedure, even if such treatment or procedure is beneficial. If a patient resident consented to a tonsillectomy, but the surgeon also removed the appendix, the surgeon may have committed a battery.

Counterclaim—A counter demand by a defendant against a plaintiff (accuser), not merely responding to the accuser, but asserting an independent cause of action against the accuser. For example, if the patient in the knitting needle illustration (see Torts) sued the orderly for damages for assault or battery, the orderly might counterclaim with a demand for damages for assault or battery.

Damages—Money awarded by a court (or jury) to a person who has been wronged by the action of another. The meaning of the terms used to describe the various types of damages available differs from state to state and depends on the type of case. Generally, actual damages, consequential damages, and incidental damages are designed to compensate the person wronged. Nominal damages are an award of a small sum of money in recognition of the invasion of some legal right of the plaintiff, which results in no actual injury, or pecuniary loss to the plaintiff. Punitive damages are designed to punish the defendant for particularly bad conduct, and to deter the defendant from such conduct in the future. Punitive damages are also sometimes called exemplary damages. Double and treble damages are a type of punitive damages sometimes provided for by particular statutes.

Defamation—The communication to a third person of that which is injurious to the reputation or good name of the victim. Oral defamation is slander. Written defamation is libel. Libel is written publication that exposes someone to public scorn, hatred, contempt, or ridicule, especially if related to an individual's profession or livelihood. Slander, because it is spoken, is more difficult to establish. The action for slander has been restricted because of the right of free speech and to avoid overloading the courts with trivial cases. Slanderous statements can only be actionable if they lead to actual damages (e.g., loss of employment), unless the words imply crime, unchastity, or relate to a person's profession or business. In the cases of both libel and slander, there must be communication to a third party, for example, showing a third party written words or speaking slanderous word in the presence of a third party.

Defendant—In criminal cases, the accused. In civil cases, the one who is sued and who must "defend" against a claim of wrongdoing brought by another.

Deposition—A statement given under oath, reduced to writing, and authenticated by a notary public. A deposition gives the attorneys for both sides an opportunity to find out what the person deposed (deponent) knows about the relevant event.

Directed verdict—A verdict given by a jury at the direction of a judge. If, for example, a plaintiff fails to make a reasonable case, or a defendant fails to make a necessary defense, the judge may direct the jury to render a specified verdict.

Discovery—Pretrial devices used by the parties' lawyers to gather information or knowledge about the case. Discovery devices include depositions, interrogatories to parties, and requests for documents and articles. The purpose of discovery devices is to facilitate pretrial settlements and to reduce surprises at trials in order that cases might be decided on their merit (rather than by ambush).

False imprisonment—See Torts.

Fraud—Intentional deception that results in injury to another.

Indictment—A formal, written accusation by a public prosecutor, submitted to a grand jury, and charging a crime. The grand jury is a body authorized to investigate crimes and accuse, that is, indict, persons within its jurisdiction when it decides a trial ought to be undertaken.

Injunction—A judicial direction to a party to do or to refrain from doing some act. Injunctions guard against future acts but do not remedy past acts. When the court issues an injunction, the party to whom it is issued is said to be "enjoined."

Litigants—The parties to a lawsuit, that is, the plaintiff and defendant.

Malice—The intentional doing of a wrongful act, without just cause or excuse, with the intent to inflict injury. Under some circumstances the law will imply evil intent. Therefore, malice (in law) does not necessarily mean personal hate or ill will. The law will imply malice to an act done with reckless disregard for another's safety, even though the actor did not dislike the injured party. For example, the law may imply malice to the act of one who shoots a rifle into a crowd of strangers.

Motion—An application to the court asking for an action favorable to one's side.

Negligence—The failure to exercise the degree of care a reasonable person would exercise under the same circumstances, which results in injury to another. Negligent conduct falls below the standard established by society (a jury) for the protection of others from an unreasonable risk of harm. Negligence may arise from either an overt act or from a failure to act. The term "negligence" is used in several different ways:

1. **Comparative negligence.** In some states one can recover damages even though they were negligent. For example, a resident slips and injures themselves partly as a result of the unreasonably slippery floors in the facility and partly because the resident had chosen very slippery shoes. The facility is negligent because it failed to warn the resident that the floors were unusually slippery. But the resident was also negligent for wearing shoes that had slippery soles. In states that have comparative negligence, the jury determines how much of the patient's injury should be blamed on the facility's negligence and how much the patient is to blame. The jury then apportions the damages (money) accordingly.

2. **Contributory negligence.** Contributory negligence is similar to comparative negligence in that the victim is partly responsible for their own injury. However, in states where the doctrine of contributory negligence applies, all recovery by the victim is barred. Contributory negligence is a favorite of defendants because they can win the case by convincing the jury that the victim was just the least bit to blame for their own injury.

3. **Negligence per se.** Conduct treated as negligence without proof. It is usually necessary to show failure to exercise a reasonable degree of care. Negligence per se is found where the act complained of is in violation of a safety statute. Negligence per se also includes acts that are so clearly harmful to others that it is plain to any reasonable person that negligence must have occurred.

4. **Criminal negligence.** Recklessness or carelessness resulting in injury or death punishable as a crime. Criminal negligence implies reckless disregard or indifference to the safety or rights of others.

Prosecutor—A public official, either elected or appointed, who conducts cases on behalf of the government against persons accused of crimes.

Res ipsa loquitur—A Latin phrase that literally means "the thing speaks for itself." The defendant's negligence is inferred from the mere fact that the event happened and that the instrumentality causing the injury was under the exclusive control of the defendant. *Res ipsa loquitur* could apply to an otherwise unexplained gas furnace explosion in a nursing facility.

Res judicata—Latin for "a thing decided." Once a court of competent jurisdiction has decided a matter, that decision continues to bind those parties in any future litigation on the same issue.

Retainer—A fee paid an attorney in advance for services on a case. In exchange, the attorney must refuse employment as the client's adversary in the case.

Risk, assumption of—The principle that a person may not recover from an injury they received when they voluntarily exposed themselves to a known danger.

Search warrant—A written order from a judge permitting certain law enforcement officers to conduct a search for and seize specified things or persons. Warrants are issued on sworn testimony or affidavits supporting probable cause. Law enforcement officers may not search or seize items or persons not within the scope of the search warrant.

Stare decisis—A Latin phrase meaning "to stand by that which was decided earlier." The doctrine of *stare decisis* means that once a court has laid down a principle of law as applicable to a certain set of facts, it will adhere to that principle in all future cases in which the facts are substantially the same. *Stare decisis* gives the law a measure of predictability. However, a court will reverse itself occasionally where considerations of public policy demand it. For example, nonprofit health care institutions were once immune from lawsuits. Public policy has demanded that such immunity no longer apply.

Subpoena—A written order issued by a court to require the appearance of a person in court. A person failing to appear may be held in contempt of court.

Subpoena duces tecum—A written court order for a person to bring to a judicial proceeding certain objects or documents in their possession. The court may, for example, require a nursing facility administrator to bring resident records to a court proceeding.

Summons—A written instrument notifying a defendant that a lawsuit has commenced against them. Failure to appear may result in a default judgment, wherein the defendant has a judgment entered against them for failure to appear.

Tort—A wrong. Literally, tort means "twisted." A tort exists when (a) a legal duty is owed by a defendant to a plaintiff, (b) duty is breached, and (c) the plaintiff is harmed as a direct result of the breach of duty. For example, the duty to provide care to residents is imposed on the nursing facility by virtue of holding itself out as a health care provider. If the facility breaches its duty to provide care for a resident, and the resident is harmed as a direct result of the breach of duty, a tort has occurred. The general term "tort" includes several specific types of bad or wrongful conduct. Assault, battery, false imprisonment, and negligence are among the types of conduct labeled by the law as torts. An assault is an attempt to inflict bodily harm on another person that creates well-founded fear of imminent peril. An assault does not require actual touching. An assault can be the basis for a civil action (actions outside criminal practice) or a criminal action (violation of criminal laws). In the civil action for assault, the person assaulted brings the action seeking to be awarded money. In the criminal action for assault, the district attorney brings assault charges of the purpose of punishment. The tort of assault is closely linked to, and often confused with, the tort of battery. Battery is the unlawful touching or application of force to another human being without their consent. For battery to occur there must be an intent to touch, actual touching, and a lack of consent. If the touching is knowingly consented to, it is not battery. Assault has been defined as a "failed battery," because an assault must cause apprehension of immediate harmful contact, without actual contact. For example, if the doctor ordered pills, and the nurse approaches the resident with a 4-inch long needle, causing apprehension in the resident of immediate contact, it is an assault. When the nurse actually used the needle (the touching), it becomes a battery (unless the resident has consented). To illustrate the differences between assault and battery consider the following. An orderly bumps into a female resident's breast. If it is purely accidental, no battery has occurred. If the orderly intended to bump into the resident's breast, it may be battery. The angry patient retaliates by throwing a knitting needle at the orderly. If the knitting needle misses, but the orderly is apprehensive about immediate harmful contact, the resident has committed an assault. If the knitting needle hits the orderly, it is battery (even if the orderly was not apprehensive of the contact). The orderly then throws a towel at the resident. If it hits the resident, it is a battery. If it misses the resident, but the resident apprehends immediate harmful contact, it is an assault. *False imprisonment* is another tort occasionally related to assault and battery; it is the confining of another human being within fixed boundaries against their will. Numerous circumstances within the nursing facility can give rise to false imprisonment. If a competent resident refuses bed (side) rails, but the nurse raises the bed (side) rails anyway, false imprisonment has occurred. If a physician leaves orders to restrain a competent resident in a wheelchair, but that resident refuses, tying the resident in the wheelchair will constitute false imprisonment. (Tying the resident in the wheelchair may also be a battery.) Another common example of false imprisonment occurs when the competent resident demands to be released from the facility, but the facility will not allow the resident to leave.

Tort-feasor—The person who commits a tort.

Warrant, arrest—A written order for the arrest of a person from a judge having authority in that jurisdiction.

Witness—A person who gives sworn testimony in a court proceeding.

3.10.4 RISKS ASSUMED BY THE OPERATION OF A LONG-TERM CARE FACILITY

The act of obtaining a license to operate and operating a long-term care facility automatically brings a set of risks to the facility. Some of these are defined here.

Employer's Liability Acts

Various states have statutes that set forth the extent to which employers are liable to their employees for injuries to them. Generally, the employer is held responsible only for injuries to employees occurring in the course of their work. Workers' compensation acts and the federal Employer's Liability Act are examples. Employer's liability acts usually pay for physician and hospital costs. These statutes removed the earlier claims by employers that the employee knew the hazards of a job and accepted them when agreeing to work for the facility.

Often these statutes also hold the employer responsible for negligent acts of fellow employees within the zone of employment. The zone of employment is the physical area within which employers are liable (legally responsible) under worker' compensation acts. This usually includes the parking areas, entryways, and other areas under the control of the employer.

Strict Liability

An employer held strictly liable is subject to liability without fault, that is, without the employee having to show employer fault.

Vicarious or Imputed Liability *(Respondeat Superior)*

The employer is held responsible for the acts of employees within the scope of their employment. For example, if a nurse's aide carelessly drops a resident from a wheelchair, causing injuries to the resident, the employer is normally held liable for the injuries. *Respondeat superior* is a Latin term literally meaning "let the master answer for the acts of their servants," or "let the employer answer for the acts of their employees."

Scope of Employment

The range of employee activities held by the courts to be the legal responsibility of the employer is called the scope of employment. Basically, it includes any acts performed in the process of carrying out one's duties. Ascertaining the scope of employment is important when determining the employer's liability for the acts of their employees.

The nurse's aide who, in the process of hurrying down the hall to aid another resident, knocks down and injures a resident on crutches, is likely to be found to be acting as a servant within the scope of employment, resulting in employer liability for the accident. An employee may be found to be acting within the scope of employment even though the employee is doing their job contrary to the instructions of the employer.

Borrowed Servant

A borrowed servant is a person under the temporary employ of another person. In a nursing facility, a nurse employed by the local community college as a nursing instructor, but temporarily working under the direction of the nursing facility's director of nurses might be found to be a borrowed servant. Using the concept of *respondeat superior,* the nursing facility might be found liable for the wrongful acts of the "borrowed" nurse.

Independent Contractor

An independent contractor agrees with another person to perform a certain job and remains in control of the means and methods of performing the job. Because an independent contractor is not an employee, the doctrine of *respondeat superior* has no application to the independent contractors. Therefore, the nursing facility would not be liable ordinarily for the negligence of an independent contractor.

Determining whether a person is acting as an employee, with the facility liable for the employee's negligence, or as an independent contractor, without this liability, depends on a number of factors:

- the extent to which the facility controls the details of the work
- whether the person is engaged in a distinct occupation or profession
- whether the work is usually done under the direction of the employer or by a specialist without supervision
- the skill required
- the portion of time the person is employed
- who supplies the equipment used
- whether the work is part of the regular business of the facility
- whether the facility and worker believe they have formed an employer–employee relationship
- whether or not the person is in business

Depending on the circumstances, physical therapists under contract to the nursing facility and private duty nurses may (or may not) be found to be independent contractors. Because facilities would naturally prefer to have a number of its employees be viewed as independent contractors in order to reduce liability, courts do give great weight to the label the facility places on the worker. Liability for injuries sustained by a resident under treatment by a physical therapist on contract to the facility might more nearly be ascribed to the facility than an injury to a resident caused by an outside painting contractor employee.

Managing Risks

How Much Risk?

How much risk is faced in an average 100-bed nursing facility over a year? Assuming that each nursing facility resident will have at least 20 contacts with staff members each day, over 2,000 staff/resident contacts occur daily in this typical nursing facility. Over the course of a month, 60,000 contacts occur. Over the course of a year nearly three quarters of a million staff/resident contacts occur. Within the nursing home industry, based on the nearly 17,000 nursing facilities certified by Medicare/Medicaid, approximately 12 billion such contacts occur each year. Each of these 12 billion annual contacts potentially incurs risks to the facility. Consider the following.

Care Decisions of a Nurse Aide

In a recent summer, an Alabama jury awarded $2.5 million in punitive damages to the family of an 86-year-old nursing home resident who was strangled to death while restrained in a Posey vest. The nurse aide, not realizing that Posey vests are color coded, chose a vest to match the resident's gown, rather than body size. She then placed the vest backwards on the resident, causing the resident to choke to death. The J.T. Posey Company, a co-defendant, was found not guilty of negligence because it had warned the nursing home that the vests' V neck should be placed in front. Nurse aides give the preponderance of hands-on care in nursing facilities.

Registered Nurse and Allied Health Professional Performance

In a Pennsylvania nursing facility, a night shift registered nurse, annoyed by the "disturbing" noise produced by a resident's respirator, turned the respirator off while she and a respiratory therapist cleared a 65-year-old man's breathing passages. Then, without turning the respirator back on, they left the room. Twenty minutes later, an alarm on the respirator sounded in the resident's room. The registered nurse returned to the room and found the patient dead in what the coroner called a "therapeutic misadventure."

Staff Performance Under Stress

At a 150+ bed nursing facility in a southern state, 9 persons died, 141 people were hospitalized, and 98 received significant injuries and treatment for smoke inhalation from a fire started by smoking materials at the foot of a resident's bed. State and local officials said the nursing facility had undergone recent inspections and was in compliance with state fire codes. An administrator for the group of facilities said the nursing facility was fully up to code, was well equipped to deal with fires, prohibited smoking in bedrooms, had fire alarms, smoke and heat detectors, and fire resistant doors. Fire, and effective or ineffective staff responses, can occur at any time (Johns & Saks, 2001, pp. 429–432).

Uncontrolled Resident Behavior

At a facility in Dade City, Florida, an 89-year-old resident beat to death his roommate and another sleeping resident with his cane, then injured four others in a room-to-room rampage sparked by squabbles with roommates.

Uncontrolled Director of Nurses Behavior

A jury awarded $15 million to the estate of a resident whose family claimed was given Darvocet (a mild painkiller) under the instructions of the director of nurses in place of morphine (a more powerful painkiller) for a period of 1 month. The jury debated less than 2 hours. Facility owners could show that the resident's physician had written prescriptions for both morphine and Darvocet to be administered as judged medically needed. The jury, nevertheless, found for the plaintiff's family.

This illustrates the growing importance of pain management as part of a facility's risk management program. Older nurses were taught a minimalist approach to pain management. In recent years there has been a movement toward more aggressive pain management regardless of the possibilities of addiction to pain medications. This is an important area to monitor, because in 2006 one out of four (24.84%) residents in facilities were on a pain management program prescribed by their physician (DHHS, 2006, F78, F133–F139).

What Is a Risk?

A risk can be defined as any event or process that can lead to actions that result, directly or indirectly, in economic losses of damage to the facility and its reputation.

Each of the events cited previously are risks to be managed. The following are six definitions of risk: (1) a program that attempts to avoid negative results; (2) liability control; (3) loss prevention; (4) reduction of patient injury; (5) avoidance of exposure to predicted and other risks; and finally, (6) minimization of malpractice claims loss.

Troyer and Salman (1986) define risk as "exposure to the chance of injury or loss; a hazard or dangerous chance." They note that there are "many considerations other than professional liability," and define loss control broadly as an attempt to prevent "financial, human or intangible harm." They include personnel and intangible resources such as position in the community as risks to be managed.

Essentially, risk management is identifying and solving problems before they get out of hand, thus preventing being sued.

For a definitive discussion of the legal aspects of risk management in long-term care see *Preventing Malpractice in Long Term Care: Strategies for Risk Management* by Marshall B. Kapp (1987). Troyer and Salman's *Handbook of Health Care Risk Management* (1986) provides a broad statistically oriented treatment of risk management.

Facilities must ensure that the environment is as free of accident hazards as possible. This is designed to prevent unexpected and unintended injury. Figure 3.13 illustrates the extensive and common exposures nursing facilities workers face ranging from slips and falls to physical violence and verbal abuse from the increasing proportion of patients who have mental impairments.

Accident Environment (F323)

F323 Facility is free of accident hazards

1993	19.7
1999	18.7
2006	21.46 3,419 facilities

External Reporting Requirements: Corporate Responsibility and Corporate Compliance

Corporate Compliance

Each facility is expected to appoint a person to be the corporate compliance officer. The Office of Inspector General of the U.S. Department of Health and Human services enforces corporate compliance.

Hazards in the nursing home environment

Accident hazards

- Slips, trips, and falls, on wet floors
- Burns and scalds from hot sterilizing equipment
- Injuries to legs and toes by falling heavy objects, e.g., food containers and medical instruments
- Acute poisoning due to inhalation or ingestion of disinfectants or sterilizing compounds or their vapors
- Acute back pain, resulting from awkward body position or when performing over-strenuous movements when handling heavy patients
- Musculoskeletal damage as a result of lifting incapacitated patients
- Acute poisoning due to accidental release of a chemical

Biological hazards

- Hazard of contacting a communicable disease from the patients
- Exposure to pathogenic microorganisms in body fluids of patients, especially for blood-borne diseases (AIDS, hepatitis, etc.)

Ergonomic, psychosocial, and organizational factors

- Fatigue and low back pain due to the lifting or other handling of heavy patients and to prolonged working while standing or walking
- Stress, strained family relations and burnout due to shift and night work, overtime work, and contact with sick patients, in particular terminal cases and their relatives
- Physical violence and verbal abuse, in particular from patients with mental impairments

FIGURE 3.13 Accident hazards in the environment of the nursing home.
Source: International Occupational Safety and Health Information Centre, International Labor Organization, 1996–2007.

Over the past few years the federal government has devoted substantial resources to investigate health care fraud and abuse. Health care providers can be found liable for submitting claims for reimbursement in reckless disregard or deliberate ignorance of the truth, as well as for intentional fraud. Because the False Claims Act authorized the imposition of damages of up to three times the amount of the fraud and civil monetary penalties of $11,000 per false claim, record level fines and penalties have been imposed against individuals and health care organizations that violate the law.

Each facility must appoint and empower a corporate compliance officer who has authority to review all documents and other information that are relevant to complying with Medicare, Medicaid and other laws. Compliance issues may range from simple overpayments to be returned to the payer to possible criminal violations. Perhaps the most difficult area for the corporate compliance officer in the nursing facility setting is to monitor the extent to which the facility is receiving all legally due reimbursement from Medicare, Medicaid, and other providers, but not claiming more reimbursement than permitted, for example, intentionally giving a resident a higher RUG score (reimbursement rate claim under Medicare and Medicaid) than is usual and customary, that is, practiced as the industry norm.

Sarbanes-Oxley Act of 2002

This act requires publicly held companies to implement internal controls over their financial reporting, operations, and assets to evaluate the strengths and weaknesses of these internal controls in official documents filed with the SEC (Securities and Exchange Commission) and to make regular disclosures concerning the viability of these controls and potential fraud or losses that may affect the company's financial position. This act covers the roughly 70% of U.S. nursing homes that are for-profit. Compliance with the Sarbanes-Oxley Act of 2002 is more of corporate concern than individual facility concern. The goals of both the Office of Inspector General of the U.S. Department of Health and Human services for monitoring facility expenses and charges is of more immediate concern for the individual nursing facility administrator.

Terms Associated With Risk Management

Civil liability—The three primary sources in health care malpractice suits are: (1) failure to obtain effective consent before intervening in the life of the resident; (2) breach or violation of a contract or promise; (3) the rendering of substandard, poor-quality care.

Claims-made policy—The insurance company pays for the claims made only during the term of the policy and only for events occurring during the term of the policy (see *occurrence policy*).

Durable power of attorney—Appointment of an agent who is empowered to act on behalf of the person creating the power in case of future incompetence (Maddox & Sussman, 2001, p. 611). (Ordinary power of attorney ends when the person creating the power becomes incompetent.)

Empty shell doctrine—View that the facility merely provides a workplace for health professionals and has no corporate liability for their actions. This doctrine was abandoned after Darling v. Charleston Community Memorial Hospital, 1965, in Illinois, in which the facility was held liable for acts of staff.

Euthanasia—A "good" or "easy" death. Active euthanasia in the nursing facility setting is involvement of facility caregivers in nonaccidental termination of a resident's life.

Guardianship—Appointment by a probate court of a substitute decision maker for a person a judge declares incompetent. Guardianship can reduce a person to the legal status of an infant—limiting a person's right to make health care and financial decisions and potentially preventing the person from voting, marrying, or entering contracts.

Malpractice system—purposes of (1) the just financial compensation of innocent, injured residents and (2) the maintenance of a high level of care by deterring undesirable provider practices.

Occurrence policy—The insurance company pays for claims for events occurring during term or policy regardless of when claims are filed (Kapp, 1987, p. 39).

Palliative care—Alleviating suffering even where "cure" of underlying disease is no longer possible (Landefeld, Palmer, Johnson, Johnston, & Lyons, 2004, p. 460; Maddox & Sussman, 2001, p. 786).

Resident's rights—sources—(1) judge-made (common) law based on society's values, (2) specific statutes, that is, legislative law resulting in rules and regulations defining resident rights.

Standard of care—The duty to have and to use the degree of knowledge and skill that is usually possessed and used by competent, prudent similar health care providers in like or similar circumstances.

Substandard care—Four elements are required for a civil lawsuit: (1) duty owed, (2) breach or violation of that duty, (3) damage or injury, and (4) causation.

The percent of accident environment deficiencies remained fairly constant at about 20% over the years 1993–2006. See Table 3.11

TABLE 3.11.   Percent of U.S. Nursing Facilities With Accident Environment
Deficiencies, 1993,1999 and Number and Percent 2006

ACCIDENT ENVIRONMENT (F323)	
F323 Facility is free of accident hazards	
1993	19.7
1999	18.7
2006	21.46; 3,419 facilities

3.10.5 BUSINESS-RELATED CONCEPTS AND TERMS

In the health care field the nursing home industry is second in size only to
the hospital industry in total dollars received and spent each year. The gross
income of the larger nursing home chains is in the billions. The following is
an introduction to some of the vocabulary of the business of running what is
a $100 billion+ plus industry.

Accounting Concepts (additional)

Activity-based costing—An accounting method that assigns identifiable
costs and allocates common costs to specific activity areas in the facility,
sometimes known as departmental area costing. This allows the facility
to identify the profit contribution of each activity or departmental area.
Similar to or the same as the step-down accounting method described
previously.

Agency—A relationship in which one person acts on behalf of and under
the control of another. The acts of the agent are binding on the person
or business the agent represents. The nursing home administrator is
the agent of the facility, thus the facility is bound by the agreements the
administrator makes on behalf of the facility.

Allowance for bad debts—A provision a facility makes for uncollectible
accounts receivable. On the balance sheet, net receivables—the amount
the facility realistically expects to collect from resident billings—is calculated by reducing the accounts receivable by the allowance for bad
debt.

American Institute of Certified Public Accountants (AICPA)—A national organization of certified public accountants. This organizations
develops standards for its members and offers advice to such governmental agencies as the Securities and Exchange Commission (SEC).
Decisions of this group usually become the standard of practice.

Annual report—A detailed statement of the facility's financial position at the end of its reporting year—either fiscal or calendar. Annual reports contain the facility's income statement, balance sheet, statement of cash flows, statement of owners or shareholder's equity, management's discussion and analysis of operations, notes to the financial statements, audit opinion, and other selected data. The Financial Accounting Standards Board (FASB) also requires reporting on all other financial activities, for example, pharmacy holdings, or any other business activities that affect the facility's financial status (Argenti, 1994, p. 41).

ARR Accounting Rate of Return—A method of measuring the potential profitability of an investment. ARR is calculated by dividing the net income by the amount (or average amount) of the investment: *Net income* = ARR.

Audit—An examination of a facility's compliance with accounting standards and policies. There are four types of audit: financial, internal, management, and compliance. In the financial audit an independent certified public accountant examines the facility's financial records and gives an audit opinion. In the internal audit the internal financial officer studies the financial records to assure they meet facility policies. The management audit examines management's efficiency. The compliance audit determines whether the facility is meeting specific rules and regulations (Argenti, 1994, p. 48).

Audit opinion—A report given by an independent certified public accountant that gives the auditor's opinion as to the reasonableness of the facility's financial statement (Argenti, 1994, p. 48).

Big Six—A term given to the six largest CPA firms in the United States. The rankings change over time, depending on criteria used, such as billings or number of staff. In alphabetical order, the most recent listing is Arthur Andersen and Co., Coopers and Lybrand, Deloitte and Touche, Ernst and Young, Peat Marwick Main and Co., and Price Waterhouse (Argenti, 1994, p. 64).

Certified Public Accountant (CPA)—A title given to accountants who pass the Uniform CPA examination administered by the American Institute of Certified Public Accountants and who satisfy the experience requirements of each given state (not unlike the licensing of nursing home administrators through the NAB exam). CPAs are licensed to issue an audit opinion on a facility's financial statements (Argenti, 1994, p. 93).

Change in accounting estimate—A revision of an accounting forecast or assumption about the facility's expected or experienced performance (Argenti, 1994, p.94).

Cumulative Effect of a Change in Accounting Principle—In accounting, the income statement account showing the effect of switching from one accounting principle to another. Cumulative effect shows the difference between the retained earnings reported at the beginning of the year under the old method and the retained earnings that would have been reported at the beginning of the year had the method never been changed (Argenti, 1994, p. 129).

Extraordinary item—In accounting, an economic item that is both unusual and infrequent (such as the replacement of the emergency power generator, which might occur once every 15 years; Argenti, 1994, p. 181).

Financial Accounting Standards Board (FASB)—The independent institution that establishes and disseminates the generally accepted accounting principles (GAAPs) and recording practices. The American Institute of Certified Public Accountants (AICPA) and the Securities and Exchange Commission (SEC) both recognize the statements of the FASB. All practicing CPAs are required to adhere to FASB guidelines (Argenti, 1994, p. 185).

Generally Accepted Accounting Principles (GAAP)—The policies, standards and rules followed by accountants in the preparation of financial statements and in recording and summarizing transactions (Argenti, 1994, p. 207).

Materiality—In accounting, the relative importance of an accounting error or omission in a facility's financial statements. A $200 error in an earnings statement of $2 million income would be immaterial, while a $500,000 error would clearly be material (Argenti, 1994, p. 278).

Qualified opinion—An auditor's report of a facility's financial statement pointing to some particular limitation, for example, inability of the CPA to obtain objective evidence of a certain transaction that might directly or inversely affect the facility's financial standing (Argenti, 1994, p. 326).

Unqualified opinion—Sometimes known as a clean opinion, that is, the report meets all the GAAP requirements (Argenti, 1994, p. 385).

Assets-Related Terms

Attachment—A legal procedure in which a defendant's property is seized by court order pending the outcome of a claim against the defendant. The purpose is to gain control over property that may be used to satisfy payment of a judgment if the plaintiff's suit is successful.

Bad faith—generally implies a design to mislead or deceive another. Good faith means being truthful and faithful to one's obligations in business dealings.

Brand mark—The portion of a brand in the form of a symbol, design or distinctive coloring or lettering; also called a logo (Argenti, 1994, p. 72). Life Care Centers of America, for example, has a caregiver standing over a person in a wheelchair, Hillhaven (Vencor) has a rose or flower symbol above their logo.

Intangible asset—An item or right that has no physical substance and provides an economic benefit. The reputation of a nursing facility as the best caregiver in the community is a valuable intangible asset, for example.

Liquidity—The ability of current assets to meet the financial obligation of current liabilities. Having high liquidity enables a facility to take advantage of investment opportunities and to borrow capital or receive a line of credit at a more favorable rate.

Long-term asset—An asset with future economic benefits that are expected for a number of years. Long-term assets are reported on the balance sheet as noncurrent assets and include buildings and equipment. A new central building for a life care community may have a long-term expected asset value for perhaps 40 or more years to come.

Net present value—In corporate finance, the present value (i.e., the value of cash to be received in the future expressed in current dollars) of an investment in excess of the initial amount invested (Argenti, 1994, p. 286). When a proposed project, such as building a new wing has a positive net present value, it should perhaps proceed; when a proposed wing shows a negative net present value, it should perhaps be delayed or abandoned.

Note receivable—A contract to receive money at a future date. Notes receivable are reported on the balance sheet as either current assets (less than 1 year) or noncurrent assets (more than 1 year).

Off-balance sheet—An item reported in financial statements that nevertheless has an impact on the operations of a facility. An example might be an estimate of the monetary value of a strong reputation for quality of a recently purchased facility.

Present value—The current value of a future payment or stream of payments (Argenti, 1994, p. 311). Present value is calculated by applying a discount (capitalization) rate to future payment(s). This is sometimes referred to as the "discounted cash flow method" or the "discounted earnings method" (Argenti, 1994, p. 311). Its purpose is to estimate the fair market value of a potential investment.

Competition / Risk-Related Terms

Bankruptcy—Inability to pay one's debts, insolvency. Also refers to the legal process of Chapter and of the federal Bankruptcy Code, under which the assets of the business or individual(s) are liquidated, creditors paid, and the debtor given a fresh start. In a Chapter 11 reorganization, the dominant form (Argenti, 1994, p. 94), under the Bankruptcy Code, the debtor's assets are not liquidated. Instead, the debt structure and business are rearranged, creditors are paid some or all of what they are owed under a "plan," and the business continues to function without serious interruption. Under Chapter 7, the conventional form under the 1978 Bankruptcy Reform Act, all the assets must be auctioned or sold in order to pay creditors. A court appointed trustee gathers, liquidates all assets, then distributes the proceeds to the creditors. In most cases, debts remaining after liquidation distribution are discharged. Generally, debtors at the bottom of the creditor ranking receive little of nothing. Attorneys usually refer to a Chapter 7 bankruptcy as a "straight" bankruptcy.

Better-off test—A method of evaluating the strategic impact of an acquisition or business venture on the facility's financial standing. The better-off test stipulates that the new venture must either (1) gain a significant competitive advantage through its functioning, or (2) offer a significant competitive advantage to the facility (Argenti, 1994, p. 64).

Cannibalization—The reduction of income in the sales of a product caused by the introduction of another similar product by the same facility or company (Argenti, 1994, p. 82). A facility may decide to offer newer forms of physical therapy that reduce use of currently used physical therapy methods. If the total combined income using the new method of physical therapy and the reduced use of the old method yields a higher final income, cannibalization is justified.

Caveat emptor—Latin expression for "let the buyer beware." The purchaser buys at their own risk. In recent years, consumer protection laws and the Uniform Commercial Code have implied certain warranties in most purchases, unless the goods are bought "as is."

Competitive advantage—The elements within a facility's operations that give it an edge over its competitors. Building a new enlarged outpatient physical therapy wing might give facility A competitive advantage over its competitors. If, however, a competing facility B counters by building an even larger and more attractive state of the art outpatient physical therapy wing, facility A is placed at a competitive disadvantage.

These are calculations used in developing the corporate strategy to be followed by facility A.

Competitor analysis—The evaluation of the intent and actions of one's competitors (Argenti, 1994, p. 104). This is part of corporate strategy. The information gained in competitor analysis is used to estimate the probable future actions of competitors such as their future goals and assumptions about the marketplace.

Cost of entry test—A method of evaluating the strategic impact of the acquisition or start-up of a new business venture for the facility (Argenti, 1994, p. 121). This test specifies that the cost of entering the new venture must not exceed the future profits generated by that venture.

Debt-to-assets ratio—A measure of the relative obligations of a facility (Argenti, 1994, p. 136). Generally, the lower the debt ratio, the more financially sound the facility is believed to be. The ratio is calculated by

$$\frac{\text{Current liabilities} + \text{Noncurrent liabilities}}{\text{Total assets}}$$

Differentiation—The emphasis a facility places on some important product benefit or set of benefits that is valued by the entire market, but not offered by the competition (Argenti, 1994, p. 149). Numerous facilities sought to differentiate themselves by being the only facility to offer, for example, subacute care or an Alzheimer's unit. These competitive advantages through differentiation (Johns & Saks, 2001, pp. 458–459) are usually short lived as competitors emulate and begin to offer the same services (Hitt et al., 2001, pp. 78–79).

Externality—Any incidental by-product(s), both positive and negative, associated with a particular course of action chosen by a facility (Argenti, 1994, p. 180). A positive externality for a facility that chooses to admit subacute patients from local hospitals might be an increased census. A negative externality associated with this course of action would be the necessity to hire additional staff and provide additional training for present staff.

Inflation—An increase in the general price level (Argenti, 1994, p. 223). Inflation can be viewed as an increase in the cost of doing business or an erosion of the value of the facility's income. Inflation rates usually force facilities to offer higher salary increases in years of higher inflation.

Management's discussion and analysis of operations—A section in the facility's annual report required by the Securities and Exchange Commission that summarizes the reasons for changes in operations, liquidity, capital resources, and working capital available to the facility. The purpose is to assist readers of the financial statements to understand the effects of changes in activities and accounting procedures (Argenti, 1994, p. 267).

Perfect competition—A market that is so competitive that all its participants have virtually no control over the price (Argenti, 1994, p. 305). Characteristics of a perfect market are thought to be (1) a large number of relatively small buyers and sellers, (2) easy entry and exit from the market, (3) a standardized product, and (4) complete information about market price. Few, if any health care markets meet these requirements.

Price elasticity of demand—The effect price change has on income (Argenti, 1994, p. 313). This is calculated by:

$$\frac{\% \text{ change in quantity demanded (sales)}}{\% \text{ change in price}}$$

Each facility, in setting its rates for private paying residents, for example, must calculate the impact on census of any rate increases. Potential private paying persons might go to a competitor if rates at Facility A are raised significantly higher than rates at facility B, other things being equal.

Return on assets (ROA)—Calculated by dividing the net income after any taxes by the average total assets:

$$\frac{\text{Net income after any taxes}}{\text{Average total assets}}$$

where average total assets are calculated by adding the ending balance of total assets of the previous year and the ending balance of total assets for the current year and dividing by 2.

Return on invested capital (ROIC)—Tells how well a facility has used the funds given to it for a long time period. Invested capital equals noncurrent liabilities plus owners' equity.

$$\frac{\text{Net income after any taxes}}{\text{Noncurrent liabilities + owner's equity}}$$

Return on investment (ROI)—A measure of the earning power of a facility's assets (Argenti, 1994, p. 335). A high return on investments is desirable whether a for-profit or a not-for-profit operation. Return on investment is broadly thought of as net income divided by investments, but may be calculated using three different figures: return on assets, return on owner's equity, and return on invested capital.

Return on owners' equity (ROE)—Measures the return that a facility has earned on the funds invested in it. These funds may be invested by shareholders (public or private) or may be, for example, the funds invested by a church in its own facilities. The ratio is calculated by dividing net income after any taxes by investor's equity:

$$\frac{\text{Net income after any taxes}}{\text{Inverstor's equity}}$$

Benefits/Pensions

401(k)—An employee retirement plan, sometimes called a salary reduction plan (Argenti, 1994, p. 182). This plan allows employees to set aside up to a government and company specified percentage of their salary in a special retirement investment account. The IRS does not count contributions to a 401(k) plan as income. Contributions and earnings accumulate tax free until they are withdrawn. Early withdrawals (before age 59 1/2) are subject to full taxation plus a 10% withdrawal penalty. Companies sometimes match contributions. Some long-term care chains use 401(k) plans in lieu of a defined pension plan as a cost saving device. A drawback to the 401(k) approach is that workers, especially when changing companies, often cash in their 101(k) plan for present *needs*.

Accumulated benefit obligation (ABO)—The present value of the amount a facility would owe to its pension plan if its eligible employees retired during that accounting period (Argenti, 1994, p. 23).

Charter—A document issued by a state or other sovereign government establishing a corporate entity (same as article of incorporation).

Contract—An agreement between two or more persons that creates legally enforceable rights and remedies. Contracts must have the following elements:

- Competent parties (of majority age and of sound mind)—In the case of some nursing home residents, the courts decide on their competence to enter into a contract.
- Consideration—Something of value given in return for performance of an act or the promise to perform an act. A promise to

refrain from an act, that is, giving up a legal right, may qualify as consideration.

- Mutuality of agreement—The parties must agree willingly. Often stated as a "meeting of the minds."
- Mutuality of obligation—All parties must be bound to some reciprocal performance. A promise by one person to do something at the will of another person without any consideration (benefit) to the first person is not a contract.

An oral contract is an enforceable agreement that is not in writing or signed by the parties. Oral contracts are enforceable, but are subject to limitations. Various state statutes impose monetary limits on oral contracts for the purchase of goods, and almost every agreement dealing with real estate must be in writing to be enforceable.Normally, no punitive damages are available for breach of contract. A person or facility suing for breach of contract can recover only what would have been received had the contract been fulfilled. Generally, the nonbreaching party can recover money damages, but cannot command performance of actual work. Ordinarily, attorney's fees cannot be recovered by the successful party.

Contractor—One who agrees to do work for another and retains control over the means, method, and manner in which the work is done. Concerning building, a general contractor is one who contracts with the owner of a property to accomplish agreed-on construction. A subcontractor is one who deals only with the general contractor for performance of some portion of the work to be accomplished by the general contractor.

Defined benefit pension plan—A program of pension benefits that employees will receive when they retire. Normally benefits are based on a formula involving years of service and compensation levels as employees near retirement (Argenti, 1994, p. 143). Whenever a facility establishes a defined benefit pension plan it must assure that its pension fund has enough assets to pay the promised benefits. Delivering promised health benefits has become a major liability to pension plans in recent years because of the escalation of health care costs. A majority of companies are moving to reduce or eliminate this type of obligation.

Defined contribution pension plan—A program designating the annual dollar amount an employer contributes to a pension plan. Under a defined benefit pension plan specific benefits such as dollar amounts and other benefits are promised. Under a defined contribution pension plan, in contrast, the employer makes no guarantee of future benefits beyond the value of the dollar amount of the funds set aside in the pension fund each year (Argenti, 1994, p. 143; Noe et al., 2000, p. 458). This is now the favored pension approach among most U.S. businesses preferring 401(k)s, IRAs, and the like as a replacement for a defined benefit.

Employee stock ownership plan (ESOP)—An employee benefit plan that gives employees shares in the facility. These may be voting shares, but more often are a special class of nonvoting common stock. ESOP rules change with revisions to the Internal Revenue Service (IRS) code. Employers are allowed a tax deduction for part or all of their donations to ESOPs. Sometimes ESOPs are used as the acquiring mechanism, via bank loans to the ESOP, to achieve management buyout of part or all of a company (Argenti, 1994, p. 169). ESOPs may borrow from banks and acquire additional shares in the company.

Minimum pension liability—In accounting terms, an obligation recognized when the accumulated benefit obligation of a pension plan is greater than the fair market value of plan assets (Argenti, 1994, p. 281). This must be shown on the balance sheet as a pension liability. This became so great among American corporations in recent years that the Financial Accounting Standards Board instituted a new rule for accounting for pensions that resulted in companies taking millions or billions of "losses" on their balance sheets to show this obligation.

Pension funds—The money set aside by an employer to meet the obligations under the pension plan. A pension fund is administered by trustees who actually pay the retirement benefits (Argenti, 1994, p. 303; Noe et al., 2000, p. 457).

Cost-Related Terms

Acceptable quality level (AQL)—The actual percentage, specified by administration, of goods in a lot of incoming materials that a facility will allow to be defective and still accept the lot as "good" (Argenti, 1994, p. 18). This applies to such areas as dietary where large deliveries of items such as baked goods or canned goods are received.

Alternative work schedules—A method of increasing worker flexibility by offering a number of different job scheduling options. Job sharing by two or more employees is such an option (Johns & Saks, 2001, p. 189). Nurses have for some years been offered plans such as the "Baylor Plan" under which a nurse may work long hours over a full weekend and receive a regular "week's" pay.

Cost-benefit analysis—A method of determining whether the results of a particular proposed course of action are sufficient to justify the cost of undertaking it (Argenti, 1994, p. 121). If a facility wished to purchase a similar facility 50 miles away a cost-benefit analysis would assist in deciding whether the purchase should be undertaken.

Default—A failure to perform an act or obligation. A common example is a default on mortgage payments due.

Deferred expense—An expense incurred in one accounting period that will benefit future accounting periods, also called a deferred charge. Insurance prepaid, as mentioned previously, is a good example.

Economic order quantity (EOQ)—A method of determining the optimum amount of materials that needs to be ordered on a regular basis (Argenti, 1994, p. 158). The costs of possession (storing, pilferage, becoming too old to use) are compared with the cost of acquisition.

Just-in-time (JIT)—An approach to dealing with materials inventories that emphasizes the elimination of all waste and the continual improvement of the production process. This concept was developed in the 1970s by Toyota Motor Company in Japan (Argenti, 1994, p. 242) to assure that materials are replenished exactly when they are needed and not before or after. JIT is so widespread that traditional materials and supplies inventory is sometimes referred to as "just in case." In the nursing facility, however, nursing supplies for wound care, IVs, oxygen tanks, and the like are of critical importance vis-à-vis availability when needed.

Marginal costs—The increase or decrease in the total costs that results from the output of one more unit or one less unit; also called the incremental cost (Argenti, 1994, p. 268). In a nursing facility, for example, adding one more bed might trigger a state requirement for an additional RN on a shift, dramatically increasing the marginal cost of adding one more bed to a wing.

Materials requirements planning—A system of materials or supplies management designed to reduce or eliminate the need for excessive inventories of supplies by analysis of product needs and lead times.

Methods-time measurement (MTM)—A system for measuring individual motions called micromotions, such as reach, grab, and position (Argenti, 1994, p. 281). One method of changing a resident's bed may take significantly less time than a second method, for example. Or designing a facility to have no bed further than "X" feet from a nursing station might produce more care time.

Price controls—The use of government powers to keep the price either above or below its equilibrium point. When the government tries to keep what is paid for a product above the equilibrium, it is establishing a "price floor," such as the price paid for a bushel of wheat being set to assure that farmers continue to raise wheat. In the nursing facility situation, however, the government has sought to keep the price of a product below its equilibrium level, that is, a "price ceiling." By paying only the lesser of usual, customary, or actual health care charges in Medicare, the government establishes a price ceiling. This normally results in cost shifting from Medicare or Medicaid residents' costs to charges made to private paying residents.

Queue time—The time a job or activity has to wait before a particular facility is available. The amount of time it takes housekeeping and nursing to "turn a room" to make it available for the next resident to move into it is a queue time that affects the occupancy rate a *facility* can achieve.

Financing: Forms, Terms

Additional paid-in capital—An accounting concept of the excess amount over par value that shareholders pay for a company's stock; usually treated as a donation (Argenti, 1994, p. 27).

Arm's length transaction—A business transaction at market-established prices between two unrelated parties (Argenti, 1994, p. 43). For example, a chain establishes and operates its own pharmacy to provide drugs to its own facilities. To be reimbursable as an arm's length transaction that chain must sell drugs to other nursing facility chains and disinterested other purchasers at the same price it "sells" drugs to itself.

Bonds—A debt obligation of a facility or corporation or other body to pay a specific amount on a stated date (Argenti, 1994, p. 66). Facilities usually issue bonds to raise capital for building or renovation projects. Not-for-profit facilities may often be allowed to issue tax-free bonds. Issuing bonds usually involves a very detailed and expensive Prospectus conforming with SEC required information. Junk bonds are debt securities rated below investment grade by credit-rating agencies (Argenti, 1994, p. 242). Long bonds are 30-year U.S. treasury bonds or other bonds that mature beyond 10 years. Interest charges used to measure the market in corporate bonds are reflected in basis points: 100 basis points equal one percentage point of interest (Argenti, 1994, p. 59).

Borrowing base—The facility assets used as collateral to secure short-term working capital loans from banks and other lenders (Argenti, 1994, p. 70).

Capital—The amount on the balance sheet that represents ownership in a business; also called equity or net worth (Argenti, 1994, p. 83); or available funds or cash, as in working capital; or financing, as in "raising capital."

Capital asset—An asset purchased for use rather than resale, including land, buildings, equipment, goodwill, and trademarks (Argenti, 1994, p. 84).

Capitalize—To classify an expense as an asset because it benefits the facility for more than 1 year (Argenti, 1994, p. 87).

Capital market theory—A set of complex mathematical formulas that strive to identify how investors should choose common stocks for their portfolios under a given set of assumptions (Argenti, 1994, p. 85).

Commercial paper—Short-term securities (2 days to 270 days) issued by corporations, banks, and other borrowing institutions to raise short-term working capital. Investors buy commercial paper as a very short-term investment (Argenti, 1994, p. 99). Commercial paper is unsecured debt that can be sold at a discount or bear interest.

Cost of capital—The rate of return available in the marketplace on investments that are comparable both in terms of risk and other characteristics such as liquidity and other qualitative factors (Argenti, 1994, p. 120).

Disclosure—A necessary explanation of a company's financial position and operating results (Argenti, 1994, p. 151). Impending lawsuits and other liabilities must be part of disclosure.

Federal Trade Commission Act of 1914—The act that established the Federal Trade Commission (FTC) and gave it responsibility for promoting "free and fair competition in interstate commerce in the interest of the public through the prevention of price-fixing agreements, boycotts, combinations in restraint of trade, unfair acts of competition, and unfair and deceptive acts and practices" (Argenti, 1994, p. 183).

Leases—*Capital lease*—A lease in which the lessee acquires substantial property rights (Argenti, 1994, p. 85). *Finance lease*—A long-term rental commitment by both lessor and lessee that usually runs for the entire useful life of the asset (Argenti, 1994, p. 184). Usually the total of the payments approximates the purchase price plus finance charges. Most leases are net leases, under which the lessee is responsible for the maintenance of the property, taxes, insurance, and the like. In the nursing home industry most leases are known as net net net, or triple net leases under which the lessor's role is strictly that of a financier whose responsibility extends solely to financing the facility, assuming no liability from the operating of the facility. *Leasehold improvement*—Any refurbishment made to leased property, for example, painting, reroofing, redoing the interior, etc. (Argenti, 1994, p. 255). Leasehold improvements (if a for-profit facility) must be amortized over the life of the improvement. *Sale/leaseback*—A transaction in which a facility sells some or all of its hard assets to a leasing company for cash and then leases them back over a period of time (Argenti, 1994, p. 345). This allows for raising immediate capital while retaining control over the assets. A cash poor small chain might, for example, use this mechanism to obtain money to purchase additional facilities.

Letter of credit—A bank instrument stating that a bank has granted the holder the amount of credit equal to the face amount of the letter of credit (L/C). This transfers collection risk from the seller to the bank. A "standby L/C" cannot be drawn unless the payee fails to perform or pay as agreed upon by the contract.

Leverage—In accounting and finance, the amount of long-term debt that a company has in relation to its equity (Argenti, 1994, p. 256).

Leveraged buyout (LBO)—Purchase of controlling interest in a company using debt collateralized by the target company's assets to fund most or all of the purchase price (Argenti, 1994, p. 256). This has allowed small nursing facility chains to purchase much larger nursing facility chains.

Leveraging—The advantage gained by using debt financing to create asset appreciation (Argenti, 1994, p. 257). This is used by most purchasers or builders of nursing facilities, which in today's market cost upwards of $4 million for a 120-bed facility. Someone buying a condominium with a small down payment and a large mortgage is leveraging, as are persons buying a nursing facility(ies) with a small amount of cash and a large loan.

Mortgage—A use of the value of a purchase to borrow money for the purchase of that property by promising to repay the debt on a scheduled basis. The interest rate on most mortgages is set in reference to the prime rate, that is, the interest rate established by money center banks as a measuring base against which to calculate customer interest charges. Banks define prime rate as the rate of interest charged to their best commercial customers (Argenti, 1994, p. 313).

Notes—A borrowing of money for an agreed upon purpose between a lender and borrower. A demand note is a promissory note with no set maturity date; the holder may require payment at any time. Notes spell out the principal amount of the loan and the interest rate and may identify a final date for liquidation of the note (Argenti, 1994, p. 145). Promissory notes with a term of 5 to 6 years are regarded as medium-term notes (Argenti, 1994, p. 280).

Recapitalization—The revision to a company's capital structure (Argenti, 1994, p. 329). May involve exchange of debt obligations for equity interests, or exchange of one type of debt for another. Some reasons to recapitalize are to reduce debt service that will allow additional borrowing, to clean up a balance sheet prior to a sale or merger, or to increase tax deductions (by for-profit facilities) by substituting interest payments for dividends.

Securities and Exchange Commission (SEC)—The federal agency responsible for regulating financial reporting (Argenti, 1994, p. 350). The SEC monitors the use of accounting principles, trading activities, and auditing practices of publicly held companies. SEC requirements are issued as Accounting Series releases and Staff Accounting Bulletins.

Stocks

Arbitrage—The process of simultaneously buying a stock, currency, or commodity on one market and selling it in another (Argenti, 1994, p. 41). The price difference between the two markets gives the arbitrageur their profit.

Blue chip—A common stock with a long history of dividend payments and earnings (Argenti, 1994, p. 65).

Book value per share—The assets of a company available to common shareholders, that is, what each share is worth based on the historical stockholders' equity costs maintained in a company's accounting books (Argenti, 1994, p. 68).

Capital stock—The shares representing ownership of a company. In the mid-1990s, Beverly had 85 million shares outstanding and Manor Care had 62 million shares.

Common stock—Certificates that represent ownership in a corporation. A variety of types of stock exist and are used by most nursing facility chains such as common stock, or preferred stock.

Common stock equivalent—A security that is not currently in common stock form but can be converted to common stock. Executives, for example, are often given stock options, that is, the right to purchase stock at a stated price over a specific time period, as a benefit.

Convertible security—Stocks and bonds that can be converted into capital stock at some future date (Argenti, 1994, p. 113).

Debenture—An unsecured bond, normally in a subordinated position (Argenti, 1994, p. 133). Debentures often have convertible features or warrants attached that permit the holders to exchange their debenture or the warrants for common stock on a stated date or when specified events occur (Argenti, 1994, p. 133).

Garnishment—A legal process through which a plaintiff can obtain goods or money belonging to a defendant, held by a third party, that are due or will become due to the plaintiff. Garnishment is similar to attachment.

A person who receives notice to retain assets belonging to a defendant is the garnishee. Thus, the nursing home may be the garnishee when a court directs the nursing home to pay over a portion of an employee's salary to a plaintiff to repay a portion of an employee's debt.

Grandfather clause—Provision whereby persons already engaged in a business or profession receive a license or entitlement without meeting all the conditions new entrants would have to meet.

Option—A right that is granted in exchange for an agreed-upon sum to buy or sell property, for example, a set amount of stock during some specified time period.

Penny stocks—Stocks of young public companies that are not listed on any stock exchange and typically sell at a very low price ranging from pennies to $10 per share (Argenti, 1994, p. 303). One major nursing facility chain did a reverse split in the mid-1990s to escape being viewed as a penny stock.

Preferred stock—A type of capital stock giving its holder preference over common stock in the distribution of earnings or rights to the assets of the company (Argenti, 1994, p. 311).

Price/earnings (P/E) ratio—A measure of the company's investment potential, literally how much a share is worth per dollar of earnings:

$$\frac{\text{Market price per common share}}{\text{Primary earnings per common share}}$$

Reverse split—A procedure whereby a company "buys back" a portion of its outstanding stock (Argenti, 1994, p. 339). One major nursing home chain in the mid-1990s reduced the number of outstanding shares dramatically by giving one new share for each four old shares held, thereby increasing the value of each remaining share.

Stock dividend—A dividend consisting of stock rather than of cash paid to shareholders (Argenti, 1994, p. 365).

Stock exchanges—There are three major U.S. stock exchanges: the New York Stock Exchange (NYSE), the National Association of Securities Dealers Automated Quotation System (NASDAQ), and the American Stock Exchange (ASE). The minimum listing requirements for the NYSE are (1) publicly held shares of $1 million, (2) market value of $16 million for those shares, (3) annual pre-tax net income of $2.5 million, (4) at least 2,000 shareholders, and (5) net assets of $18 million. In addition the company must engage a registrar and a transfer agent in New York City. The ASE requires (1) 300,000 publicly held shares, (2) market value of $2.5 million for those shares, (3) annual pre-tax net income of $750,000, (4) 900 shareholders of which 600 must own 100 shares or more, and (5) net assets of $4 million. The minimum listing requirements for the NASDAQ are (1) 100,000 publicly held shares, (2) minimum of 300 shareholders, (3) net assets of $2 million, (4) net worth of $1 million, (5) two or more market makers, and an (6) annual fee of $2,500 or $.0005 per share. These stock listing requirements are given because most nursing facility chains strive to move up the ladder to the NYSE. One mid-sized nursing facility chain, for example, was forced to list initially on the ASE, but worked diligently to become listed on the NYSE, which afforded it more status and net worth growth potential.

Treasury stock—Shares of common stock that have been issued to the general public, but are repurchased by the issuing company (Argenti, 1994, p. 382). A nursing home chain might choose to repurchase some of its stock in order to increase the value of its remaining shares.

Value Line Investment Survey—An investment advisory service that tracks over 1,700 stocks in 91 industries (Argenti, 1994, p. 387). There are a number of such investment services available, most of them at public libraries. Considering going to work as an administrator for a particular chain? Go to the library and learn all you can about their financial position! This information can help you decide whether to interview with the company, and if so, to appear well informed during the interview.

Income-Related Terms

Annual percentage rate (APR)—A measure of the true cost of credit (Argenti, 1994, p. 39). APR yields the ratio of the finance charge to the average amount of credit used during the term of a loan, or during the time money is owed to the facility in accounts receivable on which interest is charged by the facility after a specified due date.

Cash cow—A facility or product that generates cash (Argenti, 1994, p. 88). The term, according to Argenti, was coined by the Boston Consulting Group as an element of its growth/market share matrix. The outpatient physical therapy department may be a cash cow for the facility if a large volume of private paying patients use the facility.

Cash equivalent—Any asset, such as a bond or easily sold stock, held as an investment that can easily and quickly be converted to cash (Argenti, 1994, p. 89).

Cash flow—The cash receipts less the cash disbursements from a given operation or set of operations for a specific time period. If a facility has $300,000 cash income from accounts receivable for a month and operating costs of $275,000, there is a $25,000 cash flow for that month.

Contribution margin—The amount by which sales exceed the variable costs (such as supplies and labor costs) of a service. The resulting money left over is available to cover fixed costs, such as mortgages, insurance, and the like. A contribution margin can be calculated for each income producing area of the facility.

Lien—A claim on the property of another person(s) as security for a debt owed. A lien does not give any title (ownership) to the property; it is a right of the person holding the lien to have a debt satisfied out of the property to which the lien applies. If a general contractor building a nursing home is not paid money due under the terms of the contract, they may seek to have a lien placed on the facility until the indebtedness is satisfied. Similarly, regular creditors of the nursing facility, if not paid within a specified period of time, might seek to have a lien placed against the facility.

Net profit margin—Also known as return on services rendered, the net profit margin shows the percentage of net income generated by each service billed dollar in for-profit facilities. It is

$$\frac{\text{Net income after tax}}{\text{sales}}$$

Perceived value pricing—A pricing approach based on the buyer's perception of value rather than the seller's cost (Argenti, 1994, p. 304). A facility with a strong reputation for quality care may choose to price daily room rates above the prevailing market rate in its community.

Profit margin—The ratio of income to sales (Argenti, 1994, p. 321). There are two types of profit margin: gross profit margin and net profit margin. Gross profit margin shows the percentage return that the facility is earning over the cost of providing services. It is calculated as

$$\frac{\text{Gross profit}}{\text{sales}}$$

Rate of return—The annual percentage of income earned on an investment (Argenti, 1994, p. 328). There are numerous ways to calculate rate of return. These are variously termed return on investment, return on equity, return on total assets, or return on sales. Rate of return on fixed-income securities is usually calculated as the current yield, that is, the annual interest or dividend payments divided by the price of the security. Some bond, for example, may have been purchased at above or below the face value and may or may not have an additional pay out at maturity or when called before maturity. In such cases a *yield to maturity* rate of return is calculated, which assumes the asset is held until maturity.

Ownership-Related Terms

Article of incorporation—The instrument that creates a corporation under the laws of a state.

Business combination—The process of associating two or more different companies (Argenti, 1994, p. 77). According to Argenti, there are three forms of business combination: statutory merger, statutory consolidation, and acquisition. A statutory merger occurs when two separate companies combine in such a way that one of the companies will no longer exist: $X + Y = X$. A statutory consolidation occurs when two or more separate companies combine such that both companies no longer exist and a new company is formed: $X + Y = XY$. A number of hospital mergers are of this nature, for example, Columbia-HCA is a combination of two hospital companies. An acquisition occurs when two separate companies combine in such a way that both keep their separate identities: $X + Y = X + Y$.

Core competence—The particular capabilities of a company that separate it from competitors and serve as the basis for growth or diversification into new lines of business. One nursing home chain, Manor Care, has been particularly successful in attracting and maintaining a large share of the private paying patient market in communities that they serve, possibly being that company's core competence (Hitt et al., 2001, pp. 113–114).

Corporation—An association of shareholder(s) (even one shareholder) created by statute and treated by the law as a "person." In effect, it is an artificial person with a legal existence entirely separate from the individuals who compose it. A corporation may have perpetual existence: buy, own, and dispose of property; sue and be sued; and exercise any other powers conferred on it by statute.

Normally, a stockholder's liability is limited to the assets of the corporation; thus, stockholders void personal liability for their corporation's acts. Corporations are taxed at special rates, but usually stockholders must pay an additional tax on any profits received from the corporation (dividends).

A small corporation earning a modest profit may elect to be taxed as a partnership. Stockholders, in this case, avoid personal liability for the acts of the corporation and avoid double taxation. A corporation choosing to pay federal taxes as a partnership is called an S corporation. For tax purposes all income and losses of a corporation pass through to its shareholders.

To qualify for S status, a corporation and its shareholders must meet the following criteria: (1) be a domestic corporation and not part of an affiliated group of corporations; (2) not own 80% or more of the stock of another corporation; (3) not have more than 35 shareholders; (4) no nonresident aliens as shareholders; (5) shareholders must be individuals, estates, or some trusts, not corporations or partnerships; and (6) only one class of stock issued. Voting and nonvoting shares of stock are permitted (Argenti, 1994, p. 343).

Each state enacts its own corporation laws. Some states, such as Delaware, give the officers and board of directors more freedom from minority shareholder controls and thereby attract unusually large numbers of groups to incorporate under their state's laws.

De facto corporations are those that exist in fact (de facto) without actual authorization by the law. Three conditions must be met: (a) a statute exists under which it could be incorporated, (b) it behaves in such a way as to appear to be functioning as a corporation, and (c) it assumes some corporate privileges.

Public corporations are created by authorization of the federal government and the states to accomplish certain purposes. They include towns, counties, water and sewage districts, and radio and television stations. The U.S. Postal Service and the Corporation for Public Broadcasting are two such entities.

Private corporations are corporations created by private individuals for nongovernmental purposes.

Professional corporations are professional associations of one or more professionals, for example, physicians, dentists, physical therapists, and nurses, who form themselves into a corporation.

Courts may choose to ignore the protection provided to stockholders from personal liability, typically when it can be shown that the purported corporation is found to be the "alter ego" of a principal (person). When, for example, it can be shown that the purported corporation does not hold stockholder meetings or generally ignores the duties and activities associated with operating a corporation and neglects other corporate formalities, the courts may ignore the stockholders' usual immunity from personal liability and assign personal liability to the stockholders for acts of the corporation. If the incorporation itself was undertaken to defraud, the courts may hold the stockholders and officers personally liable for acts of the corporation.

Decentralization—The diffusion of authority, responsibility, and decision-making power throughout different levels of a company (Argenti, 1994, p. 137). Beverly Enterprises, long the largest publicly owned nursing home chain, chose, a few years ago, to move its national offices from the West Coast to a central U.S. location and to give each region decision-making power formerly reserved to the national office.

Horizontal integration—A growth strategy in which a company buys a competitor at the same level of services (Argenti, 1994, p. 215; Hitt et al., 2001, p. 535). Several nursing chains have purchased others in recent years, thus increasing the amount of horizontal integration of the industry.

Joint venture—A legal form of business organization between companies whereby there is cooperation toward the achievement of common goals between entities that were, prior to the joint venture, separate. A *contractual joint venture* is joint venture not created as a separate legal corporate entity. It is an unincorporated association set up to attain specific goals over a specified time period. An *equity joint venture* has two or more partners based on the formation of a legal corporation with limited liability and the joint management of it by the partners. Profits and losses are shared on the basis of their equity in the joint venture. There are, in addition, *hybrid joint ventures*, which take a variety of shapes.

Limited liability company, or limited liability corporation—Limited liability companies or corporations provide the flexibility of a partnership with the same kind of financial protection offered by a corporate structure. Wyoming passed the first state law allowing this form in 1977, and over 40 states are now following suit. In 1988, the Internal Revenue Service (IRS) ruled that it would treat limited liability companies as partnerships for tax purposes. The limited liability company provides liability protection for its owners similar to that of a corporation, but allows the limited liability corporation or company to be taxed as a partnership.

Limited liability partnership—A new form of partnership used by professional groups such as physicians, nurses, and physical therapists to limit a partner's liability to the partnership's general contractual debts, the partner's individual malpractice, and the wrongful acts of persons acting under the partners' direct supervision. Unlike the standard partnership, there is no individual liability for the malpractice of the other partners. About half the states have adopted this form of business formation. In some states, protection extends even to the partnership's contractual debts that exceed the value of the partner's interest (Lasser, 1995, p. 6).

Merger—A combination of two or more companies (Argenti, 1994, p. 281). The combination may be accomplished by the exchange of stock, by forming a new company to acquire the assets of the combining companies, or by a purchase.

Minority interest—An ownership interest of less than 50%. In consolidated financial statements, minority interests are shown as a line item in the noncurrent liability section of the balance sheet (Argenti, 1994, p. 281).

Partnership—A contract between two or more persons to pool resources and efforts for the purposes of conducting a business operation. Normally, partnership status requires an agreement to divide profits and assume indebtedness in some proportionate share. Unlike stockholders in a corporation, the partners do not have limited liability, unless it is a limited partnership—an entity in which one or more persons are designated general partners (who assume unlimited personal liability for the acts of the partnership) and one or more persons are designated limited partners (whose liability is limited to their investment). Limited partners do not share in the management of the partnership (Argenti, 1994, p. 258).

Privately held company—A company whose ownership shares—unlike publicly held companies—are not publicly traded (Argenti, 1994, p. 315). A privately held company may be of many forms including corporations, partnerships, proprietorships, limited partners, joint ventures, and limited liability corporations. The same accounting principles apply to privately held companies as publicly held companies. However, reporting requirements from regulatory agencies such as the Securities and Exchange Commission and public stock exchanges do not apply to them. Hence, in most reports on nursing home chains and ownership, privately held companies' financial statements are usually not shown, because they choose not to make them available to the public at large. Privately held companies do make their financial statements available to lenders, private investors, and, as required, some state agencies.

Product liability—The liability of manufacturers and sellers for products they place on the market that cause harm to a person because of defects.

Sole proprietorship—Ownership of a business by one individual. Before incorporation became popular among physicians, most of them were the sole proprietors of their office practices.

Vertical integration—Expansion by moving forward or backward within an industry (Argenti, 1994, p. 390). For example, nursing home chains frequently integrate backwards by owning and operating their own pharmacies. Some chains are integrating forward by owning and operating home health agencies.

3.10.6 INSURANCE TERMS

Actuary—A person who computes insurance costs, usually for the purpose of determining rates to be charged—an especially important function for the Continuing Care Retirement Communities that take life-time responsibility for their residents.

Annuity—A fixed amount of money payable periodically by an insurer under the terms of an insurance contract. Normally, the annuitant (the person receiving the payments) has no rights other than entitlement to payments for a fixed period of time. Often, nursing facility residents have insurance annuities that can be applied to their costs of care.

Beneficiary—The person named in an insurance policy to receive the proceeds or benefits under the policy.

Binder—A contract for temporary insurance until a permanent policy can be issued.

Co-insurance—A division of responsibility for losses or risks between the insurer and the insured. The insured individual might agree to pay, for example, the first $50 of any claim.

Life insurance—Insurance that may be one of several types. Whole life insurance policies can build cash value (i.e., can be turned in by the insured for cash) and normally pay dividends (i.e., interest on the cash value). Term insurance, on the other hand, has no cash value; hence, no dividends. When term insurance expires, no value is left. Whole life insurance costs more than term insurance. With computers, an almost infinite variety of types of policies can now be offered as variations on these two basic forms of life insurance.

Types of insurance:

- fidelity or bond coverage of key employees
- pharmacy

- vehicle and driver
- workers' compensation
- property damage—coverage against fire, flood, earthquake damage to buildings, furniture, fixtures, building contents
- furnace and machinery
- business interruption
- accounts receivable—protection against loss of income from destruction of financial records
- comprehensive general liability or casualty against losses sustained by residents, visitors, and others resulting from negligence not related to rendering professional services
- directors' and officers' coverage for acts done in their official capacities
- malpractice or professional liability coverage protecting against losses sustained by others, resulting from negligence related to the rendering of professional services (Kapp, 1987, pp. 37–38)

3.10.7 TERMS ASSOCIATED WITH ADVANCED DIRECTIVES, WILLS, AND ESTATES

Advanced directives are increasingly important for nursing home residents. Each state regulates the legal status and processes associated with advanced directives. It is important that upon admission each resident set up an advanced directive regarding such matters as end of life care such as whether to be a code (send the resident to the hospital when it is needed) or a no-code (give only palliative care). It is important in advanced directives to determine who has control over care under varying circumstances and how the resident views the directive, for example, whether a no-code means don't send me to the emergency room or hospital for my primary diagnosis, emphysema for example, but do send me for other events, or not. In 2006, 61.14% of nursing home residents had written advanced directives (DHHS, 2006, F78, F143–F145).

Administrator—A person appointed to transfer the property of one who dies *intestate* to those who succeed in ownership. To die intestate is to die without leaving a will. The estate (or property) of persons who die testate (with a will) is administered by an *executor* of the estate, usually named in the will.

Codicil—See Will.

Competence—The capability of a person to make a will. A person is judged capable or competent if they understand the nature and extent of their property, the identity of the property owned, and the consequences of the act of making a will.

Decedent—The person who has died.

Estate—A term that originally referred to ownership of land, but now refers broadly to all real and personal property a person owns or leaves at death.

Holographic will—An entirely handwritten will. In some states a will may be handwritten and need not be witnessed to be valid. A *codicil* is a supplement or amendment to a will. *Codicil* literally means "to say along with." A codicil must meet the same formal requirements as the will.

Incompetence—Inability to function within limits judged normal by a court of law. A *guardian* must be appointed if a person is found to be incompetent. The guardian must handle the incompetent person's affairs until the court determines that competency has returned, in which case the guardian is discharged.

Living will—Some nursing facility residents make a "living will," which governs the type(s) of treatment to be given the resident in the event the resident becomes comatose or in a similar condition. Several states have passed laws establishing living wills as valid legal instruments. A living will has nothing to do with disposition of property (Maddox & Sussman, 2001, p. 611).

Probate—The process of proving that an instrument presented as a will is in fact the valid and duly executed will of the deceased person. Some states have special courts, called probate courts, to conduct theses procedures.

Will—A person's declaration as to how they wish their real and personal property to be disposed of after their death. A will may call for actions desired by the decedent (testator), but must dispose of some property, real or personal, to be valid. Originally *will* referred to real estate and *testament* to personal property. *Last will and testament* refers to the most recent valid will left by the decedent.

REFERENCES

Argenti, P. A. (1994). *The portable MBA desk reference.* New York: Wiley.
Department of Health and Human Services. (2005). Centers for Disease Control and Prevention, National Center for Health Statistics. Hyattsville, MD: Author.
Department of Health and Human Services. (2006). Centers for Medicare and Medicaid Services, Oscar Form 672: F78–F145.

Harrington, C. H., Carrillo, M. S., Thollaug, S. C., Summers, P. R., & Wellin, V. (2000). *Nursing facilities, staffing, residents, and facility deficiencies, 1993 through 1999.* San Francisco: University of California at San Francisco, Department of Social & Behavioral Sciences.

Hitt, M. A., Ireland, R. D., & Hoskisson, R. E. (2001). *Strategic management: Competitiveness and globalization* (4th ed.). Cincinnati, OH: South-Western College Publishing.

Johns, G., & Saks, A. (2001). *Organizational behavior* (5th ed.). Toronto: Addison Wesley Longman.

Kapp, M. B. (1987). *Preventing malpractice in long-term care.* New York: Springer Publishing Company.

Landefeld, C. S., Palmer, R. M., Johnson, M. A., Johnston, C. B., & Lyons, W. L. (2004). *Current geriatric diagnosis & treatment.* New York. Lange Medical Books/McGraw-Hill.

Lasser, J. K. (1995, July). *Monthly tax letter.* New York: J. K. Lasser's Tax Letter, p. 4.

Maddox, G. L., & Sussman, S. W. (2001). *The encyclopedia of aging* (3rd ed.). New York: Springer Publishing Company.

Noe, R. A., Hollenbeck, J. R., Gerhart, B., & Wright, P. M. (2000). *Human resource management: Gaining a competitive advantage* (3rd ed.). Boston: McGraw-Hill Companies, Inc.

Troyer, G. T., & Salman, S. L. (1986). *Handbook of health care risk management.* Rockville, MD: Aspen.

PART IV

Environment

The Industry: Its Laws and Regulations

4.1 Origins Overview and Current Profile of the Nursing Home Industry

4.1.1 ORIGINS OF LONG-TERM CARE—A 400-YEAR TRADITION

Long-term care administration is not a new phenomenon. It did not, as is sometimes perceived, spring suddenly into existence after the 1965–1966 passage of Titles 18 and 19 amending the Social Security Act in 1966.

Every nation has its own tradition of providing care for the aged, chronically ill, and disabled that reflects the demands of the particular culture. Like other American institutions, the U.S. health care system was modeled on the English, just as our legal system has its foundation in English common law.

Early Nursing Home Administration

Throughout most of English and American history, until about 1850, there was little distinction made between the long-term care facility and the hospital. The long-term care facilities in England were called hospitals, but their functions were much more nearly what is now considered those of a nursing home. From the 12th through the 15th centuries nearly 700 shelters for the aged, the destitute, and pilgrims were built in England (Dainton, 1961, p. 21). These institutions housed populations similar to those deemed long-term (or custodial) residents in today's nursing homes: the aged, those without means of support in their own homes, and the disabled.

State Medicaid officials are concerned about inappropriate or unnecessary placement of persons in nursing homes. This has probably been the complaint of many a community that has found it necessary to look after those who cannot do so for themselves. Before 1453 all of these facilities were associated with monasteries, in theory, but were administered by men appointed jointly by the king and the local bishop (Freymann, 1980, p. 21). Did administrators receive training for their jobs in those days? Probably so, in an apprenticeship system not unlike our administrator-in-training programs of today.

In 1536, King Henry VIII, in a dispute with the Catholic Church, closed all the monasteries and their health care facilities simultaneously. One of the most famous, St. Bartholomew's "hospital" (St. Bart's as it was called) in London, had been operating since 1123 A.D. There are no records, however, that St. Bart's had any medical staff during those first 400 years. Pressures to provide care for the poor forced the king to allow St. Bart's to be reopened 10 years later (1546). He took responsibility for management from the bishops and appointed local citizens to direct such facilities throughout England. In this process of removing health care from the Church's charge the king appointed what is believed to be the first recorded board of citizen directors of a public hospital, consisting of 30 leading citizens. This board decided that the reopened St. Bart's could accommodate 400 aged, 650 decayed householders (Medicaid-eligible persons who have gone through today's Medicaid spend-down for eligibility requirements), 200 idle vagabonds, 350 poor men overburdened with children (no mention of the women!), and 20 sore and sick persons (Freymann, 1980, pp. 21–22).

In sum, the board viewed the "hospital" as providing 99% long-term care and 1% acute care. The shift from chronic to acute care slowly evolved over the next 400 years.

During those years, physicians had little or no contact with what were being called hospitals. Medical care, such as it was, was provided on a solo practitioner basis to those who could afford to pay. In essence, physicians served primarily the upper classes in the patients' homes or in their private clinics. Times have not changed much. The majority of nursing home patients today are recipients of Medicaid assistance; they are aged, chronically ill, and poor; and they have lost the ability to earn an income to support themselves or have not saved enough during their lifetimes to sustain them in old age. The well-to-do usually remain in their homes or move to a continuing care retirement community that admits only persons who have ample means to pay.

Nursing homes, like the hospitals, gained the ability to "cure" or offer effective restorative care to patients in the same way as hospitals did during the late 19th and early 20th centuries.

Home Health Care Versus Institutional Care: A 400-Year Old Debate

For the average person in most societies, to live to be very old or to be chronically ill is to eventually be without means of a steady income. These conditions are becoming ever more closely linked. It is as much an economic condition as one of health.

An issue hotly debated in the U.S. Congress and the state legislatures is nursing home versus home health care. Which is better and less expensive for the state? Is health care provided to older and chronically ill persons in their own homes better and less costly? Or, is it more frugal and at least as desirable to institutionalize them in a long-term facility and pay for their care where economies of scale prevail?

This controversy has its roots in the Elizabethan Poor Law of 1601. The first Queen Elizabeth required each local community to care for its poor through providing them cash and in-kind help to enable them to remain in their own homes. In the century that followed, the major mode of assistance to the elderly and chronically ill and disabled was a program to allow them to stay in their own homes as long as possible in England and in its colonies in the New World.

Our present-day state legislatures and the Congress are now warning that the projected increases in the number of older and chronically ill Americans by the early part of the 21st century may bankrupt federal funded programs and state treasuries. The English government and our colonial predecessors, when faced with the same issue early in the 18th century, decided to provide public welfare and health assistance only in institutional settings. In 1722, England enacted a new Poor Law that established almshouses, or workhouses, where it was hoped the aged, chronically ill, and disabled, as well as other persons receiving assistance, could be cared for less expensively (Hunter, 1955, p. 27). This was emulated in Philadelphia (1722), New York City (1734), and Charleston, South Carolina (1735).

1830 to 1930: Nursing Home Care Is Out—Home Health Care Is In

During the early 19th century the pendulum swung back toward provision of in-home assistance to the aged, chronically ill, and the poor. In England this was known as the Speenhamland System (Freymann, 1980, p. 30), in which a minimum annual income was guaranteed to everyone—what the Democratic party has call the "minimum annual income" and the Republican party has called the "safety net" below which or through which no one should be allowed to fall. But these programs are expensive and suspected by many to be abused by persons who are not truly needy. As a result, the pendulum swung back toward a requirement that persons needing assistance move into institutional settings, where care was believed to be less expensive and less subject to abuse.

Between 1830 and 1930, when America was a land of great economic opportunity for all, the predominant mood was to insist that aid to the aged, chronically ill, and disabled be available only in what were called public workhouses.

These institutions fostered two trends that are important in the history of long-term care in the United States. First, they had infirmaries for the ill among their population that were the origins of the early public hospitals in this country. Second, as care for subpopulations in the workhouses moved steadily toward specialization, the basis for the current long-term nursing home population was established.

Separating Long-Term Care From Acute Care: Precursors of the 20th-Century Nursing Home in the United States

To understand the process by which long-term care facilities and acute care hospitals evolved from the same institution, let us consider the Philadelphia Almshouse (1734). Their operations included an infirmary from their inception. It was not until 19 years later that the first American private or voluntary hospital, the Pennsylvania Hospital, was opened in the same city. By 1795, 114 of the 301 residents of the Philadelphia Almshouse were classified as sick (Freymann, 1980, p. 28). Its medical functions were finally recognized in 1935. At that time a reorganization was undertaken and the name changed to Philadelphia Hospital and Almshouse (read: long-term care facility for Almshouse). In 1903, the hospital section became the Philadelphia General hospital.

By 1920, the Philadelphia Almshouse and the Philadelphia General Hospital were officially separated (Freymann, 1980, p. 28). From the original combined facility, two separate institutions had emerged: an acute care hospital and a long-term care organization.

Emergence of Specialization

The Publick Workhouse of New York City (1734) illustrates the slow emergence of health care services specialization from an early nonspecialized long-term care facility. It had been established in 1734, thus predating the New York Hospital, which opened in 1769. By 1825, the medical functions of the workhouse infirmary, until then without medical personnel, had been given administrative recognition when the first resident physician was appointed to its staff. The name was simultaneously changed to Bellevue Hospital (Freymann, 1980, pp. 28–29). Then began a process of specialization of care leading to the current structuring of our nursing home long-term population. In 1831, the blind were removed to specialized care; in 1848, the hospital assumed care of the acutely ill in addition to responsibility for the mentally retarded, children, the insane, epileptics, the infirm, the aged, and the chronically ill.

Subsequent removal of certain categories of patients to facilities delivering specialized care occurred in the second half of the century, so that by 1900 the Bellevue Hospital had evolved into an institution providing care to persons with infectious diseases, the aged, the chronically ill, and the infirm.

20th Century

The dual functions of (a) short-term acute care and (b) long-term care for the aged and chronically ill had evolved as the primary functions remaining from what had begun nearly two centuries earlier as the public almshouse. This process laid the groundwork for the dual development of short-term acute care hospitals and of long-term care institutions in the 20th century. This was a response to the great strides in clinical medicine in the early years of the 20th century. When physicians were actually able to cure their patients of many diseases, separation of short-term acute care and long-term care into distinct facilities seemed indicated.

The first specific remedy in the pharmacopoeia of modern 20th-century medications—Salversan, for an infection, syphilis—was discovered by Paul Ehrlich In 1907. In 1912, L. J. Henderson observed that "a random patient, encountering a random physician with a random disease has, for the first time, a better than even chance of profiting from the encounter" (Blake, 1959, p. 13). Astonishing progress was to be made over the next century.

Separating Long-Term Care From Short-Term Care—20th Century

From 1900 to 1954, the age-adjusted death rate in the United States fell by 57%. This occurred in three identifiable stages: From 1900 to 1919 engineering and preventive measures accounted for a 1% drop per year; from 1920 to 1935 mortality decreased 0.7% per year; and between 1936 and 1954, with the introduction of sulfonamides and antibiotics, the rate of decline became 1.5% per year.

With the capacity to cure many common diseases, the typical hospital rapidly evolved into an institution focused primarily, if not exclusively, on short-term acute care. Some of them specialized in long-term care, and some assigned a wing to long-term care, but the time had come for a fuller separation of the long-term care functions.

During these years deaths due to infection were reduced from 33% to 4% (Freymann, 1980, p. 13), with dramatic implications for channels of health care delivery. Until the appearance of AIDS the health community thought infectious diseases, in the United States, at least, had been conquered.

Genesis of the Current Nursing Home Industry: Federal Government Reimbursement

With hospitals focusing more and more exclusively on short-term acute care, pressures mounted for long-term support to the aged, the chronically ill, and the disabled. In response the United States once more tried giving financial support to persons in their home instead of having them occupy a nursing home or other institutional bed. It began when the New York Old Age Security Act of 1930 was enacted under the leadership of Franklin Delano Roosevelt.

Like its federal successor, which would not appear until 1935, the New York Act provided cash income to persons in need of economic support in their old age. But it excluded those who were in public and private institutions. Similarly, its health care provisions emphasized short-term acute episodic care to the exclusion of direct payments for long-term care in institutions. Persons needing such care were expected to pay for this out of direct cash assistance made to them through the Act. This was a step in the right direction, but these cash payments were usually not large enough to support the resident in a full-time institutional setting. In any case, few institutions at the time were able to deal with this population.

Short-term hospital beds were far more available than long-term ones. More and more acute care beds were being built to match the ever-increasing capacity of the medical profession to effect cures. Not much thought was given to the needs of patients with chronic diseases.

Their care had traditionally been the responsibility of the states and of the cities and counties within those states. As life expectancy increased, so did pressures to develop a care system for this burgeoning sector of the population (Maddox & Sussman, 2001, pp. 3, 599).

The states, cities, and counties were unwilling to assume the economic burden generated by the development and searched for resources other than their own tax bases to meet the cost of this care. A partial solution was to come through judicial interpretations of a seemingly minor provision of the federal Social Security Act passed in 1935.

The Social Security Act of 1935

As a response to the growing numbers of aged persons who could not afford to pay the costs of living out of their savings, Congress passed the Social Security Act of 1935. It amounted to an old-age insurance policy. Old people then were able, if they chose, to use the cash to pay for the first small nursing homes that sprang up. Today this legislation, primarily through the 1965 Title 19 and Title 19 amendments, provides a substantial proportion of the cash flow that supports the modern nursing home industry (Maddox & Sussman, 2001, p. 947).

Like the New York Old Age Security Act after which it was in part patterned, the U.S. Social Security Act sought to enable the aged, and subsequently the chronically ill and disabled, to stay in their homes through funding to support them. It also enabled them to choose to enter the small "mom and pop" type of nursing home that became available. In its earliest form the Act was almost entirely a cash assistance program. The monthly Social Security check was to be the extent of federal governmental participation. This explains why, like the New York legislation, the framers of the federal Act excluded payments to persons who were institutionalized. Similarly, no home health program, such as exists currently, was set up or envisioned.

Legislative and Judicial Origins of Today's Nursing Home Industry

By limiting Social Security payments to noninstitutionalized persons, the federal Social Security Act left to the states, counties, and cities the onus of paying for long-term institutional care for the aged, chronically ill, and disabled. This seems to have been the intention of the Congress. However, the Act did make federal dollars available for up to half of costs for noninstitutionalized care for the long-term care population. Local officials, under pressure to provide assistance for institutional care, sought ways of making this sector of the community eligible for federal dollars, despite the original intent of the federal lawmakers.

Backing Into the Current Solution

The solution (for the state and local officials) came in a series of court cases concerning persons in need of long-term institutionalization, who had been placed by local officials in private homes for care. Often these were the homes of retired nurses or other persons seeking supplemental income. The courts ruled that these private homes/boarding houses were *nonpublic* institutions and therefore eligible for federal dollar reimbursement. In this way state and local officials were successful in shifting a significant portion of the costs of long-term care from the local and state governments to the federal government. Once the federal government began systematically paying for long-term institutionalized care through the Social Security Act, the nursing home industry began an expansion phase that appears likely to last through the aging of the baby boomers—some time past the period 2010–2025.

4.1.2 OVERVIEW / CONTEXT OF THE NURSING HOME INDUSTRY

Profile of the Current Nursing Home Industry

Every day over 5,000 Americans celebrate their 65th birthday and join the "elderly" sector of the population. In 1900, 4% of the population were aged 65 or older; in 1980, 11% were in that group; in 2030, 18% are expected to be 65 years or older (see Table 4.1).

Increased Life Expectancy

Increased life expectancy accounts for much of the change in the elderly population that is of the most direct concern to the nursing facility administrator and staff. Since 1900, life expectancy has increased from 46 years to 75+ years. A greater number of people are reaching age 65 (Department of Health and Human Services [DHHS], 2005, Data table for Figure 26, p. 116). Contrary to what one might predict, life expectancy in the United States ranks 26th among nations for men and 15th among nations for women. It is believed that these data reflect the uneven access to health care among the U.S. population (DHHS, 2005, p. 165).

Increased Proportions of the "Old–Old"

As a group the elderly are growing older all the time. The 64–74 cohort, now referred to more and more often as the "young–olds" increased at approximately

TABLE 4.1. U.S. Population 65 Years of Age and Older and Percentage of Total Population: Selected Years and Projections, 1950–2030

Year	No. 65 or over in thousands	% of U.S. population
1950	12,397	8.1
1970	20,087	9.9
1980	24,927	11.2
2000	31,822	12.2
2010	34,837	12.7
2020	45,102	15.5
2030	55,024	18.3

Source: U.S. Bureau of the Census as referenced in Doly, P., Korbin , L., and Wiener, J. "An Overview of Long Term Care," *Health Care Financing Review,* Spring 1985, Vol. 6, No. 3, p. 69.

the rate of the general population during the 1980s and 1990s. Those 74–84 and 85 and older are increasing at twice the rate of the general population (Liu, Manton, & Allston, 1982, p. 84). Thus, by the year 2000, a full quarter of the elderly were old–old (see Table 4.2 and Figure 4.1). The striking increase in health care needs of the age group 85 and older is dramatically changing the face of the nursing home facility population. Active life expectancy continues to rise.

Fewer Men, More Women

As the elderly grow older, their age group becomes more and more dominated by women. In 1900, men in all age groups outnumbered women 102 to 100, but by 1975 the ratio had reversed, with fewer men than women: 69 men for every 100 women. In the 1990s this was even further reduced to 66 men for every 100 women. The preponderance of women is even more pronounced in the 75+ age group: The ratio of men to women for 1900 in this age group was 96 men for every 100 women; in 1975, this had decreased to 58 men per 100 women; and today, even fewer—54 men—are expected to be alive for every 100 women (Evans et al., 2000, p. 14). No wonder that most of the residents in nursing facilities are women!

Aging Baby Boomers: The 21st Century's Major Challenge to the U.S. Health Care System

From 2004 to 2050, it is anticipated that the percent of the population 55 years and over will increase substantially. The population age 55–64 years of age is projected to be the fastest growing segment of the adult population

TABLE 4.2.   Percentage Increases in U.S. Population for 10-Year Intervals, by Age Groups: Selected Years and Projections, 1950–2010

Year	All ages	65–74 years	75–84 years	85 years or over
1950–1960	18.7	30.1	41.2	59.3
1960–1970	13.4	13.0	31.7	52.3
1970–1980	8.7	23.4	14.2	44.6
1980–1990	10.0	13.8	26.6	20.1
1990–2000	7.1	−2.6	15.6	29.4
2000–2010	6.2	13.3	−2.4	19.4

Source: U.S. Bureau of the Census as referenced in Doty, P., Korbin, L., and Wiener, J. "An Overview of Long Term Care," *Health Care Financing Review*, Spring 1985, Vol. 6, No. 3, p. 69.

Total Population and Older Population, selected years, 1950-2050 (rounded)

	All ages	65 years and over	75 years and over
1950	150,000,000	12,000,000	4,000,000
2004	284,000,000	36,000,000	18,000,000
2010	304,000,000	40,000,000	19,000,000
2020	336,000,000	55,000,000	23,000,000
2030	364,000,000	71,000,000	34,000,000
2040	392,000,000	80,000,000	45,000,000
2050	420,000,000	87,000,000	49,000,000

FIGURE 4.1 U.S. population group aged 65 and over from 1950 to 2050.
Source: HEALTH, U.S., 2005, Data table for, p. 95.

during the years 2005 and 2015. In future decades both the population age 55–64 and the population age 65 years and over will increase dramatically as the baby boomers, born in the post-World War II period of 1946 through 1964, age. By 2029, all of the baby boomers will be age 65 and over. Between 2004 and 2050, the population 65–74 years of age will increase from 6 to 9% of the total population, and the population 75 years and over will increase from 6 to 12%. By 2040, the population 75 years and over will exceed the population 65–74 years of age! (Robbins & Coulter, 2007, p. 43).

The aging of the population has important consequences for the health care system, especially nursing facilities. As the older fraction of the population increases, more services will be required for the treatment and management of chronic and acute health conditions. Providing health care services needed by Americans of all ages will be a major challenge in this 21st century (DHHS, 2005, Figure 2, p. 21).

Medicaid Spending Trends

As illustrated in Figure 4.2 Medicaid, the major funding source for nursing home care days, is shifting its focus away from institutional spending, down 5% from 1990 through 2002 for nursing homes and down 13% for intermediate care. During these years noninstitutional spending for personal care increased by 1% while home health Medicaid expenditures remained a steady 3%.

Increasing Dependency Levels Among the Aged

As individuals age, they become susceptible to chronic conditions (explored in depth in Part 5). Therefore, it is no surprise that older Americans also dominate the dependent population. Of people relying on others for eating, bathing, dressing, getting to and using the bathroom, getting in or out of a bed or chair, and mobility in general, approximately 7 in every 10 are elderly (Weissert, 1989, p. 11). These are called the activities of daily living (ADL). Persons more able to care for themselves are described in the concept of instrumental ADL (see Figure 4.3).

Medicaid Spending Trends

1990   2002

Institutional

Nursing homes ↓

61%   57%

Intermediate care
For mentally retarded ↓

26%   13%

Noninstitutional

Personal care   ↑

6%   7%

Home health   ↕

3%   3%

FIGURE 4.2 Need for institutional- and community-based long-term care: Medicaid spending trends, 1990 and 2002.
Source: Centers for Medicare and Medicaid Services, 2004.

The elderly have higher dependency rates than the nonaged population, and aged women are much more likely to have dependency in mobility and personal care than aged men. Old–old nonwhite females are especially hard hit. Their dependency rates are double those for white males and triple those of nonwhite males. The population at risk for institutionalization is most probably those elderly who need personal care assistance. Studies have shown that nearly 20 times as many nursing home residents need this type of assistance compared to those needing mobility assistance (Weissert, 1989, p. 13).

Over the next few decades there will be a dramatic need for all types of senior housing, both institutional and noninstitutional, as illustrated in Table 4.3 and Table 4.4.

Expect High Occupancy and to Be Overwhelmed

The total number of nursing homes in the United States has changed too little over the past several years to meet these increasing needs, as illustrated by the following:

Nursing Homes, Nursing Home Beds, Percent Occupancy 1995–2003, U.S. (rounded)

	Homes	Beds	% OCCUPANCY
1995	16,389	1,750,000	84.5
2000	16,886	1,795,000	82.4
2003	16,323	1,756,000	82.6

(DHHS, 2005, p. 355)

The actual impact on the nursing facilities of the United States is difficult to predict due to governments shifting reimbursements toward in-home care

ADL	Activities of Daily Living	Generally includes eating, bathing, dressing, getting to and using the bathroom, getting in and out of a bed or chair, and mobility.
IADL	Instrumental Activities of Daily Living	Generally includes going outside the home, keeping track of money or bills, preparing meals, doing light housework, using the telephone, and taking medicine.

FIGURE 4.3 Definitions of activities of daily living and instrumental activities of daily living. Source: Rose, J.L. (April, 1995). Long-Term Care: Current Issues and Future Directions. United States General Accounting Office: Report to the Chairman, Special Committee on Aging, U.S. Senate. GAO/HEHS-95-109, Long-Term Care Issues, p. 5.

TABLE 4.3.   Estimated Percent Increase in Need for Care in Long-Term Care Institutional Settings, 2010, 2020, and 2040

	2010	2020	2040
Nursing Homes	10	20	30
Assisted-Living Facilities	20	30	40
Multiunit Senior Housing	15	25	50

Source: Based on CMS OSCAR estimates of current capacities and projected increases in proportion of persons 65 years of age and older in the U.S. population.

and similar alternatives. Even so, increasing demand for nursing home beds by aging baby boomers will likely fill all nursing home beds by 2020, thus potentially alleviating cash flow problems experienced in the early years of this century. In early 2007, the incoming Federal Reserve Bank Chairman, Ben Bernake, observed that the right time to start dealing with the budgetary strains posed by an aging population that could lead to economic harm was about 1997. In short, the United States faces an unprecedented challenge to meet the needs of the aging baby boomer group.

TABLE 4.4.   Projections of Daily Volume of Long-Term Assistance by Source of Assistance, 1980–2040

Year	Institution[a]	Source of assistance			
		Spouse[b]	Offspring[b]	Other relative[b]	Nonrelative[b]
		Number in thousands			
1980	1,187	1,442	1,438	1,213	655
1990	1,623	1,801	1,950	1,610	880
1985	1,411	1,612	1,701	1,414	771
1995	1,861	1,953	2,232	1,814	1,003
2000	2,081	2,049	2,484	1,989	1,110
2020	2,805	2,976	3,392	2,728	1,530
2040	4,354	3,900	5,172	4,028	2,298

[a] These Projections refer to a full day of care in an institution.

[b] These Projections refer to the number of episodes of caregiving on a given day.

Source: Preliminary data from the Department of Health and Human Services, 1982 National Long-Term Care Survey, 1977 National Nursing Home Survey, National Center for Health Statistics, and Social Security Administration projections as referenced in Duty, P., Korbin, L., and Wiener, J. "An Overview of Long Term Care" Health Care Financing Review , Spring 1985, Vol. 6, No. 3, p. 71.

Resident Rates (Proportion of Population in Need of Being Served) Are Going Down

1995	404
2000	349
2003	308

Resident rate is the number of nursing home residents (all ages) per 1,000 resident population 85 years of age and over. The decreasing rate at which nursing homes are serving persons 85 years and over is going down, not up. While a number of persons 85 and over may be moving to assisted living and other types of multilevel housing and thus getting served, the primary issue is that the number of U.S. residents 85 years and older is growing faster than the increase in capability of nursing home beds to care for this population (DHHS, 2005, p. 356).

Ability to Perform the Activities of Daily Living

The nursing home resident population is heavily dependent on the nursing home staff, especially the nursing assistants. Across the United States, residents are dependent on staff for assistance with nearly 4 (3.94) of the 5 activities of daily living of eating, dressing, toileting, transferring, and bathing (DHHS, 2006, F78–F93).

4.1.3 NURSING HOMES

Facility Characteristics: Do Size and Ownership Matter?

In a word: no. Researchers have been unable to establish whether size or ownership affects process and outcomes in terms of quality of care (Harrington, Carrillo, Thollaug, Summers, & Wellin, 2000, p. 17). Many researchers have unsuccessfully attempted to demonstrate that not-for-profits deliver consistently better care.

Average Monthly Charges for Privately Paying Patients in U.S. Nursing Homes, 1985, 1999

Monthly Charges

	For-Profit Monthly Charge	Not-for-Profit Monthly Charge
1985	$1,444	$1,462
1999	$1,462	$3,903

(DHHS, 2005, p. 377).

The monthly per capita expenditures on nursing home care trended upward at an average of 5.9% each year between 1991 and 1998, charging an average of $290 in 1991 and $433 in 1998 (DHHS, 2005, p. 408).

Facility Trends

Trends in chain ownership increased from 1993 to 1999 then decreased slightly by 2006. Hospital-based facility ownership peaked in 1999 at 13.2% and has been steadily decreasing during the years 1999 through 2006.

Number of Facilities: Slightly Increasing

The total number of Medicare and Medicaid certified nursing facilities declined very slightly over the years 1994–1999: from 15,288 in 1994 to 15,086 in 1999. This trend reversed itself in the early 2000s with 15,933 facilities in 2006 (DHHS, 2006, F78–F93). There are an unknown number of noncertified nursing facilities. Some of these are fully private pay, stand alone facilities while some are in, for example, continuing care retirement communities, but the number, though unknown is small and may range possibly from 100 to 300.

Number of Beds: Mostly Steady

The number of certified beds in the United States varied slightly around the figure of 1,570,000 (Harrington et al., 2000, p. 21).

Number of Residents

In June, 2006, the average number of residents in U.S. nursing facilities was 1,432,864 suggesting that most facilities were not filled to capacity (DHHS, 2006, F78–F93).

Trends in Total Number of Nursing Home Residents 65 Years of Age and Over, U.S. Various Years (rounded)

1974	961,000
1985	1,318,000
1995	1,400,000
1999	1,500,000

(DHHS, 2005, p. 339)

With the total number of facilities and beds relatively constant over recent years, due mostly to Certificate of Need requirements not permitting much new construction, it is not surprising that the number of nursing home residents has varied little.

Patient Profiles

In the National Nursing Home Survey the following characteristics of the nursing facility population were documented.

Age

Under 65 years	11.6%
65–74 years	16.4%
75–84 years	35.1%
85 years and over	36.8%

Sex

Male	38.4%
Female	61.6%

Race

White only	85.3%
Black and other	12.3%
Unknown	2.0%

National Center for Health Statistics, 1999, p. 5.

Average Size of Nursing Facilities

With some slight variations upwards and downwards in the interval, facilities averaged 104 beds in 1994 and 104 beds in 1999 (Harrington et al., 2000, p. 23).

Average Occupancy Rates: Declining

Figure 4.4 and Table 4.5, Number of residents and facility occupancy rates, 1993, 1999, and 2006 demonstrate a slight dip between 1993 and 1999 with a slight increase by the year 2006. Correspondingly, occupancy rates dipped slightly between 1993 and 1999 then rose slightly to 85.4% in 2006. As can be seen in Figure 4.5, during the years 1993 through 2006 the percentage of chain-owned facilities remained relatively constant at approximately half of all facilities while hospitals' nursing home ownership dipped slightly.

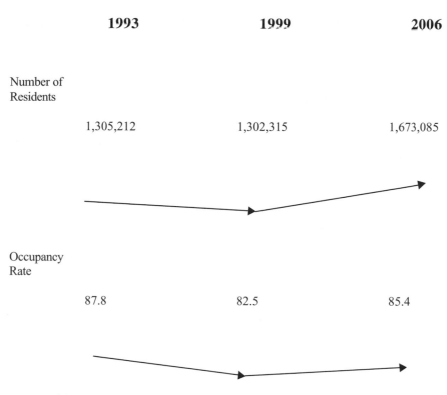

1993   **1999**   **2006**

Number of
Residents

        1,305,212   1,302,315   1,673,085

Occupancy
Rate

        87.8   82.5   85.4

FIGURE 4.4 Trends in number of residents and facility occupancy rates in the United States, 1993, 1999, and 2006.
Source: DHHS, 2006, F78–F93, F75–F78.

4.1.4 OVERVIEW OF THE LONG-TERM CARE CONTINUUM

The American long-term care system, insofar as it can be called a system, is loosely interconnected. Each agency and program is separately authorized by various pieces of legislation. No single agency or program is authorized, or indeed able, to coordinate the various efforts on behalf of the elderly. Although the Older Americans Act calls for and authorizes coordination, in reality offi-

TABLE 4.5. Trends Among Total Number of Residents and Facility Percentage Occupancy Rates for Certified U.S. Nursing Facilities, 1993, 1999, and 2006

	1993	1999	2006
Total number of residents	1,305,212	1,302,315	1,673,085
Occupancy rate percentage	87.8	82.5	85.4

Source: DHHS, 2003, L18, L38, L39; DHHS, 2006, F78.

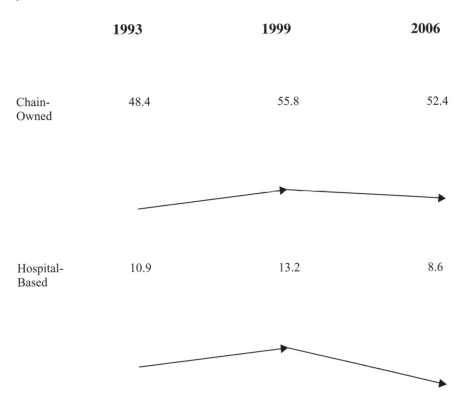

	1993	**1999**	**2006**
Chain-Owned	48.4	55.8	52.4
Hospital-Based	10.9	13.2	8.6

FIGURE 4.5 Trends in percent of chain-owned and hospital-based nursing facilities in the United States, 1993, 1999, and 2006.
Source: DHHS, 2003, F10, F13.

cials of the Older Americans Act have not been empowered to bring this about (Maddox & Sussman, 2001, p. 763).

A result has been that the elderly must largely fend for themselves in seeking services in most communities. One proposed remedy for this situation is called "case management," which is the assignment of each elderly person in need of an assistance program to a specific caseworker, who will help that individual plan and carry out a care program composed of services from a number of different agencies (Maddox & Sussman, 2001, p. 162; Steinberg & Carter, 1983, pp. 1–111). This is, in fact, what employees in departments of social services and the Area Agencies on Aging attempt to do. However, funds are insufficient to employ enough staff to assist all older Americans who need this type of assistance, and most of them are left to fend for themselves. In any event, case management can occur primarily if the clients can reach or come under the guidance of an agency in the first place.

Figure 4.6 describes the major sources of services available to older Americans moving from the least restrictive to the most restrictive.

HOME-BASED LONG-TERM CARE	COMMUNITY-BASED LONG-TERM CARE	INSTITUTION-BASED LONG-TERM CARE

• FRIENDLY VISITING   AAA
• MEALS ON WHEELS   AAA
• CHOREWORKER   AAA
• HOMEMAKER   AAA
• HOME HEALTH AIDE
    MEDICARE OR MEDICAID
• SOCIAL WORKER VISITS DSS
• PROTECTIVE SERVICES AAA
• HOME REHABILITATION AAA
• HOME HEALTHY AGENCY
    MEDICARE OR MEDICAID-DSS
• HOSPICE CARE   MEDICARE
	• CONGREGATE MEALS AAA
	• SENIOR CITIZENS CENTER
	           AAA
	• COMMUNITY MENTAL
	  HEALTH MENH
	• ADULT DAY CARE MEDICAID
	• GERIATRIC DAY HOSPITAL
	• RESPITE CARE
	    MEDICARE, IF HOSPICE CARE
		• LOW INTENSITY — VARIOUS HOUSING
		  ARRANGEMENTS — GROUP PERSONAL
		  CARE, FOSTER CARE, DOMICILIARY CARE
		  REST HOME DSS AND OTHERS
		    CONGREGATE HOUSING DSS,AAA, HUD
		    WITH MEALS
		    WITH SOCIAL SERVICES
		    WITH MEDICAL SERVICES
		    WITH HOUSEKEEPING
		
		  LIFE OR CONTINUING CARE
		  COMMUNITIES
		      NO PUBLIC PROGRAM SUPPORT

AAA = AREA AGENCY ON AGING
        (OLDER AMERICANS ACT)

DSS = DEPARTMENT OF SOCIAL SERVICES
        (ADMINISTERS MEDICAID)

MENH = DEPARTMENT OF MENTAL HEALTH

HUD = DEPARTMENT OF HOUSING & URBAN
        DEVELOPMENT

• HIGH INTENSITY: NURSING FACILITY
                           DSS – MEDICAID
                           MEDICARE

LEAST RESTRICTIVE ◄——————————————————————————► MOST RESTRICTIVE

FIGURE 4.6 Overview of the long-term care continuum.

The nursing facility (NF) plays at least two major roles in this continuum. First, it may be simultaneously providing rehabilitative services to almost anyone receiving a combination of long-term services. It is estimated that 25% of all older persons use the services of a nursing facility at some point. Second, the nursing facility is the major provider of intensive services for persons no longer able to care for themselves and in need of nursing care on a 24-hour basis. It is estimated that at any one point in time, 5% of all the elderly are residents in nursing facilities.

Home- and Community-Based Long-Term Care Options

Table 4.6 provides an overview of various types of services offered under home- and community-based services in 1995. Dramatic growth in the number of home health agencies during the years 1990–1997 increased competition for the typical nursing home patient. However, the number of home health agencies declined after the Balanced Budget Act of 1997 required prospective payments for care given thereby drastically reducing cash flow to home health agencies.

Home-Based Options

Friendly Visiting

Both the Area Agency on Aging and local volunteer groups arrange for regular visits to the elderly living alone. This offers both needed social contact and continuous monitoring of these individuals.

TABLE 4.6.   Examples of Home- and Community-Based Services

Case Management

Assists beneficiaries in getting medical, social, educational, and other services.

Personal Care

Includes bathing, dressing, ambulation, feeding, grooming, and some household services such as meal preparation and shopping.

Adult Day Care

Includes personal care and supervision and may include physical, occupational, and speech therapies.

Respite Care

Provides relief to the primary caregiver of a chronically ill or disabled beneficiary. Allows the primary caregiver to be absent for a time. Often a nursing facility will admit a person over the weekend thus providing respite care.

Homemaker

Assists beneficiaries with general household activities and may include cleaning, laundry, meal planning, grocery shopping, meal preparation, transportation to medical services, and bill paying.

Source: Older Americans Act.

Meals on Wheels

As can be seen in Table 4.7 a variety of federal programs funded care for the elderly in 2005.

Title 3c of the Older Americans Act pays for home-delivered meals. To qualify, an organization must deliver meals (usually only the noon meal) on each of 5 days or more per week and meet certain standards, including providing one-third of daily nutritional requirements. As a rule, the Area Agency on Aging contracts with groups to provide these meals. Nursing facilities frequently offer meals on wheels, both as a public service and as a contact mechanism with potential applicants. The dietary department of the nursing facility automatically meets the various requirements of the program through preparing food for its residents.

Choreworker—Homemaker

Area Agency on Aging subcontractors offer the services of persons who will come into older persons' homes to perform specific tasks. Choreworkers usually do window washing or other less routine tasks. The homemaker visits

TABLE 4.7.   Major Federal Programs Supporting Long-Term Care for the Elderly in 2005

Medicaid

The major source of reimbursement for nursing facility days of care.

In 2003, 1,058,419 were aged, receiving 7.8% of total Medicaid expenditures.

In 2006, the average daily nursing facility reimbursement was	$152.14
In 2006, the average daily shortfall for actual costs was	$13.10
In 2006, the total Medicaid national shortfall for actual costs was	$4,495,000.

Medicare: Title 18 of the Social Security Act

Administered by Centers for Medicare and Medicaid (CMS).

Pays for home health services, limited nursing facility costs.

In 2005, total Medicare expenditures were $324,864 billion, of which $16,976 billion (5.2% of total Medicare expenditures) were on nursing facility care.

Older Americans Act

Provides noninstitutional care help to the elderly, e.g., nutrition services, home- and community-based social services, protective services, and the long-term care ombudsman program.

In 2004, the following appropriations were made by Congress.

Supportive services	$354 million
Congregate meals	$386 million
Home delivered meals	$180 million
Elder rights	$19 million
Caregiver initiative	$153 million

Sources: AARP.org/research, The State of Long-Term Health Care Sector 2005, Reimbursement and Research Department, American Health Care Association, August 29, 2006

on a more regular basis and performs housekeeping tasks such as dusting, dishwashing, and laundry.

Home Health Aide

The home health aide, in contrast to the homemaker and chore worker, is expected to perform only health-specific tasks, such as administering medicines, changing bandages, and the like. The home health aide is paid from Medicaid or Medicare funds, not by the Area Agency on Aging. A home health agency, discussed later, can send such an aide if the older person is receiving Medicare services in the home for a specific illness or injury. Over the past few years local Medicaid offices have increasingly been permitted to use Medicaid funds to pay for services designed to prevent or postpone institutionalizing older persons. Originally, these were called Title 19 waivers, for which states had to apply.

Since 1984, the DHHS authorized all Medicaid programs to offer a variety of services similar to those available under the Older Americans Act if they were conducive to postponement or prevention of institutionalization. Usually, these services are funded up to three quarters of the costs of institutionalizing the client.

Social Worker Visits

The local department of social services, under Title 20 or other authorizations, is permitted to pay for social worker visits to the homes of the elderly. This is similar to a social worker or case worker visiting any other client.

Protective Services—Home Rehabilitation Services

The Area Agency on Aging or its subcontractor is authorized to assist elderly persons to bring their homes up to minimum standards and to provide added security measures to reduce the possibility of break-ins.

Home Health Care

Home Health Agencies are affording increasing competition to freestanding nursing facilities. In the mid-1960s the federal government fueled an exponential growth in nursing facilities through its funding legislation. Currently, federal (and state) support is resulting in increasing numbers of home health agencies on the assumption, probably erroneous, that they can provide care more inexpensively than the nursing facility.

An older person is entitled to receive home health care through any one of three programs, all under the Social Security Act: Medicare Plan A, Medicare Plan B, and Medicaid.

Services Under Medicare Plan A

Unlimited home health visits at no cost are available to any Medicare recipient hospitalized under Plan A and evaluated to need post-hospital home health care for the final DRG diagnosis.

Services Under Medicare Plan B

Unlimited visits, at 80% of cost, are available to persons covered by Medicare Plan B who are found to need part-time health care in their home for the treatment of an illness or injury. No prior hospitalization is required, but four conditions must be met: (a) the care must include part-time nursing care, physical therapy, or speech therapy; (b) the client must be confined to their home; (c) a doctor must diagnose the need and design the plan; and (d) the agency must participate in Medicare.

Medicare does not cover general household services, meal preparation, shopping, assistance in bathing or dressing, or other home assistance to meet personal, family, or domestic needs. Thus, to keep an ailing older adult who requires various types of home assistance functioning, several agencies, with separate priorities and interests, must be coordinated by the client or by a friend or a caseworker acting in the older adult's behalf. During the period from 1966 (the year Congress authorized Medicare to pay for home care) to 1988, the number of home health care agencies rose from 1,000 to 10,850. Home health care agencies are increasingly able to care for persons as nearly disabled as at the skilled nursing facility (Simon-Rusinowitz & Hofland, 1993, p. 159). A cost effectiveness study by Greene, Lovely, and Ondrich found that 41% of persons studied could be effectively cared for outside the nursing facility (1993, p. 179). There has been a steady movement toward increasing utilization of home health care (Manton, Stallard, & Woodbury, 1994, p. 155). In 1995, the American Academy of Medical Administrators formed a division for home health care executives, a further recognition of the maturing of this field (Shriver, 1995, p. 35).

In 1982, 1.1 million Americans were receiving home health care. The number of home health agency patients peaked at 2.4 million in 1996 and was 1.3 million in the year 2000, close to the 1982 level (DHHS, 2005, p. 322).

While home health care is expected to remain a significant competitor for the nursing home patient its growth is difficult to predict. With virtually no requirements for opening and operating a home health agency in place many opened home health agencies with no health background. When the federal government passed more effective regulations the number of home health agencies decreased (DHHS, 2005, p. 322).

The trajectory of the home health care industry can be seen here:

Millions of Patients Served

1988	1.1
1992	1.2

1994   1.8
1996   2.4
1998   1.8
2000   1.3
(DHHS, 2005, p. 322)

In 2000, diseases of the circulatory system (heart 11%, cerebrovascular disease 7%) were the most common primary admission diagnosis (DHHS, 2005, p. 322).

By 1993, there were 7,400 home health agencies of which 37% were proprietary, 43% nonprofit, and 20% government and other. A high percentage were certified by Medicare (84%) and Medicaid (83%; Strahan, 1994, p. 2). Of all patients receiving home health care the proportion publicly paid for is even higher: 89% on Medicare and 91% on Medicaid. In short, when compared to nursing home care payment sources, a dramatically higher percentage of costs of home health care patients are paid by Medicare and Medicaid. The same is equally true of hospice patients, 90% of whom are both Medicare and Medicaid eligible (Strahan, 1994, p. 3). It has been estimated that between 5% and 10% of physician time is spent in home health care, some of them are full time (Council on Scientific Affairs, 1990, p. 1244). By 1998, some 20,000 providers were delivering home care with annual expenditures of over $40 billion (Maddox & Sussman, 2001, p. 494).

Medicaid Services

If a Medicaid recipient is found apt to need full-time institutional care, Medicaid can pay for nearly any of the types of in-home services available through either Medicare or the Area Agency on Aging.

The economic rationale of this program is to reduce public expenditures by offering services that allow people to function in their own home where they, or often their family, will be sharing the financial burden, thus reducing public costs. The care rationale to encourage them to remain at home is based on the positive psychological and emotional benefits.

Hospice Care

Hospice care is given to persons usually believed to be at the end of their lives, with perhaps 6 months or less to live, who mainly seek alleviation from pain rather than intensive technological medical treatment. Hospice care is usually provided at home. There is a trend for hospice agencies to attend such patients in nursing facilities. Hospice is also offered in freestanding hospice centers for inpatients and patient wards in hospitals designated as hospice units, as well as for individual patients on other wards.

Medicare Plan A pays for hospice care if three conditions are met: (a) medical certification that the patient is terminally ill; (b) patient's choice is to receive care from a hospice instead of the standard Medicare benefits; and (c) the program must be provided by a Medicare certified hospice. People who choose hospice can be given Medicare Plan A hospitalization care for events unrelated to their terminal illness, for example, a bone broken during an accidental fall (Maddox & Sussman, 2001, p. 494).

The Centers for Medicare and Medicaid Services defines hospice as a public agency or private organization that is primarily engaged in providing pain relief, symptom management, and supportive services to terminally ill people and their families. Medicare pays 100% of all hospice services except for 55% of outpatient drugs and respite care.

By 1998, 540,000 terminally ill persons were receiving hospice care through 2,287 agencies. About 68% of hospice patients were 65 and older, and 71% listed cancer as the major disease. By the year 2000, the percent of hospice patients with cancer as the primary diagnosis had dropped slightly to 52% (DHHS, 2005, p. 323). About 90% of hospices are not-for-profit. In 1998, 39% were independent agencies, 25% were hospital programs, 35% were part of a home health agency, and 1% were managed by nursing facilities (Maddox & Sussman, 2001, p. 494).

Conventional wisdom suggests Medicare is wasteful, spending about 30% of its total on people in the last year of their lives, most of it during their last month. However, a Medicare program self-study of those expenditures when compared with costs for survivors differed little during 1976, 1980, 1985, and 1988. Payments during the last month do not differ as dramatically as believed (Burke, p. 36). Burke concluded that any evidence that people in the last year of life account for a larger share of expenditures than beneficiaries who are younger is inconclusive. One study suggests that when all of medical services are included the costs for the "older old" might be somewhat less during their last year of life (Burke, p. 36).

Report of a costly investigation by the Robert Wood Johnson Foundation involving 9,000 patients in five large hospitals in the *Journal of the American Medical Association* (November 22, 1995) revealed that an aggressive effort to improve counseling and communications between doctors and terminally ill patients and their families had no impact on the cost and intensity of their end-of-life experience. In short, managing the costs of dying is proving to be a complex social phenomenon with which nursing home personnel and the medical care community will be wrestling for some time to come.

In 2006, 3.42% of residents in nursing facilities were receiving care both from the facility and a hospice care program (DHHS, 2006, F78–F93).

Community-Based Long-Term Care

Congregate Meals at Nutrition Sites and Senior Citizens Centers

Under Title 3c of the Older Americans Act, an effort has been made to make congregate meal sites available to as many elderly as possible in both urban and rural areas.

To accomplish this the Area Agencies on Aging contract with many thousands of groups who serve such meals 5 or more days a week. Often these nutrition sites, as they are called, are rural schools or churches that are usually centrally located. Transportation is usually provided as well as counseling, nutrition education, recreation, and referral services at the same site and time.

Senior Citizen Centers Activities and In-Center Services

The Area Agencies on Aging offer a variety of activities and services at these centers, and usually congregate meals as well.

Community Mental Health Centers

Mental health legislation over the past two decades has resulted in the establishment of an extensive network of community mental health centers to which older persons may refer themselves or be referred. However, the utilization rate of these centers has tended to be disproportionately low among the elderly.

Adult Day Care

An adult day care program is a community organization providing daytime health or recreational services to groups of impaired older adults in a centralized protective environment, often for long periods of time (Landefeld, Palmer, Johnson, Johnston, & Lyons, 2004, p. 38). Nursing facilities are uniquely positioned to offer adult day care programs, and some do. Payments for adult day care can come from various sources, including federal revenue sharing programs, Title 4 of the Older Americans Act, Title 6 of the Social Security Act, and Medicaid.

People enter an adult day care program for a variety of reasons, such as need for the caregiver to be at work during the day. Its primary function is to allow older persons with various kinds of disabilities to remain in the home setting longer.

Often the adult day care participant in a nursing facility eventually becomes a resident there. This earlier exposure to the environment serves to reduce the trauma usually involved in the transition to institutional care.

Adult day care began in the mid-1970s. The National Institute of Adult Day Care was established in 1979. The average day care program cares for about 22 persons, between 9:00 A.M. and 3:00 P.M. at an average cost of $43 per day in 1997 (Maddox & Sussman, 2001, p. 19). Day care programs normally offer a structured day including social interaction, exercise, and a hot noontime meal. Some offer case management, health assessment, nutrition education, and therapeutic diets (Weissert, 1985, pp. 640–646).

A majority of adult day centers are located in nursing homes. The majority of such participants are functionally dependent elderly white women. Most are unmarried and about a third are mentally impaired. Compared to the nursing home resident, they tend to be younger, less dependent, and have less mental impairment. Few, if any, adult day care programs are physically located in a hospital (Weissert, 1985, p. 648).

Geriatric day rehabilitation hospitals are a medical model of the adult day care program. Adult day care programs range from offering recreation with no health care to nearly full health services similar in intensity to those of the nursing facility. Several studies have concluded that stand alone adult day care centers and day care hospitals achieve the same outcomes (Maddox & Sussman, 2001, p. 20).

Adult Foster Care

This form of care is typically defined as care for no more than six unrelated persons in a community-based residence (Maddox & Sussman, 2001, p. 24). Twenty-four hour supervision and care are offered. Sponsorship can be individuals or public of similar agencies. There are no accurate estimates of how many such facilities exist (Maddox & Sussman, 2001, p. 26).

Respite Care

Respite care is a relatively new program under Medicare Plan A, where it is defined as a short-term inpatient stay that provides temporary relief to the person who regularly assists with home care (DHHS, 2005, p. 20; Maddox & Sussman, 2001, p. 882).

Under Medicare, respite care is available only to caregivers of hospice patients. Medicare will pay 95% of the costs and 100% of the costs after the patient has paid a specified number of dollars of coinsurance. Medicare limits inpatient respite care to stays of no more than 5 consecutive days.

Depending on occupancy level, nursing facilities have offered respite care over the years. Some organizational obstacles to their ability to do so are (a) costs involved in the extensive paperwork required at each admission and discharge, regardless of whether the patient is a regular or a hospice resident, and (b) costs associated with keeping beds empty for hospice type admissions, which by definition are of short duration and therefore incur higher administrative costs to the facility.

In late 2006, Congress authorized the Lifespan Respite Care Act, which for the first time reimbursed family members (not just unrelated persons).

Informal Caregiving

Estimates are that 2.6 to 22 million active caregivers are assisting the noninstitutionalized elderly in the United States. An estimated additional 1.69 million persons are informal caregivers in the nursing homes and similar settings (Maddox & Sussman, 2001, p. 541). By one estimate, that of the National Caregiver Support Program, that had increased to 44 million persons providing unpaid care by 2006.

New Web resources for persons seeking elder care help include:

- Eldercare Locator (www.eldercare.gov): connects seniors to federal state and local resources.
- National Association of Professional Geriatric Case Managers (www. caremanager.org): helps design care plans and determines when nursing home care is needed.
- National Academy of Elder Law Attorneys (www.naela.com): helps prepare documents such as health care power of attorney, wills, and estate planning.

The economic value of noninstitutional caregiving in the top 10 states ranged from $30 billion in California to $7.5 billion in North Carolina in 2003.

Institution-Based Care

Low-Intensity Institutional-Based Arrangements: Housing

An almost infinite range of housing options faces the elderly attempting to decide where and how to live out their final years. Numerous group housing arrangements exist. These are variously called group homes, family homes, personal care homes, foster care homes, domiciliary care homes or, often, rest homes. The number of older adults involved varies from three or four in a group or foster home to as many as several hundred in "rest" homes. The major source of public support for these housing arrangements is the local department of social services that administers the Medicaid program. A new variety of care giving for elderly persons is emerging that is variously named but most often referred to as assisted living. Definitions vary confusingly from state to state (Landefeld et al., 2004, p. 38).

Congregate care housing arrangements exist in many forms. These usually are publicly supported housing sites for elderly and disabled persons. Support can come from numerous public sources, including local tax moneys.

These housing arrangements range from no services to a progressive array that includes meals, social services, housekeeping, and medical care. Often they are high-rise buildings or small complexes that offer the low-income person an approximate equivalent to the services offered to middle- and upper-income Americans in what are called life care or continuing care communities.

Life or continuing care retirement communities (CCRCs) are a relatively new phenomenon, at least on the scale on which they are now being offered. This type of setting can be a microcosm of the community at large with its diverse services.

Continuing Care Retirement Communities (CCRCs)

This text focuses on the nursing facility. However, professional preparation as a nursing home administrator offers simultaneous preparation for becoming the administrator of a continuing care retirement community (CCRC).

The original CCRCs, often called life care communities, were usually set up and managed by religious communities. In return for all their worldly possessions, participants were promised care for the rest of their life. Today, the typical resident pays a one-time entrance fee plus monthly fees.

The CCRC that offers life care is, in essence, an insurance pooling. The entry and monthly fees are set based on actuarial calculations to cover the expected lifetime costs of each resident. In exchange for the entry and monthly fees residents of life care communities are guaranteed care no matter how long they live, even if one's personal funds run out. Not every resident will need expensive nursing facility care, but the fees paid by all residents pay for those who do. As with an insurance annuity, those who live longer receive more benefits than those who die earlier.

Normally, the new resident initially occupies either a detached (garden) apartment or moves into an apartment building. As the need arises for more protected and assisted living, residents may move progressively from a detached unit, to an attached apartment, to "sheltered" care (assisted living), and as needed, into full-time nursing care.

In 1990, CCRCs were serving some 230,000 residents whose average age was 82, 79% of whom were women. Average age at entrance was 77 (a second retirement for most). The average age in their nursing centers was 86. Currently, the number of CCRCs is estimated to be between 1,200 and 1,800.

The CCRC is predominantly a middle-class, elderly housing phenomenon—the rich have assistance brought into their homes. Entry fees usually are set to collect 25% of projected lifetime costs with the monthly service fees collecting the remaining 75%. Few, if any facilities place a cap on monthly service fees: These fees must fluctuate to account for inflation and other costs. CCRC administrations prefer to admit only persons capable of independent living. The relationship between the resident and the administration is lengthy—24 hours a day, 12 to 14 years. The administrators guarantee a service package with no time constraints and no limit on cost in the full-featured CCRC.

Array of Facilities

A broad array of financial arrangements have emerged. Three types of CCRCs are identified in the literature (Landefeld et al., 2004, p. 39).

Type A, or all-inclusive (about 33% of CCRCs) guarantee fully paid nursing care for as long as needed at no extra cost beyond the resident's monthly fee. Many services are "bundled" or included in the monthly fee (e.g., two or more meals each day, cleaning, laundry, linen, utilities, and recreation facilities). Fees vary by geographical area and size of living unit with entry fees averaging $70,000 to well over $500,000 and monthly fees averaging $900 to well over $3,000.

Type B, or modified CCRCs (about 26% of facilities) usually offer nursing care at no substantial increase in monthly fees, but include fewer services. Fees, for example, may be charged for cleaning or laundry, and only one or two meals may be included. Residents in this type of community assume some of the financial risk of extended nursing care costs. Entry and monthly fees are commensurably reduced.

Type C, or fee-for-service CCRCs (about 38% of CCRCs) usually offer no meals or personal care service in the monthly fee. Access to nursing care, onsite (usually) or off-site, is normally guaranteed, but the resident using the service bears the full costs.

Originally entry fees were usually nonrefundable. Competition for residents has spawned an array of approaches varying from no refund to 100% refund upon resale of one's unit.

Eighty to 90% of all CCRCs are not-for-profit, most of them also having a church affiliation. However, for-profit corporations have been eager to enter the field.

Regulation

Resident contracts vary. By 1990, 31 states had some type of regulation in effect, but little uniformity existed among them. Some states regulate through the insurance department, others through the health department, offices on aging, or even departments that supervise securities and corporations.

Successfully building and operating a CCRC is a complex business venture. The most common reason for failure is low occupancy rate—major costs are fixed.

4.1.5 HOSPITAL TRENDS: UNDERSTANDING THE CHANGING NURSING HOME CASE MIX

Hospitals may be regarded as the weather vane for where health care industry providers such as nursing facilities and home health care agencies may be heading. This tends to be true because ultimately the behavior of the health care industry is driven by cost and new technologies. Generally, to understand hospital trends is to understand nursing facility trends.

U.S. Hospital Trends 1975–2003

	1975	1990	2000	2003
Number of all hospitals*	7,156	6,649	5,810	5,764
Community	5,875	3,191	3,003	2,984
For-profit	775	749	749	790
Admissions (in thousands)	36,157	33,774	34,891	36,611
Average length of stay in days, all hospitals	11.4	9.1	6.8	6.6
Average length of stay in days, 65–74 years old	10.7	8.7	6.0	5.7
Average length of stay in days, 75 years and older	11.4	9.2	6.2	5.8
Days of care per 1,000 pop.	1,297	819	557	574
Outpatient visits (thousands)	255,000	368,000	593,000	649,000
Outpatient surgeries in percent of total surgeries	16	50	63	63
Occupancy rates in percent, 1960 75%	76	67	64	66
Community	77	69	65	68
For-profit	66	53	56	60

*includes federal and state–local government owned hospitals
(DHHS, 2005, pp. 338, 354, 351)

Changes in the Wind

These hospital data reveal a number of trends in the health care field most of which impact the nursing facility. From 1965 (federal Medicare reimbursement legislation) until 1985 (federal Diagnostic Related Group reimbursement legislation) hospitals simply billed the federal government whatever they wished and were reimbursed. Beginning in 1984, hospitals were paid a fixed fee on a per admission basis based on what the federal government was willing to pay for the admitting diagnosis no matter whether the patient stayed 2 days or 10 days. This change in how hospitals were paid for their services dramatically changed how hospitals cared for patients and when nursing homes received discharged hospital patients (sooner and sicker).

Number of Hospitals, Ownership Changes

From 1975 to 2003, the total number of hospitals in the United States dropped from 7,156 to 5,764. With the federal government no longer paying whatever not-for-profit community hospitals billed, their numbers dropped dramatically from 5,875 in 1975 down to 2,984 in 2003. County and city hospitals became a county or city tax burden once the federal government limited payment beginning in 1984. For-profit hospital chains bought several of these not-for-profits increasing their number from 775 in 1975 to 790 in 2003. Still, community (not-for-profit) hospitals deliver the majority of care.

Admissions

Admissions remained relatively steady from 1975 to 2003: In 1975 there were 36,157 admissions; in 2003 there were 36,611 admissions. What happened to these admissions has undergone dramatic changes, most of which have affected the nursing facility case mix.

Average Length of Stay, Days of Care Drop Dramatically

While admissions remained relatively constant the average number of days patients stayed once admitted dropped from 11.4 days in 1975 to 6.6 days in 2003, a response to receiving a single pre-set federal reimbursement per patient stay regardless of length of stay and improved technologies allowing for less invasive techniques and faster patient recuperation. Thus, the days of care per 1,000 population dropped from 1,297 down to 574. By 2003, patients were being discharged to nursing homes (and similar settings) at twice the rate as they had been in 1975.

Average Length of Stay for Persons 65 and Older

Typically, older persons stayed in the hospital longer, but the new reimbursement system (paying a fixed number of dollars per admission no matter how many days the patient stays) had a similarly dramatic effect on when patients were discharged to nursing homes: after 11-day hospital stays in 1975, after 5-day stays in 2003. In effect, hospitals currently use nursing homes to provide the subacute care provided in 1975, but no longer provided in the hospital by 2003.

Changes in How Hospitals Do Business

With lowered federal reimbursement and improving technology and drugs hospitals began emphasizing outpatient visits: 255,000 in 1975 and 649,000 in 2003—thus avoiding the more costly inpatient days for which reimbursement was more limited.

Outpatient surgery experienced a similarly dramatic trend: 16% outpatient surgery in 1975 and 63% outpatient surgery in 2003. A significant portion of surgical patients that were being cared for post-operatively in the hospitals were being discharged to the nursing home setting for subacute care once given in the hospital.

Hospital Expenses in the United States

Hospital care remains the largest single source of health care expenditures, increasing from $92 billion in 1980 to $498 billion in 2003. The average annual percent change in hospital costs from 1980 to 1990 was 9.8%, decreasing only slightly to 8.0% during the years 2000–2003 (DHHS, 2005, p. 376). Per capita expenditures for hospital care increase each year rising from $1,109 in 1991 to $1,405 in 1998 (DHHS, 2005, p. 405).

What Is the Least Expensive Level of Care?

Health care systems facility usages are cost driven. Hospital care costs thousands of dollars per day; nursing home care costs hundreds of dollars per day. Health care payers, whether government entities or private entities, prefer lower daily rates for health care. The acuity level in nursing homes is increasing in response to the dramatically high cost per hospital day of stay.

Occupancy Rates as Behavioral Influences

Even though admission rates have held steady over the past several decades, occupancy rates have gone down because the relatively same number of patients admitted to U.S. hospitals each year were staying fewer days per admission. Occupancy rates dropped in response to the advent of federal preset reimbursement rate regardless of length of stay and improving technologies. In the 1960s and 1970s, community hospitals enjoyed 75% and 76% occupancy rates . . . high enough to be a sustainable business model. By 2003, occupancy rates in not-for-profit (community) hospitals had dropped to 66%, and for-profit hospitals occupancy rate of 60% resulted in strained finances.

Hospitals and home health care agencies are vying for many of the same residents sought by the freestanding nursing facility. As a result of lowered occupancy rates, hospitals are adding hospital-based nursing facilities at an alarming rate. By 1991, 767 hospitals had 56,292 beds and were serving 51,897 patients. The trend for hospitals to build and operate their own nursing homes is continuing. The economic incentive for hospitals to own nursing home beds is simple. Placing a hospital resident in a hospital-owned nursing home bed begins a new and otherwise unavailable flow of cash to the hospital for nursing home care days (hundreds of dollars per day) and ends the thousands of dollars of actual cost to the hospital for which they receive only a single reimbursement rate regardless of how many days the patient stays. (Note: The total picture is much more complex, of course, because Medicare and Medicaid with their fixed reimbursement rate per admission are not the only providers that pay for hospital days of care. However, the reality is that most non-Medicare/Medicaid providers negotiate reimbursement rates to hospitals based primarily on published Medicare and Medicaid reimbursement rates.)

The effect on the nursing home case mix is thus similar: Patients are being discharged by hospitals to the nursing home quicker and sicker to lower the daily cost of care to the payers such as Medicare and Medicaid.

Hospitals are building nursing facilities for several reasons. They want to assure an immediately available nursing facility bed to place their patients. With this maneuver their DRG costs can be capped for each admission by means of an early discharge. Simultaneously, a new income stream from Medicare can begin by placing a new patient in a skilled nursing bed. This trend is likely to intensify as long as hospitals are forced to seek new revenue streams to supplement their losses incurred on daily charges. A study by Lagore (1994, p. 327) showed a 53% decrease in hospital nonacute census when nursing home beds were made readily available, sensitizing hospitals to possible income losses. Hospitals themselves are moving toward increased specialization under pressures from the DRGs. Duke University Health System has begun referring to itself as a hospital offering "quarternary" care, one specialization level beyond the previous tertiary care level of sophistication (Duke University Medical Center, 1995, p. 2).

Hospitals are seeking alternative sources of income because their occupancy rates and average length of stay are continuing a downward trend. Between 1989 and 1993, median occupancy rates decreased from 49% to 47%, and average length of stay decreased from 4.34 days to 3.83 days (Lutz, 1994, p. 68).

Roles of the Nursing Facility in the Long-Term Care Continuum

Institutional nursing care is prescribed by physicians for persons in a stable or unstable condition who require continuing medical supervision and services of licensed nursing personnel around the clock.

Outside Resources of the Nursing Facility

The nursing facility staff alone is physically and emotionally incapable of meeting the complete psychosocial and medical needs of its residents. Churches, schools, and other community groups, along with individual volunteers, are necessarily a part of caregiving in a nursing facility.

Outliving one's peers is one of the more difficult adjustments in old age. For persons living to the age of 80 and beyond, the deaths of most of one's friends and peer family members is a saddening reality. In every facility there is a portion of the resident population with no one left who is interested in their welfare.

There is simply not enough money in the average nursing home budget to staff at a level sufficient to provide all the human contact and caring that is needed by the residents. Even in those few instances where there are funds, there remains a qualitative difference between care offered by a paid staff member and what a volunteer from the community brings to the situation. If the nursing home experience is to be fully humanized, this will occur only when there is sufficient contact between the residents and the community.

Major Organizations in the Long-Term Care Field

The following are some of the outside groups and organizations that will directly or indirectly impact the lives of nursing home administrators.

American Association of Homes and Services for the Aging (AAHSA)—
The national not-for profit industry group. Represents approximately 5,000 nursing homes, life care communities, assisted living and senior housing, and community services organizations; www.aahsa.org.

American Association of Retired Persons (AARP)—Over 33 million Americans aged 50 and over. Represents aging Americans' interests on a number of dimensions; www.aarpwebplace.org.

American College of Health Care Administrators—The professional organization for nursing home administrators. About 6000 members (of about 40,000 administrators); www.achca.org.

American College of Healthcare Executives—28,000 members, mainly hospital executives; www.ache.com.

Administration on Aging—www.aoa.gov.

American Federation for Aging Research—National voluntary organization focusing on biomedical research in aging; www.afar.org.

American Geriatrics Society—Major society for aging interests. About 6,000 members; www.americangeriatrics.org.

American Health Care Association—The for-profit national nursing home association. Has 50 state affiliates, 12,000 members, mostly representing the for-profit nursing home interests; www.ahca.org.

American Society on Aging—Broadly representative of professionals interested in the aging field; www.asaging.org.

Assisted Living Federation of America—Over 6,500 members and growing rapidly as the major national professional association of assisted-living facilities; www.alfa.org.

Gerontological Society of America—Broad array of 6,500 persons interested in aging; www.geron.org.

Gray Panthers—8,000 active, 40,000 membership organization to further the interests of older women. Chapters in 35 states (Maddox & Sussman, 2001, p. 449); www.graypanthers.org.

U.S. Administration on Aging—A major resource on legislation, policy, and funding; www.aoa.gov.

National Institute on Aging—Maintains an informational Web site; www.nih.gov.

National Association of Boards of Examiners for Long-Term Care Administrators—The required national nursing home administrator exam is offered by NAB, as well as a new assisted-living national exam; www.nabweb.org.

National Citizens' Coalition for Nursing Home Reform—The major national coalition for new legislation in the long-term care field; www.nccnhr.org.

National Council of Senior Citizens—4.5 million members in 4,500 local clubs; www.ncsinc.org.

National Council on Aging—Nonprofit group helping community service organizations to enhance lives of older adults; www.ncoa.org.

4.2 The Social Security Act: Medicare and Medicaid

4.2.1 THE SOCIAL SECURITY ACT: MEDICARE

The nursing home industry is molded by the Social Security Act and owes the large scale of its economic existence (passing $100 billion per year mark in 2000) to this original legislation and its later amendments. This one Act is mainly responsible for generating the financial support for older persons that has enabled the nursing home industry to become perhaps the second largest segment of the health care industry, after hospitals.

Origins of the Social Security Act

When the Social Security Act came into existence in 1935 it was a response to a fundamental societal change in American life: our evolution from an agrarian to a highly industrialized form of society. Growing old suddenly became visible nationally during the shift from an agricultural form of society in which the aged were normally cared for by the family in the home to a society where the workplace was a factory. Industrialized society workers are controlled by economic conditions beyond their influence. Urbanization and industrialization brought increased problems to the aged, such as unemployment and economic survivorship of the dependents when the wage earner died.

The event that brought these problems to the attention of America in dramatic terms was the Great Depression of the 1930s. By 1935, 50% of the aged were indigent. Within 5 years, the proportion had grown to 66% (Clement, 1985, p. 21).

Impacts of the Social Security Act

Although additional factors are involved, a comparison of the number of aged persons receiving Social Security checks and the percentage of them living at the poverty level reveals a clear association. By 1959, the proportion of aged Americans who were indigent had fallen to 35%. Although this reflected some improvement, it still constituted a major social problem. As Social Security benefits during the 1950s and 1960s continued to expand, the percentage of aged living in poverty declined to 14% of older persons by 1978 (Kaplan, 1985, p. 5). According to the U.S. Census Bureau, during the inflation and recession period from 1979 to 1982, the elderly receiving Social Security checks based on Cost of Living Adjustments (COLAs), which began in 1975, were the only group studied whose poverty rate did not increase.

In 1985, the President's Council of Economic Advisors declared that older Americans were no longer disproportionately poor and that the percentage of the general population in poverty (15.2%) was slightly higher than that of the same segment of the elderly population (Kaplan, 1985, p. 7). Today nearly all Americans are covered by Social Security, although on occasion a person will apply for admission to a nursing home who has no Medicare eligibility. In 1950, only 1 of 4 persons received Social Security checks, but by 1977, 9 out of 10 did.

Many factors, such as the political activism of the aged, general improvements in the economy, the Older Americans Act of 1965, and related actions have led to general improvement in the economic condition of the elderly. Even so, while direct measurement is not feasible, it appears that a significant number of older Americans have little more than their Social Security check for income—a poverty level income.

Aspects Affecting the Nursing Home Industry

The nursing home industry owes its size to Social Security checks and reimbursement of Medicare and Medicaid bills for residents.

The Original Social Security Act and Its Amendments

The original Social Security Act, as passed in 1935, consisted of 11 titles enacting the program, authorizing the necessary taxes, and establishing the administrative mechanisms of the Act. Numerous amendments have been added to the Social Security Act over the years. Only those more directly affecting the nursing home industry are mentioned here.

In 1950, permanently and totally disabled persons, who might at some time need nursing home care, were added as beneficiaries. In that same year, federal matching money was made available to states to pay for medical care for persons on public assistance—a precursor of Medicaid, which was to come in 1965. States were required to establish licensing programs for nursing homes. Some already had done so.

By 1956, the Social Security program was known as OASDI—old age (OA), survivors (S), and disabled (D) insurance (I). It was not until 1960 that the H (for health) was added, and it became OASDHI. The next step toward the Medicaid program, so critical to the nursing home industry, came in 1960 with the Kerr-Mills Act, which amended the Social Security Act to provide Medical Assistance to the Aged (MAA). This amendment offered 50% to 84% in matching funds to states, depending on the per capital income of each state. However, during the following 5 years, only 25 states implemented this program to assist their aged.

The major amendments affecting the nursing home industry were added in 1965, with the passage of Title 18, known as Medicare, and 1 year later, Title 19, known as Medicaid.

Amendments in 1967 called for the licensure of nursing home administrators and recognized the category of "intermediate care facility." The 1972 amendments established the definition of the skilled nursing facility (SNF) and dropped the term *extended care facility* (ECF), which had been causing some confusion. In 1990, the federal designation *intermediate care nursing facility* (ICF) and *skilled nursing facility* (SNF) were replaced by the single term *nursing facility*.

Title 20 was added in 1974, supporting, among other things, in-home services to the elderly. In 1977, antifraud amendments were passed to minimize abuse of the program. Numerous additional amendments were passed during the 1980s. The primary focus has been containment of costs, rather than expansion of services since the mid-1970s.

In general, it appears that from 1935 to about 1975 the federal government sought to expand benefits under the Social Security Act, whereas since 1975, the thrust has been reduction in the rate of cost increases and the units of service for which payment is made.

The Conditions of Participation

After an extended implementation period and several additional amendments (described later) the Social Security Administration prepared an extensive set of rules, or minimum conditions, which it required any nursing facility receiving federal funds to meet (Freymann, 1980, p. 32; Miller, 1982, p. 7042; Rosenfeld, Gaylord, & Allen, 1983, p. 57; Smith, 1981, pp. 8, 10).

Proposed rules were published in the *Federal Register* on July 12, 1973. So many comments were received that the usual 30-day period for public comment was extended to 60 days, ending September 13, 1973. Officials made several changes in response to public comments and on January 17, 1974, published final rules (*Federal Register,* 39(12), Part 3, pp. 2238–2249).

Importance to the Nursing Home Industry

Federal rules are of overriding importance to the nursing home industry because, directly or indirectly, most nursing homes must comply with them, especially if they expect to be reimbursed for services to Medicare or Medicaid patients (Boling, Vrooman, & Sommers, 1983, pp. 198–199; Freymann, 1980, p. 31; Miller & Barry, 1979, p. 32).

Nursing homes are licensed by the states (Wilson & Neuhauser, 1982, p. 41). However, most states relied very heavily on these earlier federal Conditions of Participation in drawing up their own standards for licensing nursing homes (Smith, 1981, p. 10). The net effect is that nearly every nursing home, directly or indirectly, is obligated to comply with the federal standards (Miller & Barry, 1979, pp. 22–25; Wilson & Neuhauser, 1982, p. 41).

These new rules did bring some clarity to the industry. Nomenclature for the various levels of nursing care facilities had been a source of confusion at the federal level (and still is at the state level). States use different designations for nursing home levels of care. To further complicate matters, the development of continuing care retirement communities and the concept of assisted living, which is used in a number of states, suggests that we may be moving into a period of multiple designations for nursing home and nursing-home-like services.

States, using federal money in part, conduct on-site inspections of nursing home facilities to determine whether it meets state, and usually, federal requirements.

Not many months after the 1974 Conditions were published the Department of Health Education and Welfare (currently DHHS) commissioned "Operation Common Sense" involving a group of federal regulation writers who committed themselves "to revise and recodify (these) regulations to produce clear, readable and helpful documents" (DHHS, 2006, p. 7042). In the process of making the regulations more easily understood, these federal employees attempted to introduce "needed" policy changes at the same time (DHHS, 2006, p. 7042).

By 1976, a drive called the "Long-Term Care Facility Improvement Campaign" (LTCFIC) was on within the Department of Health Education and Welfare. It began by issuing a monograph supporting the idea of a comprehensive patient-assessment mechanism.

Out of this grew a 3-year project called the Patient Care Evaluation Project (PACE). PACE staffed tested two versions (PACE I and PACE II). Criticisms were that the instrument brought "burdensome paperwork," that it put "too much emphasis on the medical model" (for the nursing home), and that "evidence was lacking that PACE produced either cost effectiveness or benefit" (DHHS, 2006, p. 7043). However, the federal government was preparing to move.

In response to rumblings received from its regional offices, state agencies, and the general public, Centers for Medicare and Medicaid Services (CMS) published a general notice in the June 8, 1978, *Federal Register* that it planned to revise these federal regulations. It invited public comment.

The response by 1,200 organizations, individuals, and providers was impressive. Hearings were held in California, Georgia, the District of Columbia, Maryland, and Illinois. In addition, 620 written comments were received. "Most commentators," CMS reports, "urged us to find ways to ease the burdens of regulation" (DHHS, 2006, p. 7044). In the summer of 1980, CMS published what it assumed to be the new requirements destined to replace the long criticized 1974 amendments.

CMS officials ran into heavy seas. President Carter, in whose administration all of these changes had been proposed, lost the election to Ronald Reagan, who rejected the proposed revisions, using the Tax Equity and Fiscal Responsibility Act of 1981 as his vehicle.

Several years of unrest followed. The executive branch, to deflect Congressional criticism, suggested that the Institute of Medicine appoint a 20-person panel to study nursing home care. This panel issued a 400-page report in the summer of 1986. They found the quality of care and quality of life in nursing homes to be "unsatisfactory" and called for a new federal government regulation effort (Committee on Nursing Home Reform, 1986, p. 21). The panel members sought a strengthening of the federal requirements, with a new emphasis on inspections based more on quality of patient care actually delivered, that is, to focus on the outcomes of care. Patients' rights, they argued, should be given more attention.

A coalition of more than 40 concerned, long-term care organizations successfully lobbied for new legislation that embodied much of the 200-page Institute of Medicine report. Medicare and Medicaid long-term care amendments were passed in the 1987 Omnibus Budget Reconciliation Act (OBRA). This legislation, and new federal requirements proposed by CMS in the February 2, 1989, *Federal Register,* were implemented during 1989 and 1990. This ended a 15-year period during which the federal regulations (called Conditions of Participation) remained static despite constant attempts at reform.

We turn now to an examination of the basic components of the Medicare and Medicaid legislation after which we will examine several other pieces of legislation that affect and constitute what may be called the long-term care continuum.

Medicare

As of this printing, these were the basic Medicare and Medicaid coverages; we use the past tense although they may still be current. See also the current edition of *Nursing Home Federal Requirements: Guidelines to Surveyors and Survey Protocols, 6th ed.* from Springer Publishing Company for any new changes. Attempts have been made to modify them during each session of Congress, and these attempts continue.

Plan A

Everyone receiving Social Security was automatically covered under Plan A.

Hospital Costs

Covered hospital-related costs were paid on the following basis: During the first 60 days of hospitalization for each period of illness (defined later), the patient pays for the equivalent of the first day, and Medicare pays for the other 59. During the years of Medicare coverage, the cost of this first day rose from an initial cost of nearly $100 to almost $1,000.

During days 61 to 90 of hospitalization, the patient paid for about 25% of the daily rate. Medicare picked up the remaining costs. Inpatient days were covered only during the first 90 days of any spell of illness. Each Medicare recipient had a lifetime reserve of 60 days, which could be used after the 90th day of hospitalization. During days 91 to 150 the patient paid for about 50% of the daily rate. In addition, each Medicare recipient was eligible for up to 190 days of inpatient psychiatric care during their lifetime. Determining a spell of illness became so complex that in early 2007 Centers for Medicare and Medicaid issued chart "Skilled Nursing Facility (SNF) Spell of Illness Quick Reference Chart," which may be found at the CMS Web site, www.cms.hhs.gov/MLNGeninfo.gov.

Prospective Payment: The Era of DRGs

Beginning with federal fiscal year 1984, the federal government began to pay hospitals for Medicare patient costs on the basis of 467 diagnostic/reimbursement categories (Prospective payment, 1983, pp. 1–6). Each year, Medicare officials prospectively (ahead of time) decided on the amount of reimbursement for each Medicare hospital admission based on the principal diagnosis, that is, the condition established after study to be chiefly responsible for admission of the patient.

DRG stands for Diagnostically Related Group (of diseases). There are 9,000 disease codes listed in a book called *International Classification of Diseases*. Using the 9th edition's clinical modifications (called ICDM9CM), the federal government identified 467 diseases for reimbursement to hospitals for care of Medicare patients based on their principal diagnosis and the severity of the disease for which the Medicare patient was admitted.

The theory was that some patients' length of stay was shorter than average and some longer. Medicare reimbursed on the average length of stay for each disease, based on the level of severity experienced by the patient. At the end of each year, Medicare made adjustments, using up to approximately 6% of its total funds to reimburse hospitals for especially expensive cases (called outliers).

Payments varied for each of the nine U.S. geographical regions established by Medicare and by whether the hospital was rural or urban. For example, an urban hospital in New York City would be reimbursed at a higher rate than a rural Georgia Hospital for treating a patient with the same principal diagnosis. The basis of each hospital's reimbursement rate was based 25% on whether it was rural or urban and 75% on the cost experience of that hospital during the first year it was in the program, called the base year. New "base" years were designated as time passed.

One impact for the long-term care industry was that because payment was by disease, no matter how extended the length of stay of each patient, hospitals sought to place Medicare patients into a nursing home, home health agency, or "nursing home bed equivalent" for what is currently called *sub-acute* care. This is the phenomenon of hospitals discharging Medicare patients "quicker and sicker." As has already been seen, hospitals often opened their own "nursing home equivalent," that is, Medicare certified beds in the hospital itself, in order to start up a new stream of cash income for themselves for that same patient.

Nursing Facility Costs

For each spell of illness, Medicare paid 100% of "reasonable costs" during the first 20 days. During days 21 to 100 the patient co-paid a required amount, set usually at well over half the daily cost. Medicare paid nothing beyond 100 days of nursing facility care during any one spell of illness. A number of wheel and chart devices are available from medical supply companies, such as Briggs and Med-Pass, Inc., that assist the facility in accomplishing the requirements based on and dating from the Assessment Reference Date (ARD) from which all subsequent dates are calculated.

In 1960, the United States spent 800 million dollars on nursing home care. By 2003, the United States was spending $110 billion on nursing home care each year (DHHS, 2005, 363).

Nursing Facility Average Annual Percent Change From Previous Year

1960	17%
1980	15%
1990	11%
2000	5%
2003	4%

Nursing facility costs average annual percent change from previous year have faced constraints as the federal and state governments have attempted to rein in exploding health care costs.

Home Health Care Costs

Medicare paid 100% of all home health care costs associated with any one spell of illness (care provided for a diagnosed illness for which 3 or more days of hospital care was given).

It is important to realize that Medicare was intended to cover brief periods of illness. Medicare provided short-term acute care. It was not intended to cover long-term care patients. Medicaid is the vehicle for covering long periods of illness, but only after the individual had spent all but about $2,000 of their total resources (discussed in more detail later).

In 1960, the United States spent $1 million on home health care. By 2003, the United States was spending $40 billion on home health care per year, an even more dramatic increase in rate of spending than on nursing facility care (DHHS, 2005, p. 363).

Home Health Average Annual Percent Change From Previous Year

1960	6%
1970	14%
1980	27%
1990	18%
2000	.7%
2003	9.5%

The reduced average annual increase in 2000 reflects the federal restrictions placed on operators of home health care agencies (DHHS, 2005,p. 363).

Eligibility for Nursing Facility Care

To be eligible for inpatient nursing facility care, at least four conditions had to be met by the Medicare patient.

1. The patient had to have spent three consecutive days in a hospital (not including the day of discharge).
2. The patient had to have been transferred to a nursing facility, because treatment for the original cause of hospitalization is required.
3. The patient had to have been admitted within 14 days of hospital discharge (leeway is generally allowed up to 30 days).
4. The patient had to have been certified by a physician to be in need of and receiving nursing care or rehabilitation services on a *daily* basis (Aetna Life Insurance Company, p. 1).

Plan B

Plan B was voluntary. The Medicare recipient had to pay a small monthly premium—determined every 2 years and based on the benefits paid and administration costs of Plan B. General funds from the U.S. Treasury paid one-half of the costs of Plan B and the participants paid the other half.

Three major expenses were covered under Plan B:

1. Medical expenses (including physician services; inpatient and outpatient medical services and supplies; physical and speech therapy; ambulance, diagnostic X-ray, laboratory, and other tests; dressings; splints, medical equipment, etc.)
2. Outpatient hospital treatment
3. Home health care

Payments Under Plan B

After the recipient paid an annual deductible amount, Medicare plan B paid 80% of Medicare-determined reasonable charges for medical expenses, outpatient hospital treatment, and home health care. If home health care qualified under Plan A post-hospital care, 100% of home health care costs were paid under Plan A.

Excluded From Coverage

Many health care costs associated with the elderly were excluded from payment by Medicare plans A and B. Neither plan would pay for:

- routine physical and related tests
- eyeglasses or eye examinations
- hearing examinations or hearing aids
- immunizations (except for pneumococcal shots))
- routine foot care
- orthopedic shoes or other supportive devices for the feet
- custodial care
- preventive care, filling, removal, or replacement of teeth

Plan D

Under Plan D, which was implemented in 2006, some relief for medication expenses has come to nursing facilities through increased Medicare payment for drugs. In 2006, 8.23% of all nursing facility residents were receiving antibiotics, some of which can be quite costly (DHHS, 2006, F78, F133–F139). Prescription drug use among the general U.S. population 65 years of age and over was 85% in 2002 (DHHS, 2005, p. 316). In the nursing facility nearly all residents use prescription drugs. Nationally, 96% of persons aged 65 and over used prescription drugs at an annual cost (in 2002) of $8,000 (DHHS, 2005, p. 367).

Some Definitions

Intermediaries and Carriers

Medicare payments were actually made by private insurance organizations that had contracted with the federal government to do so. Organizations handling claims from nursing facilities, hospitals, and home health agencies were called intermediaries. Organizations dealing with claims from doctors and other medical suppliers covered under the medical insurance (Plan B) were called carriers.

Approved Charges

Under Plan B, approved charges were those determined as follows: The carrier in each geographic area annually reviewed the charges made by physicians and suppliers during the previous year. Suppliers were persons or organizations other than physicians who furnished equipment or services, such as ambulance transportation laboratory tests, and medical equipment, for example, wheelchairs.

To calculate an approved charge, the carrier determined the customary charge, that is, the one most frequently made by each physician and supplier during the previous year. Then the carrier found the prevailing charge for each service and material supplied during that year. The prevailing charge was an amount sufficient to pay for the customary charges in three out of every four bills that were submitted in the previous year for each service and supply (limited by an economic index ceiling). When a claim was received from a physician or supplier, the carrier compared the actual charge with the customary and prevailing charges for that service or supply and paid 80% of the lowest of the three. The Medicare recipient paid the remaining 20%, either out of pocket or through a small insurance policy (called Medigap insurance), which was designed to pay the remaining 20%.

Assignment

When a physician or supplier accepted an assignment of the medical insurance payment under Plan B, they agreed that the total charge to the patient would be the one approved by the carrier. In this case, Medicare paid the physician or supplier directly, after subtracting any part of the annual deductible not met.

Assignment was voluntary and had to be agreed to by both the provider and the patient. It guaranteed that the physician or supplier would not charge the patient more than the 20% of approved charges not paid by the carrier.

In 2004, 35 million Americans were receiving Medicare, which made the following payments:

Billions of Dollars

Nursing facilities	17	to approximately 16,000 providers
Home health agencies	6	to 6,926 providers in 2003
Hospice	7.6	to 2,323 providers in 2003
Hospitals	116	to 5,000+ providers

(DHHS, 2005, Table 139, p. 394)

4.2.2 TITLE 19: MEDICAID

Medicaid and Medicare were both passed as amendments to the Social Security Act. Medicare has been essentially an insurance program for recipients of Social Security benefits. Medicaid has not been insurance. Medicaid, as designed, has been literally medical aid for persons receiving welfare and for comparable groups of persons who were defined as medically indigent.

Whereas Medicare was a federally run program, Medicaid was a program of federal grants to the states to enable them to provide medical assistance to four categories of persons:

- families with dependent children (AFDC)
- the aged—persons receiving Old Age Assistance (OAA)
- the blind—Aid to the Blind (AB)
- persons permanently and totally disabled (that is to persons receiving federally aided public assistance)
- comparable groups of medically indigent persons, not currently on welfare but who fall into the same preceding four categories. Such persons are categorized as medically needy when medical expenses reduce their income below the Medicaid eligibility level.

"Spend Down"

Research by Sloan and Shayne (1993) suggests that, using a community simulation model, the majority of nursing home residents were, at entry, either already financially qualified or would have been so immediately had they been institutionalized (p. 585). After undertaking similar research, Adams, Meiners, and Burwell (1993) concluded that (1) one in four persons admitted as private paying stayed long enough to become Medicaid recipients, (2) approximately one in three persons eventually covered by Medicaid were not eligible when admitted, and (3) about 30% to 40% of Medicaid expenditures on nursing home care is attributable to individuals who spent down (p. 21). Different studies come up with different conclusions, depending on the original assumptions and geographical locations of research. Estimates from a National Nursing Home Survey were that 14% of nursing home residents were admitted as already receiving Medicaid (Short, Kemper, Llewellyn, & Walden, 1992, p. 294).

The federal share ranged between 50% to 83% of costs, depending on the state's per capita income. Each state determined its coverage above a basic minimum of at least some of each of the following services: inpatient hospital, outpatient hospital, other laboratory and X-ray, nursing, and medical.

Tightening Medicaid Rules

In the February, 2006, Deficit Reduction Act passed by Congress, the rules for qualifying for Medicaid help with long-term care after making gifts were significantly tightened. Instead of denying Medicaid based on gifts during the 3 years prior to application for Medicaid help, the "look back" period, as it is called, was increased from a limit of 3 years prior to applying to 5 years prior to applying. Under these new rules the possibility of the nursing facility being denied payment when a resident applies for Medicaid status can be significant.

In addition to these basic services, a state could include any medical care recognized under state law if it chose. No residency requirements could be established for eligibility for services. Medicaid recipients have not been subject to deductible payments, as in the case of Medicare, but state have been allowed to require some copayments for recipients for care. Some states, for example, charged copayments for prescriptions, usually 50 cents per prescription and $1 to $2 copayment for dental visits, eye visits, and similar services (Muse & Sawyer, 1982, p. 96).

Changing Congressional Goals

Originally the federal government set July 1, 1975, as the date by which all participating states were to be offering comprehensive services to all eligible persons. As cost soared under the program, Congress scaled down this goal and in the 1980s and following years moved toward containing Medicaid costs rather than expanding its services. Congress has been concerned because Medicaid has to ceiling on annual expenditures. The federal government was committed to pay its share of services the states provided to Medicaid recipients.

Buy-In Agreements

To maximize the contribution of federal dollars to state programs, participating states have signed "buy-in agreements" under which the state pays for Plan B costs for Medicaid recipients. The buy-in obligated the federal government to pay entirely for medical costs that might have been cost-shared by the states' Medicaid programs, thus reducing the total dollar costs to the states (Muse & Sawyer, 1982, p. 115). So intense has been the states' effort to shift costs from state budgets to the federal budget that several states placed a special tax on nursing homes, then used the taxes collected to help pay for Medicaid-assisted health care for older persons, shifting thereby an even larger dollar burden to the federal government.

To further contain costs, some states have obliged county governments to use their own funds to pay for a portion (usually about 3% to 5 %) of Medicaid costs. Medicaid dollars, initially committed by county social workers, became thus more carefully supervised by the county governments.

Eligibility for Medicaid has been generally determined at the county level by a social worker, and the program was usually administered by the local Department of Social Services, which assigned recipients as part of the case load of its social worker.

As mentioned elsewhere, the elderly have traditionally benefited to a great extent under the Medicaid program; they represent approximately 15% of all recipients, but received slightly more than one-third of the benefits paid out (Muse & Sawyer, 1982, p. 8).

Spending in 1997 was over $160 billion with 30% of that going to care for the elderly (Maddox & Sussman, 2001, p. 653).

Unmarried persons appeared to be five times more likely than married persons and Medicaid enrollees 10 times more likely than those without Medicaid to use nursing homes.

Both the federal and state governments have been seeking ways to reduce expenditures under Medicare and Medicaid. Consequently, details of the payment plans change constantly. The reader should obtain current information and check with the local Medicare and Medicaid offices for the latest coverages and payment mechanisms.

In 1997, the Program of All-Inclusive Care for the Elderly (PACE) was formalized as an integrated Medicare-Medicaid for managed care for the elderly (Maddox & Sussman, 2001, p. 653).

Facility Beds by Certification Category

Licensed nursing facilities may apply to be certified for participation in the Medicare or Medicaid program on a voluntary basis. Facilities may participate in (1) the Medicaid only (Title 19) program, (2) the Medicare only (Title 18) program, or (3) in the Medicare/Medicaid dually certified (Title 18 & 19) program. Since 1991, the Medicare program classified facilities as skilled nursing facilities (SNFs) while the Medicaid-certified facilities are designated as nursing facilities (NFs). Federal Medicare certification allows for all or part of a facility to be certified.

Over the years 1993–1999, about 3% of facilities were certified Medicare only, and 50% were certified Medicaid only with an increasing trend toward dual certification, increasing from 34% in 1993 to 43% in 1999, due to a relaxing of Medicare reimbursement rules that reduced payment for unfilled Medicare beds.

Residents by Payer Source

Who Pays for Nursing Home Care?

Over the past several decades Medicare and Medicaid have been the predominant payers for nursing home care given in the United States. The typical profile has been:

	Medicare	Medicaid	Other Payer
2000	24%	68%	8%
2006	13%	65%	22%

The predominant payer has been and is likely to remain Medicaid. Medicare reimbursement policies, together with Medicaid reimbursement policies, typically determine the profitability of the average facility. The role of private payers has been slowly increasing, but not as quickly as expected. Long-term care insurance has not become a significant payer source due to its high annual premiums.

In 2006, Medicare was paying for 188,976 residents' care, Medicaid was paying for 934,402 residents' care, and Other Payers were paying for the remaining 309,486 of the 1,432,864 residents in facilities that were receiving Medicare and Medicaid payments (DHHS, 2006, F75, F78).

The profile varies among the multifacility chains and stand alone facilities. Many facilities have veterans administration beds, some contract with local hospitals to reserve beds, some have managed care, some workman's compensation, and the like. On the whole, facilities resemble this profile with some variations one way or the other. It is a complex picture inasmuch as any single patient may be consecutively on Medicare, then private paying while in Medicaid spend down, then become a Medicaid resident.

Currently the federal government is attempting to control Medicare and Medicaid costs by supply restrictions, reimbursement limitations, and tightened eligibility requirements. The Balanced Budget Act of 1997 mandated the use of a prospective payment system for both skilled nursing facilities and home health care and by allowing states to allow mandated enrollment in a managed care organization as a condition of receiving Medicaid assistance (Giacalone, 2001, p. xv). This led to the Balanced Budget Refinement Act of 1999 in which some of the draconian Medicare and Medicaid cuts mandated by the Balanced Budget Act of 1997 were mitigated. This process will continue over the next decades as need for nursing home care rises and funds for care are curtailed by the federal government and state legislatures.

In 2001, Medicaid had 46 million recipients. Only 8.3% of Medicaid recipients were aged 65 and over, but these 8.3% received 26% of all Medicaid dollars (DHHS, 2005, p. 399). Interestingly, nursing facilities received 20% of all Medicaid dollars, more than the 14% of Medicaid dollars received by inpatient hospitals (DHHS, 2005, p. 400). In dollars, nursing facilities received 21 billion in 2001 compared to inpatient hospitals' 5.3 billion (DHHS, 2005, p. 401).

4.3 Older Americans Act of 1965

The Older Americans Act (OAA) can be characterized as Congress' response to noninstitutional primarily nonhealth care needs of the elderly. Medicare and Medicaid provide primarily for their institutionalized health care needs (home health care, e.g., being the exception). Title 20 of the Social Security Act is also a response to the primarily noninstitutional needs of the elderly.

The Older Americans Act authorizes payment for almost any activity that may lead to an improved quality of life for persons 60 years and over (with some programs, e.g., "reemployment" programs for persons 55 and over). The funds and agencies authorized and generated by the Older Americans Act play major roles in shaping the long-term care industry in the United States. For this reason some of its more important features are explored in this section.

Precursors of the Older Americans Act

Events that laid the foundation for the passage of the Older Americans Act in 1965 began about 1945, when Connecticut set up a commission concerned with the needs of older individuals. By 1961, all states had established similar commissions or aging units. That same year a White House Conference on Aging was held, at which heavy pressure for a federal role in addressing the needs of the elderly was brought to bear by lobbyists. Two years later President John F. Kennedy sent a message to Congress titled "Elderly Citizens of Our Nation." He recommended federal help for older individuals who do not need institutional care, but are encountering the expected increase in difficulty of successfully performing the activities of daily living, such as bathing, dressing, and toileting. Continued lobbying for federal aid for the functional elderly led to passage of the Older Americans Act in 1965.

Grand Objectives: Title 1

Title 1 states the goals of the Older Americans Act: equal opportunity of every older individual to the full and free enjoyment of

- adequate income
- the best possible physical and mental health science can offer, without regard to economic status
- affordable, suitable housing
- full restorative services for those needing institutional care
- employment
- retirement in health and dignity
- pursuit of the widest civic, cultural, educational, and recreational opportunities
- efficient community services: low-cost transportation, choices in living arrangements, coordinated social service assistance
- immediate benefit of technologic developments
- freedom, independence, and the free exercise of individual initiative in planning and managing their own life

Other portions of the Older Americans Act authorize the Commissioner on Aging, who is the administrator of the Older Americans Act, to pay for virtually any service or activity that will foster these broadly stated goals. The goals and authorizations are sweeping; however, the economic realities of the level of funding have prevented implementing large-scale programs to achieve these goals.

Other Titles

Title 2 established the Administration on Aging (AOA) within the Office of Human Development Services (OHDS), which is in the federal Department of Health and Human Services (DHHS). A Commissioner on Aging, appointed by the President and confirmed by the Senate, is empowered to administer the Older Americans Act and report directly to the Secretary of Health and Human Services.

Title 3 authorized grants to the states to create Planning and Service Areas within which the local Area Agencies on Aging (AAAs) function. Title 3b is concerned with social services, Title 3c1 with congregate nutritional services for those 60 or over as well as their spouses, and Title 3c2 with home delivered meals. Title 4 deals with research and training. Title 5 creates the Senior Community Services Employment Program (SCSEP) for those 55 or older with limited incomes (usually 125% of poverty). Title 6 addressed grants to American Indian tribes. Title 7, passed in 1984, authorized a health education and training program for older individuals.

to accomplish the task. Whether the services under the Older Americans Act would be available without a means test to every elderly person is also in question.

One of the greatest burdens of growing old is the loneliness resulting from loss of friends and family members of the same generation (Maddox & Sussman, 2001, p. 615). Participating in the congregate meal is, for many individuals, regardless of their income level, a primary source of social contact with other people.

Have the Area Agencies on Aging been successful in establishing a coordinated service system for long-term care in their communities? Generally, no. They have had neither the funds nor the organizational authority to bring together and organize the long-term care providers in the communities. Despite the meager funding levels, and lack of authority, however, there is a network of services in place for all older Americans who need assistance to remain outside an institution. This is a major improvement over the decades before the 1960s, when such services did not exist at all. This network and the nutritional assistance to all older Americans have become integral to the long-term care system in which nursing facilities are active participants.

The Urban Institute (a private nonprofit research group in Washington, DC) estimated that in 1994, 4.9 million elderly persons were either malnourished or hungry—about 16% of the population over 60! The Urban Institute found that two-thirds of needy older persons are not being reached by food assistance projects. In New York State, 2,500 older persons are on waiting lists for home delivered meals. About 62,000 of its elderly are in the program, but officials estimate about 10,000 more are starving to death in urban high-rise buildings. The funding levels for the Older Americans Act have fallen behind with each succeeding year as inflation and a dramatically increasing elderly population outstrip funding. This is not surprising because the government funds available to feed the elderly amounted to about $0.53 per person according to a 1992 Government Accounting Office study.

4.4 Labor and Management: Laws and Regulations

What rights do nursing home administrators have when employees in the facility are seeking to form a union? What rights do the employees have? What are the basic laws and regulations governing the managers dealings with employees?

This section provides a framework to enable the reader to begin to answer these questions.

4.4.1 EARLY MANAGEMENT–LABOR RELATIONS IN THE UNITED STATES

During most of the earlier years of its history, the government of the United States strongly supported management in its dealings with employees. It was not until 1935 that American workers won government sanction of the right to form trade unions.

The passage of the National Labor Relations Act (better known as the Wagner Act) in 1935 was the first nationwide American labor legislation to favor the growth of trade unions. This was the culmination of a long slow process.

Management Preferences

Most managers would prefer not to have to deal with organized labor. Unionization is perceived as intensifying the difficulty of the administrator's responsibilities. There is a natural tendency for what organizational theorists call the "we–they" phenomenon to occur in the relationship between labor and management. Workers often perceive their interests as different from those of managers, whose task is to operate cost effectively, that is, to produce the best results for the least cost.

The administrator would be happy to pay nurses and nurse's aides the premium wages that will attract the most competent workers available, but pressures to keep costs down do not often permit this. The result is that most nursing home workers, especially the nurse's aides, and the kitchen and housekeeping staffs are paid at prevailing rates in the particular geographical area, which are usually close to the required minimum wage levels. Understandably, these workers, many of who hold second full-time jobs to make ends meet, seek to increase their personal incomes from the nursing facility and obtain the best working conditions on their jobs. Tensions between managers and workers are inevitably built into the situation. How do they deal with them? What are the manager's rights? What rights do the employees have?

The Colonial Period

So powerful were the managers in the Colonial period that workers contented themselves with forming "fraternal unions" to help each other in coping with personal economic adversity, but certainly not to act collectively for improved working conditions and more pay (Department of Labor, 1976, pp. 1–104). Employers were able to prevent effective unionization. Employers could, at their own discretion, fire any worker seeking to organize a union, refuse to negotiate with any union representative, and require each new employee to sign a "yellow dog" contract, by which the worker agreed not to join a union (Chruden & Sherman, 1980, p. 345).

During the 19th century the U.S. courts consistently sided with management. In 1806, a federal court ruled that workers who sought to combine to exert pressure on managers were participating in a "conspiracy in restraint of trade," which in effect meant that such grouping was to be treated as criminal activity (Ivancevich & Glueck, 1983, p. 533). The first hint of rights for workers did not appear until 1842, when the Massachusetts Supreme Court ruled that unions that did not resort to illegal tactics were not guilty of criminal conspiracy (Chruden & Sherman, 1980, p. 345). Still, managers could fire any worker at will for union activity, impose yellow-dog contracts, and when all else failed, obtain a court injunction against threatened strikes. The managers still retained nearly all of the power (Ivancevich & Glueck, 1983, p. 533). Despite this, the union movement grew. By 1886, skilled workers such as machinists, bricklayers, and carpenters formed the American Federation of Labor (AFL).

It was not until 1935 that another major labor force, the Congress of Industrial Organizations (CIO), emerged (Raskin, 1981, pp. 12–32) and in 1955 merged with the American Federation of Labor. It was a slow process because the government did not substantially back labor until the Wagner Act was passed in 1935.

The federal government had actually given American workers some negotiating rights earlier in the century in order to keep the nation's railroads running. The Railway Labor Act of 1926 was the first federal legislation sanctioning union organization and the right to bargain collectively with management (Chruden & Sherman, 1980, p. 353).

The first national effort to define workers' and managers' respective rights came just 6 years later. In 1932, the Norris-LaGuardia Act, also called the Anti-Injunction Act, limited the powers of federal courts to side with management through issuing injunctions, that is, court decrees that stopped or limited union efforts to picket, boycott, or strike. Yellow-dog contracts were prohibited (Ivancevich & Glueck, 1983, p. 534).

4.4.2 MAJOR LEGISLATION AFFECTING EMPLOYER–EMPLOYEE RELATIONSHIPS

The Wagner Act, 1935

The Wagner Act of 1935 is the landmark law that, for the first time in federal legislation, defined the rights of workers (Boling et al., 1983, p. 185). The Wagner Act limited the freedom of employers to give their views on proposed unionization. The Wagner Act also guaranteed employee bargaining rights: "Employees shall have the right to self-organization, to form, join, or assist labor organizations, to bargain collectively through representatives of their own choosing, and to engage in concerted activities, for the purpose of collective bargaining or other mutual aid or protection" (Chruden & Sherman, 1980, p. 354). The National Labor Relations Board was created by the Wagner Act (see www.nlrb.gov).

Proportion of Workers in Unions

In 1933, there were 3 million unionized workers in this country. By 1947, they numbered 15 million, representing about 31% of the work force. Union membership increased until about 1956 representing about 35% of employees (Noe, Hollenbeck, Gerhart, & Wright, 2000, p. 498), then declined until 1963, when it resumed a slow growth. In 1980, about 20 million workers were in unions—approximately 20% of the total work force and 29% of nonagricultural workers (Ivancevich & Glueck, 1983, p. 547). Today unions represent about 10% of private sector employees, and some analysts foresee membership continuing to trend down to 5% (Noe et al., 2000, p. 498). One estimate is that the percentage of nursing home employees in unions declined steadily from 17% in 1983 to 11% in 1998 (Giacalone, 2001, p. 76).

The period from 1935 to 1947 was one of dramatic growth in union membership. The power given to unions through the Wagner Act resulted in what Congress in 1947 viewed as abuses. This led to the Taft-Hartley Act, which placed limitations on unions, just as the Wagner Act had placed limitations on managers 12 years earlier.

The Taft-Hartley Act, 1947

In the provisions of the Taft-Hartley Act unions were prohibited from the following actions (Chruden & Sherman, 1980, p. 355; Ivancevich & Glueck, 1983, p. 534).

Unions Are Prohibited From:

1. Restraining or coercing employees in the exercise of their right to join a union or not (unless an agreement existed with management that every worker must be a union member). Union members could not physically prevent other workers from entering a facility, nor act violently toward nonunion employees, nor threaten employees for not supporting union activities.
2. Causing an employer to discriminate against an employee for anti-union activity, nor could unions force employers to hire only workers acceptable to the union.
3. Bargaining with an employer in bad faith. They could not insist on negotiating "illegal" provisions, such as the administration's prerogative to appoint supervisors.
4. Participating in secondary boycotts or jurisdictional disputes. Unions may not picket a nursing home in an attempt to force it to apply pressure on a subcontractor (e.g., a food service contractor) to recognize a union, nor can a union force an employer to do business only with others, such as suppliers, who are unionized; nor can one union picket for recognition when another union is already certified for a nursing home.
5. Charging excessive or discriminatory membership fees. They may not charge a higher initiation fee to employees who did not join the union until after a union contract was negotiated.
6. Coercing or restraining employees in the selection of the parties to bargain on management's behalf. The manager is free to hire the best labor lawyer available to represent the facility.
7. Forcing managers to hire employees when they are not needed (called featherbedding).

However, when the Wagner Act was amended by this promanagement act (the Taft-Hartley Act), certain employee's rights were retained (Ivancevich & Glueck, 1983, p. 535).

Managers May Not:

1. Interfere with, restrain, or coerce employees in the exercise of their rights. Managers may not, for example, give wage increases timed to discourage employees from joining a union or threaten with loss of their jobs employees who vote for a union.
2. Interfere with or attempt to dominate any labor organization, or contribute financial or other support to a labor organization. For example, managers cannot take an active part in union affairs or permit a nursing home supervisor to participate actively in a union, or show favoritism toward one union over another.
3. Discriminate in hiring or giving tenure to employees or set any terms for employment so as to encourage or discourage union membership. For example, they cannot fire an employee who urges others to join a union or demote an employee for union activity.
4. Fire or discriminate against any employee who files charges or gives testimony under the Wagner Act.
5. Refuse to bargain collectively with the duly chosen representatives of its employees. For example, the nursing home administrator must provide financial data to a union if the facility claims to be experiencing financial losses, must bargain on mandatory subjects such as hours and wages, and must meet with union representatives duly appointed by a certified bargaining unit.

An important consideration for nursing home administrators is the denial of legal protection to supervisors seeking to form their own unions, thus keeping the management roles of these persons (usually department heads in nursing homes) clearly managerial in function and identification.

Probably the single most important provision of the Taft-Hartley Act for nursing home administrators is the restoration of the right of managers to express their views regarding unions and unionizing efforts. This means that administrators are free to express their opinions about their employees voting for a union in the work place and judgments about unions in general. Administrators are still prohibited from threatening, coercing, or bribing employees concerning their union membership or their decision to join or not to join a union.

The National Labor Relations Board

A major aspect of the Wagner Act was its creation of the National Labor Relations Board (NLRB), which plays a dominant role in U.S. labor-management relations. It has the following responsibilities (Chruden & Sherman, 1980, p. 355):

- To determine what the bargaining unit or units within an organization shall be. (A unit contains those employees who are to be represented by a particular union and are covered by the agreement with it.)
- To conduct representation elections by secret ballot for the purpose of determining which, if any, union shall represent the employees within a unit.
- To investigate unfair labor practice charges filed by unions or employees and to prosecute any violations revealed by such investigations.

The Board is empowered to initiate action against illegal strikes or unfair labor practices by unions. In a typical month as many as 4,000 new cases are filed with the NLRB.

One of the more controversial features of the Taft-Hartley Act is a provision allowing the President of the United States, through the Office of the Attorney General, to seek an injunction for a period of 80 days against strikes or walkouts affecting the nation's welfare or health. Some labor leaders have called this "slave labor" (Chruden & Sherman, 1980, p. 356).

The Landrum-Griffin Act, 1959

Officially designated the Labor-Management Reporting and Disclosure Act of 1959, the Landrum-Griffin Act seeks to protect the interests of the individual union member against possible union abuses. Specifically the Act gives to each union member several rights (Ivancevich & Glueck, 1983, p. 536).

Each union member has a right to

- Nominate candidates for union office
- Vote in union elections
- Attend union meetings
- Examine required annual financial reports by the union to the Secretary of Labor.

In addition, employers are required to report any payments or loans made to unions—the officers or any members—to eliminate what were called "sweetheart contracts," under which union officials and the managers benefited, but the rank and file of union members did not.

Special Dispute-Settling Rules for Nursing Home and Hospital (Health Care) Administrators

The NLRB had jurisdiction over health care institutions. However, until 1974 the Board was expressly forbidden by the original Taft-Hartley law to hear cases in the nonprofit sector. Because the vast majority of nursing homes and hospitals operated in the 1950s and 1960s were nonprofit, this meant that most of the health care industry was not subject to these labor laws.

In 1973, Congress began talking of having the law apply to not-for-profit nursing homes and hospitals. Nursing homes and hospitals pressed for the following benefits (American Hospital Association, 1976; Rosmann, 1975, pp. 64058):

- Special protection against strikes
- Priority for rapid NLRB action on disputes
- Mandatory mediation requirements (Johns & Saks, 2001, p. 425)
- Limit on the number of bargaining units to one each for professional, technical, clinical, and maintenance and service workers

The nursing homes and hospitals were successful on the whole.

In 1974, Congress amended the Taft-Hartley Act to bring nursing homes and hospitals under its regulations (1974 Non-Profit Hospital Amendments, Public Law 930360; Wilson & Neuhauser, 1982, p. 89). However, special provisions were made (Pointer & Metzger, 1975, pp. 41–60):

- A nursing home, hospital, or union must give to the other party 90 days notice of a desire to change an existing contract (this is 30 days more notice than required of others).
- The Federal Mediation and Conciliation Service (FMCS) must be given 30 days notice if an impasse occurs in bargaining for an initial contract after the union is first recognized
- A nursing home or hospital union may not picket or strike without 10 days prior notice, in order to allow the facility to make provisions for continuity of care (no prior notice is required of other unions).
- The FMCS may appoint a board of inquiry to mediate the dispute if it decides a strike would imperil the welfare or health of the community. Neither the nursing home nor the union is obliged to accept the board's recommendations, but they must provide any witnesses or information sought by the Board.

For-profit nursing homes benefited from the 1974 amendment to the Taft-Hartley Act because of the four special labor relations rules (Miller, 1982, p. 49).

The Bargaining Unit

Labor unions must seek recognition as representing the majority of persons in a specific bargaining unit of a nursing home. As indicated previously, nursing homes and hospitals sought to limit the number of bargaining units in negotiations to professional, technical, clinical, and maintenance and service workers.

During most of the decade after the 1974 amendments to the Taft-Hartley Act, the NLRB ruled that in nursing homes and hospitals, service and maintenance workers, clerical staff, licensed practical nurses, registered nurses, and security guard units constitute appropriate bargaining units (Miller, 1982, pp. 49–50).

In August 1984, the NLRB issued a new ruling. In the case of St. Francis Hospital (Memphis, Tennessee) v. International Brotherhood of Electrical Workers Local 474, the NLRB ruled that a group of 39 maintenance workers did not constitute an appropriate bargaining unit. Health care workers thereafter had to represent either "all professionals" or "all nonprofessionals" rather than the particular interest groups allowed during the previous decade.

The effect of this NLRB ruling is to make union organization of nursing facility employees much more difficult. A far more diverse group of workers must be approached than before for purposes of union representation in elections. The Service Employees International Union, at that time, argued that that made it extremely difficult for health care workers to unionize.

Decisions favoring either labor or management are reflections of the political administrations in power. Nursing homes and hospitals had originally wanted to keep the number of bargaining units to no more than four. The NLRB, under more liberal (prolabor) auspices in Washington, according to Miller (1982), had permitted five. Under the more management-oriented administrations, the number of allowable bargaining units was cut back to two, which could ease matters considerably for nursing home administrators.

The unionization of nursing facilities is a complicated affair. Vigorous attempts to unionize nursing homes have been undertaken by several unions over recent years. A study by the AFL-CIO and data from 1983–1986 showed 15.9% of nursing home facilities were unionized. By the beginning of the 1990s, about 20% of U.S. nursing facilities were believed to have unions.

All regions of the United States have unionized nursing facilities. From "most unionized" to "least unionized" were the mid-Atlantic, followed by the West Coast, New England, Midwest, Southeast and South Central states. The Service Employees International Union (SEIU), for example, had organized 225 of the 1,832 nursing homes in California by 1990.

Since 1990, the SEIU has been the most active union seeking to organize nursing home workers. Since the mid-1990s, the SEIU has waged a campaign against a number of the major nursing chains including numerous attacks on the quality of care provided by nursing facilities and arguing that nurses in particular are overworked, stressed out, and sick (SEIU, 1995a, p. 11; SEIU, 1995b, p. 7; SEIU-AFL-CIO, 1995, p. 12). In some cases SEIU claimed harassment (Scott, 1994, p. 8), in others it attempted to prevent mergers of nursing home chains (Shriver, 1995, p. 18). Strikes have been called to draw attention to "patient care and demands for a new contract" (Moore, 1995, p. 12).

The largest proportion of nursing homes with unions are in the Service Employees International Union (SEIU), which is an AFL-CIO member with a membership of over 600,000 (Health Care Labor Manual). The membership in SEIU increased from 762,000 members in 1989 to 1,081,000 in 1997 (Noe et al., 2000, p. 495). In the mid-1990s the SEIU represented 60,000 RNs, 30,000 LPNs, and 400,000 health care workers overall.

By 2006, the SEIU had 1.8 million members, having added 200,000 workers in 2005. It represented 900,000 caregivers and hospital employees and was the largest union of long-term care workers serving 350,000 home care and 150,000 nursing home employees (www.seiu.org, 2006).

In 1989, the National Union of Hospital and Health Care Employees, which had about 74,000 members merged with two other unions. About two-thirds of their members joined the SEIU, and the remaining one-third joined the American Federation of State County and Municipal Employees. However, to complicate the picture, nursing homes have been organized by numerous other unions such as the United Food and Commercial Workers, the Teamsters, and the Federation of Nurses and Health Professionals, which is an offshoot of the American Federation of Teachers.

Normally employees in nursing, dietary, housekeeping, and laundry are the most likely to be unionized. A growing number of employers, particularly the larger chains, attempted to prevent unionization of nurses by arguing that all nurses (RNs and LPNs) are statutory supervisors and thereby excluded from labor law protection to join a union. The employers insisted that all nurses supervise nurse's aides, hence all nurses are supervisory personnel and therefore not covered by labor laws. In a set-back for unionization of nursing home workers, the U.S. Supreme Court, by a

5–4 decision, agreed and ruled in May, 1994, that nurses who supervise lesser-skilled employees are not protected by the National Labor Relations Act (NLRB v. Health Care & Retirement Corporation of America; Burda, 1995, p. 13).

On May 29, 2001, the U.S. Supreme Court in NLRB v. Kentucky River Community Care, Inc., again confirmed that professional employees, such as nurses, who direct other employees are supervisors and thus ineligible for union membership.

Conventional wisdom in the nursing home industry is that facilities are subject to being unionized when employee management/employee communication is low and focuses more on dissatisfaction with working conditions than on pay levels.

2005 Unionization Status

As of 2005, 12.5% of U.S. workers were union members. Unionization rate for private sector workers was 7.8% in 2005 compared to 7.9% in 2004 (*Wall Street Journal,* January 21, 2006, p. A4).

Nonunion Workers

At least 80% of the total labor workforce in this country is not unionized. What of their rights?

Over the years the federal government has enacted legislation establishing and protecting the rights of workers in general. Three of these laws are the Civil Rights Act of 1964, the Equal Employment Opportunities Act of 1972, and the Americans With Disabilities Act of 1992.

Equal Pay Act, 1963

This act requires that men and women performing equal jobs receive equal pay, covers all facilities, in effect, and is enforced by the Equal Employment Opportunities Commission (EEOC) (Noe et al., 2000, p. 77).

Civil Rights Act, 1964

Title VII of the Civil Rights Act of 1964 prohibited employers and others from discriminating against employees on the basis of race, color, religion, sex, or national origin.

Title VII also prohibits discrimination with regard to any employment condition including hiring, firing, promotion, transfer, and admission to training programs.

Consumer Credit Protection Act, 1968

Title III of this act limits the amount of an employee's earnings that may be garnisheed and protects employees from being discharged for any one indebtedness. In general, an employee's earnings that may be garnisheed is the lesser of 25% of disposable earnings or the amount by which disposable earnings are greater than 30 times the federal minimum wage. Other conditions apply. The Department of labor's Wage Hour Division administers and enforces Title III. Violations can require back pay, reinstatement, and fines up to $1,000 or imprisonment for not more than 1 year, or both.

The Equal Employment Opportunities Act, 1972

The Equal Employment Opportunities Act (EEOA) amended Title VII of the Civil rights Act. EEOA strengthened enforcement of the original Act and expanded its coverage to additional groups, such as state and local government workers and private employment of more than 15 persons.

What Is Discrimination?

Congress did not define discrimination in its legislation. Over the years the courts have established three definitions (Noe et al., 2000, p. 77):

- During World War II, discrimination was defined as harmful actions motivated by personal animosity toward the group of which the target person was a member.
- Later this was redefined as unequal treatment. Accordingly, a practice is illegal if it applies different standards or different treatment to different groups of employees or applicants. For example, minorities may not be kept in less desirable departments (different treatment); rejecting women with preschool-age children is not permissible (different standards). Point: The administrator may impose any standards so long as they are applied equally to all groups or individuals and do not result in any intended or unintended adverse treatment of any group.
- In Greggs v. Duke Power Co. (1971), the U.S. Supreme Court defined employment discrimination as unequal impact. In this case Duke Power was using employment tests and educational requirements that screened out a greater proportion of Blacks than Whites (Ivancevich & Glueck, 1983, p. 67). This is also called adverse impact.

Adverse impact is often measured (for the purposes of Title VII cases) when the selection rate for a protected minority group is less than 80% of the selection rate for a majority group.

Although the practice in the Duke Power case was not motivated by prejudice against Blacks, and the tests were all applied equally, they had the result of adverse impact, for example, unequal impact on Blacks. The job involved was that of shoveling coal into a furnace. Duke failed to prove that passing employment tests and requiring a level of education were related to success on the job. The burden of proof is on the employer to show that a hiring standard is job related.

Minority groups that are specifically protected under the Civil Rights Act are Blacks, Hispanics, American Indians, Alaskan natives, and Asian-Pacific Islanders.

Discrimination Based on Sex

Few situations exist that justify discrimination based on sex. In the current U.S. cultural setting, perhaps employment of a wet nurse is justifiable, of a woman to model women's clothes, or a woman as an attendant inside a locker room for other women. In the final analysis, the only legitimate basis for discrimination based on sex may be that the employee must use body organs specific to their sex to accomplish the job requirements, for example, wet nursing or providing semen for a sperm bank.

Sexual Harassment

Sexual harassment has been defined in the EEOC guidelines as follows:

> Unwelcome sexual advances, request for sexual favors, and other verbal or physical conduct of a sexual nature, constitutes sexual harassment when (1) submission to such conduct is either explicitly or implicitly a term or condition of an individual's employment, (2) submission or a rejection of such conduct by an individual is used as a basis for employment decisions affecting such individual or (3) such conduct has a purpose or effect or reasonably interfering with an individual's work performance, or creating an intimidating, hostile, or offensive working environment. (Section 1604.11)

In recent years two general categories of cases have emerged: quid pro quo and hostile work environment. In quid pro quo the harassment is not only a demand for sexual favor(s), but also the adverse employment decision that results from the rejection of those demands. A hostile work environment case requires evidence of pervasive offensive conduct of a sexual nature, for example, proof that obscenities and sexual gestures, remarks, or touching were commonplace. Some "environment" cases have involved the presence of nude or partially nude women as part of the proof of discrimination (*Robinson v. Jacksonville Shipyards,* 1991).

The facility can be held strictly liable for the acts of department managers who are found to be sexually harassing employee(s). A written policy against sexual harassment containing procedures available to employees is an advisable step for facility management to take. It has been pointed out that sexual harassment laws apply equally to both females and males, to heterosexuals, homosexuals, bisexuals, and transsexuals (Argenti, 1994, p. 355). Sexual harassment laws generally are aimed at superior–subordinate relationships, but they also apply to peer relationships and those between residents and employees. The number of sexual harassment charges rose from 7,000 in 1991 to nearly 16,000 in 1997 (Noe et al., 2000, p. 94).

The Pregnancy Discrimination Act, 1978

The 1964 Civil Rights Act was amended in 1978 to end discrimination against pregnant women. The Act makes it illegal to discriminate on the basis of pregnancy, childbirth, or related medical conditions in hiring, promoting, suspending, or discharging women who are pregnant. In addition, the employer is required to pay medical and hospital costs for childbirth to the same extent it pays for other conditions.

Equal Employment Opportunity Commission: Enforcing the EEOC Laws

The Equal Employment Opportunity Commission (EEOC) was established by the 1964 Civil Rights Act. The Commission was empowered to interpret the Act and resolve charges brought under it. The 1972 amendments gave the Commission additional authority to bring lawsuits against employers in the federal courts. Since 1979, the EEOC has enforced the Age Discrimination in Employment Act of 1967, the Equal Pay Act of 1963, Section 501 of the Rehabilitation Act of 1973, and the Americans with Disabilities Act of 1990. On average, about 17,000 age discrimination complaints were filed each year during the 1990s (Noe et al., 2000, p. 80). Employers have been generally successful in finding creative ways to successfully shed older workers without being prosecuted.

Even so, the Commission still cannot directly issue enforceable orders as do other agencies such as the Environmental Protection Agency. Hence, the EEOC cannot order an employer to discontinue discriminatory practices, nor can it order back pay to victims of discrimination. It must seek action through the courts.

The average backlog of cases for the EEOC runs approximately 20,000+. It is not possible to handle all of them, of course. Only a small percentage of charges are eventually resolved by EEOC or by the courts (Ivancevich & Glueck, 1983, p. 74). Nevertheless, legal history is being made by the EEOC, and its presence is felt in employment practices (Noe et al., 2000, p. 82).

EEOC Procedures

Step 1. The EEOC has the power to require employers to report employment statistics on federal forms.

Step 2. If the EEOC feels charges are justified, it authorizes its preinvestigation division to review the complaints.

Step 3. The investigation division then interviews all parties concerned.

Step 4. If there is substance to the case, the EEOC seeks an out-of-court settlement.

Step 5. If the parties cannot be reconciled, the EEOC can sue the employer.

In cases settled by court decisions, the courts have required such actions as back pay, reinstatement of employees, immediate promotion of employees, hiring quotas, abolition of testing programs, and creation of special training programs. Some settlements have cost millions of dollars.

Specifically, the EEOC may seek any or all of the following:

- Back pay (all)
- Hiring, promotion, reinstatement, benefit restoration, front pay, and other affirmative relief (Title VII, ADA, ADEA)
- Actual pecuniary loss other than back pay (Title VII, ADA)
- Liquidated damages (ADEA, EPA)
- Compensatory damages for future monetary losses and mental anguish (Title VII, ADA
- Punitive damages when employer acts with malice or reckless disregard for federally protected rights (Title VII, ADA)
- Posting a notice to all employees advising them of their rights under the laws EEOC enforces and their right to be free from retaliation (all)
- Corrective or preventive actions taken to cure the source of the identified discrimination and minimize the chance of its recurrence (all)
- Reasonable accommodation (ADA)
- Stopping the specific discriminatory practices involved in the case (all)

Laws Affecting Federal Contractors and Subcontractors

Several laws and executive orders (orders issued by the President of the United States under their authority) govern hiring and job practices of firms that hold federal contracts of over $50,000. While it is unlikely that any nursing facility would be directly affected by these regulations, many contractors doing construction work for them are subject to these regulations (Noe et al., 2000, p. 82).

Executive Order 11246

This order by the President of the United States requires written affirmative action programs of all contractors with 50 or more employees and $50,000 or more in federal contracts.

To enforce this order, the Office of Federal Contract Compliance Programs (OFCCP) was established. This agency was later given responsibility for administering laws protecting veterans (Noe et al., 2000, p. 82).

The Vocational Rehabilitation Act of 1973

This act requires federal government contractors to mount affirmative action programs for the handicapped. It is enforced by the OFCCP. The Act also provides a measure of federal support for programs to assist in training the handicapped. By 1980, approximately half of the 15 million Americans of working age deemed to be handicapped had been able to find employment (Ivancevich & Glueck, 1983, p. 82).

Vietnam Era Veterans Readjustment Act, 1974

This act requires firms with more than $10,000 in federal contracts to have affirmative action programs for employment and advancement of Vietnam veterans.

The American With Disabilities Act, 1990

Title I of the Americans with Disabilities Act of 1990 (ADA) prohibits facilities from discriminating against qualified individuals with disabilities in job application procedures, hiring, firing, advancement, compensation, job training, and other terms, conditions, and privileges of employment.

An individual with a disability is a person who:

- has a physical or mental impairment that substantially limits one or more major life activities (e.g., walking, lifting, seeing, learning, doing manual tasks),
- has a record of such an impairment (e.g., has been treated for a mental illness), or
- is regarded as having such an impairment (e.g., a person who has extensive scars from burns).

The Act applies to any qualified individual with a disability who can perform the essential functions of the position with or without reasonable accommodation. Individuals who have HIV or AIDS are considered disabled within the meaning of the ADA. Current users of illegal drugs are not protected as disabled persons. In 1999, about 1.4% of AIDS cases occurred among persons 65 and older, with the ratio of men to women being 7:1 (Maddox & Sussman, 2001, p. 51). Residents with AIDS is a now common experience in U.S. nursing facilities. The facility may not limit, segregate, or classify a disabled job applicant or employee in any way that adversely affects their opportunities. Facilities may not fire or refuse to hire disabled persons for any cause that could be eliminated by a reasonable accommodation.

Reasonable Accommodation

May include making existing facilities freely accessible to handicapped persons; supplying readers or interpreters; modifying policies, examinations, or training manuals; restructuring jobs or changing work schedules; reassigning the individual to a vacant position; or acquiring or modifying equipment for use by the disabled.

"Undue Hardship"

The facility is required to make an accommodation to the known disability of a qualified applicant or employee if it would not impose an "undue hardship" on the facility. Undue hardship is defined as an action requiring significant difficulty or expense when considered in light of factors such as a company's size, financial resources, and the nature and cost of the proposed accommodation.

Standards

The facility is not required to lower quality or production standards to make an accommodation nor to provide personal use items such as glasses or hearing aids.

Medical Examinations

The facility may not ask job applicants about the existence, nature, or severity of a disability. Applicants may be asked about their ability to perform specific job functions. A job offer may be conditioned on the results of a medical examination if the examination is required for all entering employees in similar jobs. Medical examinations of employees must be job related and consistent with the employer's business needs (EEOC Notice 915.002, 1994, p. 28). Medical tests must contain only "normal" medical test aspects given all pre-employment applicants and contain no features that could be construed to be testing for or testing a disability. The EEOC Notice 915.002 describes a number of scenarios and illustrations concerning pre-employment medical examinations around which the facility should build its medical examination policies.

If an applicant is not hired because of post-offer medical exam results, the reason must be given and a statement made that no reasonable accommodation was available that would have enabled the applicant to perform the essential job functions or that accommodation would impose an undue hardship.

Employee/Applicant Rights

Employees and applicants are entitled to apply to the Equal Employment Opportunity Commission (EEOC). If the applicant is successful the EEOC may require that the person be placed in a position if the discrimination had never occurred. This might entitle the applicant to hiring, promotion, reinstatement, back pay or other remuneration, or reasonable accommodation including reassignment. The successful complainant may also be entitled to damages for future money losses, mental anguish, and inconvenience. Punitive damages may also be imposed on the facility if the EEOC feels it acted with malice or reckless indifference. The complainant may also be entitled to their attorney's fees. Charges can be filed at any field office of the EEOC, which are located in 50 cities.

Unanticipated Results

Over the 1990s, approximately 90,000 complaints were filed, with about 50% being found to have merit (Noe et al., 2000, p. 98). Surprisingly few (10%) concerned failure to hire. Half of these complaints dealt with firings, about one-third with failure to make reasonable accommodation. According to the National Organization on Disability, a private citizens group, fewer disabled persons (31%) were employed in 1993 than in 1986 before the act (33%; Noe et al., 2000, p. 99). Of significance to nursing homes is that the largest identifiable category of complaints allege back problems (Noe et al., 2000, p. 99). Lower back disability accounts for about 25% of all lost workdays and is estimated to cost nearly $30 billion each year (Noe et al., 2000, p. 103).

Patient Self-Determination Act of 1990

The Patient Self-Determination Act (PSDA) of 1990 was technically an amendment to the federal Medicare and Medicaid law passed as part of the 1990 Omnibus Budget Reconciliation Act. It is usually referred to, however, as the Patient Self-Determination Act.

Requirements

The Act requires that all health care facilities accepting Medicare or Medicaid moneys do the five following things:

- "provide written information" to patients/residents at the time of admission concerning "an individual's right under State law (whether statutory or as recognized by the courts of the State) to make decisions concerning . . . medical care, including the right to accept or refuse medical or surgical treatment and the right to formulate advance directives";
- "maintain written policies and procedures" with respect to advance directives (e.g., living wills and health care power of attorney) and to inform residents of the policies (Maddox & Sussman, 2001, p. 611);
- "document in the individual's medical record whether or not the individual has executed an advance directive";
- "ensure compliance with the requirements of State law (whether statutory or as recognized by the courts of the State) respecting advance directives at facilities of the provider"; and
- "provide (individually or with others) for education for staff and the community on issues concerning advance directives."

The facility may not "condition the provision of care or otherwise discriminate against an individual based on whether or not the individual has executed an advance directive."

A signed copy of each resident's acknowledgment of receipt of their information and the opportunity to act under the provisions of the PSDA should be in their file. Relevant advance directives should be prominently located in the resident's medical record.

Safe Medical Devices Act of 1990

Under the Safe Medical Devices Act of 1990 nursing homes must report to the Food and Drug Administration or the manufacturer all incidents in which a medical device caused or contributed to a resident's death, serious injury, or illness.

A medical device is any instrument, implement, machine, implant, or related article intended for use in diagnosing, treating, or preventing disease. Drugs are not medical devices. Nursing home examples are such items as blood glucose devices, blood pressure devices, catheters, hearing aids, infusion pumps, pacemakers, restraints, scales, thermometers, and wheelchairs (Carley, 1991, p. 66).

Reasonable Probability

All incidents that reasonably suggest a likelihood that a medical device has caused or contributed to a resident or patient's death, serious illness, or injury must be reported. Reports are to be made as soon as possible, but no later than 10 days.

Clinical Laboratory Improvement Act

The Clinical Laboratory Improvement Amendments of 1988 (CLIA) established quality standards for all laboratory testing to ensure the accuracy, reliability, and timeliness of patient test results regardless of where the test was performed. If a facility only does blood draws (only collects specimens and performs no testing) it does not need a CLIA number. However, most nursing facilities today do enough testing, such as glucose testing, to be required to enroll in the CLIA program by obtaining a Certificate of Waiver (COW), pay applicable certificate fees biannually, and follow manufacturers' test instructions. Of the 174,504 laboratories enrolled in CLIA, approximately 93,129 (54%) of these hold a COW. Detailed information about CLIA is available on the CMS Web site. Type www.questions.cms.hhs.gov for an effective Web search.

Civil Rights Act of 1991

This act expanded the 1964 Civil Rights Act. The 1964 Civil Rights Act only permitted back pay, and perhaps attorney's fees. The 1991 Act permitted compensatory damage such as money lost, emotional pain and suffering, and loss of enjoyment of life. Punitive damages, which are meant to discourage other employers from similar practices, were also allowed by providing payments to the plaintiff beyond actual damages suffered. This applied to the Civil Rights Act of 1964, the Americans with Disabilities Act, and the Age Discrimination in Employment Act of 1967. Maximum punitive damages per incident were set at between $50,000 for smaller employers to $300,000 for employers with more than 500 employees (Noe et al., 2000, p. 80).

The Family and Medical Leave Act of 1993

Under the Family and Medical Leave Act (FMLA), a covered employer (50 or more employees) must allow up to 12 weeks per year of unpaid leave connected with pregnancy, childbirth, and recovery, or a serious health condition affecting an employee or an employee's family member (Maddox & Sussman, 2001, p. 382).

Benefits Eligibility

The employee must have worked for at least 12 months (1,250 hours at least) prior to the leave. The 12 months need not be consecutive.

Benefits

A person is entitled in connection with: birth of a son or daughter or adoption or foster care; caring for a spouse, son, daughter, or parent with a serious health condition; or a serious health condition that prevents the employee from performing their job functions. A serious health condition does not normally include any short-term condition that could be covered under regular sick leave policies. Absence for substance abuse without a treatment program is not within the definition of a serious health condition for the purposes of this Act.

Options

The employee may ask for leave as reduced work hours or any combination of modified work schedule to accommodate covered reasons for unpaid leave under the Act.

Return

Generally, the employee is entitled to return to their former job or its equivalent at the same pay, benefits, and other equal working conditions.

In practice, only 3.7% of workers have taken advantage of this act according to one study (Maddox & Sussman, 2001, p. 383). The rate may be higher in nursing facilities, but the workers who most need the Act's benefits (the nurses' aides) can least afford to take leave without pay.

Benefits Improvement and Protection Act

Both the administrator and director of nursing need to assure facility compliance in Section 941 of the 2000 Benefits Improvement and Protection Act effective January 1, 2003, stating that the number of registered nurses, licensed practical nurses, and nurse aides directly responsible for resident care on each shift must be posted in a clearly visible place (*Quality Care Advocate,* Winter 2003 p. 7).

Health Insurance Portability and Accountability Act (HIPAA) of 1996

Effective April, 2001, the Department of Health and Human Services issued privacy standards that facilities must ensure for their residents in order to continue to be eligible for Medicare funds. Included are such requirements as:

- a policy against emailing patient records
- a written information security plan
- assurance that third-party vendors and contractors are compliant with HIPAA
- written record that all patients in the facility are informed about all the ways their records are being used
- written record that all patients have been given the opportunity to refuse to allow the facility to share their medical information

HIPAA compliance is a vast and evolving topic. The Final Rule can be accessed at www.cms.hhs.gov/regulations/hipaa/cms.

Facility Guidelines Institute and American Institute of Architects 2006 Guidelines

In July 2006, these two bodies issued a guideline that any new rooms added to the nation's hospitals be private rooms. Forty-two states follow these guidelines, and hospitals are observing these guidelines. It has been observed nursing facility guidelines tend to follow hospital guidelines, for example, hand washing precautions and similar health policies. If the future hospital room will tend to be a private room, it seems likely that the future nursing home room will be a private room.

Lifespan Respite Care Act of 2006

It is estimated that in 2006 more than 44 million Americans gave unpaid care to disabled adults in their home according to Family Caregiver Alliance, a nonprofit organization. This new law allows, for the first time, payment to relatives to give care to family members. This continues a trend away from support for nursing home care signaled in the 2000 National Family Caregiver Program, which provided aid to caregivers and patients over 60 years of age only. This new act provides care regardless of age, which may reduce the number of younger persons seeking admission to nursing facilities.

4.4.3 REGULATION OF COMPENSATION

Most states and the federal government have passed laws that regulate compensation for work done.

Federal jurisdiction covers only those workers engaged in producing goods for interstate and foreign commerce. Technically, the federal government does not have authority to regulate worker compensation within states.

More than 40 states have their own wage and hour laws and also regulate other conditions of employment, such as hours allowed per week before overtime must be paid.

The practical effect of having both federal and state regulations governing compensation is that both prevail. In reality, the federal laws are applied to most workers regardless of whether they are producing goods for interstate or foreign commerce. This breadth of application of the federal wage laws is achieved by including persons whose work is (loosely defined) closely related to any production for interstate or foreign commerce.

New overtime rules affected numerous nursing home employee categories. In 2004, the Department of Labor raised the wage payment requirements for workers who are eligible for overtime pay for working more than 40 hours a week from the 1970s level of $8,060 to the new level of $23,600.

On a day-to-day basis, this means that nursing home employee compensation and other work conditions must meet both federal and state regulations.

The original goals of federal wage and hour regulations were (a) to encourage the spreading of work among as many wage earners as feasible and (b) to establish a floor for wages for any worker regardless of the job. Requiring a rate of 1 1/2 times the regular pay rate for all overtime has helped to accomplish spreading the work. Requiring a minimum wage for all persons has accomplished the second goal.

Fair Labor Standards Act (FLSA) 29 United States C. {} 201, et seq. (Wage and Hour Act)

The Fair Labor Standards Act was originally passed in 1938, but like the Social Security Act of 1935, it has been amended many times. The four primary foci of the Act are (a) minimum wage rates, (b) overtime, (c) child labor, and (d) equal rights (Noe et al., 2000, p. 413).

Minimum Wage Rates

When first instituted, the minimum wage was 25 cents per hour. Over the decades it has risen nearly 15-fold as the value of the dollar has declined.

The new minimum wage must be calculated on the actual earning wage before any additional payments are added. For example, the employee works a 46-hour week. They received the minimum wage for the first 40 hours and are paid at 1 1/2 times that rate for the additional 6 hours. Generally, the employee must be paid in cash or in a "negotiable instrument payable at par" (a check) except that board, lodging, and other facilities regularly furnished to employees may be provided in lieu of cash wages or the cost deducted from cash wages (Noe et al., 2000, p. 413).

What Is Work?

Preparatory activities integral to the employee's job may be considered work time. If an employee performs work that is prohibited, with the knowledge or acquiescence of management, the employee must be paid, even if the work is away from the facility, if the employer has reason to believe the work is being performed. On-call or waiting time may be considered work if the employee is "engaged" by the employer to wait for the work. Travel associated with or required by the job is compensable. Bona fide meal periods are not compensable, must be 30 minutes in duration, and totally free the employee from performing any work. If meal periods are frequently interrupted, as happens often in a nursing facility setting, the whole meal period may be considered compensable work time. Rest periods and coffee breaks are compensable.

The minimum wage rates are especially important to nursing homes because many of them pay nurse's aides and housekeeping and maintenance employees at or just above the minimum wage.

Overtime

The Fair Labor Standards Act requires overtime for all hours over 40 hours per week, to be paid at one and one-half the regular rate of pay. Hospital and nursing home employees are entitled to an exception in that overtime may be calculated on the basis of a 14-day period if overtime is paid for hours worked in excess of 8 daily and in excess of 80 during the 14-day period. There must be an agreement between employees and employer to this arrangement.

Overtime must be calculated on the basis of a single work week and not be averaged over 2 or more weeks. A fluctuating work week is permitted under certain circumstances.

Whenever compensatory time is given for overtime hours worked, the employee must be given 1 1/2 hour off for every hour of overtime worked. Employees may not accumulate more than 240 hours, however.

If bonuses are paid for some other period—a month or a quarter, for example, the base for overtime wage must be recalculated to add any additional remuneration to the base rate for that period in calculating the time-and-a-half rate for all hours worked over 80 hours in each 2-week period.

Because of their exemption from coverage by the Fair Labor Standards Act, management personnel are referred to as exempt employees. Nonmanagement employees are considered nonexempt. A number of complicated definitions apply to this area.

Congress amends this act frequently, so it is important to check with the Department of Labor to keep abreast of current and upcoming regulations and changes.

Exempt/Non-Exempt

Executive, professional, administrative, and outside sales occupations are exempt from FLSA coverage. Nonexempt occupations are covered and include most hourly employees such as the nurses and nurses' aides. It is estimated that about 20% of employees are in the exempt category (Noe et al., 2000, p. 413).

Most nurses prefer to work as exempt employees because this permits them to receive overtime pay. A July 2004 Fact Sheet #17N: Nurses and the Part 541 Exemptions Under the Fair Labor Standards Act indicates that nurses qualify as learned professionals if they are paid $455 per week. Nurses who are paid on an hourly basis should receive overtime pay. However, registered nurses who are registered by the appropriate State examining board generally meet the duties requirements for the learned professional exemption, and if paid on a salary basis of at least $455 per week, may be classified as exempt.

Enforcement of FLSA

Records may be subpoenaed without a warrant at off-site locations. Normally a warrant is required for on-site inspections. Violations are subject to a penalty of up to $1,000 per violation. Injunctions may be issued regarding minimum wage, overtime, child labor, and record-keeping violations. Criminal proceedings may be brought by the Department of Justice. First offenders may be fined up to $10,000. Second offenders may be so fined and a maximum prison sentence of 6 months imposed. Wage and hour inspectors are liable to show up unannounced. In general, the word of the employee is taken most seriously by these inspectors. If an employee said they worked 2 hours per week "off the clock" for the previous year the facility may be required to pay that employee for 2 hours of overtime per week for that past year.

Child Labor

Minors under 16 may not be employed except under a temporary permit issued by the Department of Labor. Many states have regulations concerning the employment of persons between ages 16 and 18 in certain industries, such as nursing homes, where the worker can be exposed to disease or other hazardous conditions. Generally, special temporary work permits must be obtained

Equal Pay Act

In 1963 the Fair labor Standards Act was amended by the Equal Pay Act. Under that amendment:

> No employer shall discriminate between employees on the basis of sex by paying wages to employees less than the rate at which he (sic) pays wages to employees of the opposite sex for equal work on jobs which require equal skill, effort and responsibility, and similar working conditions. (Chruden & Sherman, p. 453)

Progress has been slow in this area. U.S. Department of Labor, Bureau of Labor Statistics studies have shown that women earn slightly over 60 cents for every dollar men earn in comparable positions.

The equal-pay provision of the Fair Labor Standards Act is of special concern to nursing home operators, who may employ both male and female nurses, male and female aides, and male and female maintenance and laundry persons.

4.4.4 WORKER'S COMPENSATION: ASSISTANCE FOR ON-THE-JOB INJURIES

Worker's compensation laws are based on the principle that employees themselves should not have to pay costs associated with injuries that occur at work. On-the-job injuries, the lawmakers have reasoned, are a cost of doing business and should be passed on to the consumer.

In New Jersey, Texas, and South Carolina worker compensation insurance is voluntary. In all other states it is compulsory for employers to participate in a state-sponsored or state-approved program.

Under most state laws, workers are paid a percentage of their regular wages while recovering from an injury on the job. States normally set limits to benefits and specify how long they must be paid.

Hospitalization and other medical costs are also normally covered by worker compensation insurance funds. There are usually death benefits for the worker's family. States establish commissions that handle any claims that are in dispute. Generally, the result is little cost to the injured worker and reasonably rapid assistance.

States usually take one of two basic approaches to funding worker's compensation insurance. Sometimes the state operates its own insurance system in which employers are usually obliged to participate. In other states, employers are allowed either to self-insure or to join a private insurance company program.

One characteristic of most worker accident compensation plans is that the amount the employer must pay per month is based on experience. Under this system, employers with good safety records pay less than those with large numbers of claims. In some states, benefits to the injured worker are reduced if the worker is willfully negligent in following safety procedures.

Unemployment Compensation

In 1993 alone, 216,400 employees in nursing and personal care facilities suffered work-related illnesses and injuries, an incident rate of 16.9 nonfatal injuries and illnesses per 100 full-time employees (Burda, 1995, p. 24). This was 50% higher than hospitals 10.9 rate. The nursing and personal care homes injury rate in 1993 was the second highest of all industries with 100,000 or more total injuries and illnesses, motor vehicle and equipment makers rate (17.7) being slightly higher.

In an effort to cut worker's compensation insurance costs Genesis Health Care Corporation launched a lift program. In one facility alone the $30,000 invested in lifts in 1 year reduced the number of back injuries related to moving patients to zero from six, thus dropping worker's comp claims from $97,000 to zero (*Wall Street Journal*, February 26, 2006, B1).

Employees who participate in the Social Security Act program are eligible for unemployment compensation when they are laid off by their employer. Nearly all nursing home employees are covered by the Social Security Act.

Unemployment compensation is available for up to 26 weeks through the state employment agency if the worker registers and is willing to accept any suitable comparable work offered through the agency.

Unemployment compensation is funded by a federal payroll tax based on the wages of each employee up to a certain maximum. The federal government turns these moneys over to the states for disbursement.

A separate record is kept for each employer. Once a company has paid an account equivalent to the required reserve, its rate of taxation is reduced. In actual practice, this means that nursing facilities with few unemployment compensation claims against them pay at a lower tax rate than those with a large number of such claims.

Experience has shown that, although they are discharged or let go for valid reasons (unrelated to lack of work), unless the facility has extremely good documentation on the circumstances of the dismissal, employees may be successful in claiming unemployment compensation. When this happens the costs of the unemployment compensation paid by the state are allocated to that individual nursing facility's account.

Extensive information on these labor-related topics can be accessed at www.dol.gov.

4.4.5 RETIREMENT

Age Discrimination Employment Act, 1967 (Amended 1978)

This act protects employees from being discriminated against on the basis of age. It is intended to prevent companies from replacing older employees with younger ones, whether to achieve a younger average among the working force or to avoid paying pension benefits. There are some exceptions, such as certain occupational groups and employers with fewer than 20 employees, but the practical effect is that no employees in the typical nursing facility can be forced to retire against their wishes solely on the basis of age.

During the 1960s, Congress investigated pensions for American workers and discovered that for a variety of reasons, up to one-half of American workers covered by pension plans would never receive any benefits. The largest problem was a failure of businesses to fund their pension plans adequately. For the worker the basic problem was loss of any pension benefits when leaving the company for almost any reason before retirement. The EEOC is the primary agency responsible for enforcing this act through ERISA.

The Employee Retirement Income Security Act, 1975

In reaction, Congress passed the Employee Retirement Income Security Act (ERISA) of 1975. This act sets minimum funding levels for pension funds, requires certification every 3 years of the actuarial soundness of the plan, and requires vesting of the employee's equity in the pension fund. Employers are *not* required under ERISA or any other law to provide a private pension fund for their employees (Noe et al., 2000, p. 479).

Among its regulation ERISA set up the Pension Benefit Guaranty Corporation, established in 1974, which is supported by premiums from employers to assure that employees will eventually receive retirement funds. Companies that decide to withdraw from the plan must make substantial payments into the Corporation before being permitted to do so. This and other elements of the Act create hardships for employers who otherwise are committed to providing pension benefits for employees.

One major drawback to the ERISA legislation is that its rules are so demanding that many employers choose not to offer pension plans. Also, upon implementation of the Act, many employers chose to withdraw their plans rather than try to comply with the law when it went into effect. Another unfortunate result is that many employers are electing to receive their accumulated "retirement" benefits when they leave the organization. Studies have documented that all too often these pension benefits never find their way into 401k or similar retirement mechanisms (Noe et al., 2000, p. 458).

In place of regular company created and maintained pension plans, a number of employers have opted to offer employees participation in what are known as 401k and similar plans under which employees contribute money on a tax-deferred basis for retirement purposes. The major drawback for the employee is that upon leaving the company they often receive their 401k contributions in a lump sum. Employees can roll over these 401k funds to similar tax-deferred investments within specified days and retain them for eventual retirement purpose, but, as with regular lump sum pension proceeds given to an employee at termination, for too many employees the temptation to use the funds for current expenses is too great (Maddox & Sussman, 2001, p. 331).

4.5 Workplace Safety: The Occupational Safety and Health Act (1970)

Origin and Passage

For the first 7 decades of the 20th century state governments were responsible for safety in the workplace. During that period organized labor became less and less satisfied with enforcement of state laws, variation in laws among the states, and often absence of any safety laws. In the half-decade before the passage of federal legislation, job-related accidents were causing up to 2.5 million disabilities and 14,000 deaths annually (Department of Labor, 1976, p. 1).

After 3 years of intense lobbying by employees and the unions, Congress passed the Occupational Safety and Health Act (OSHA) in 1970 (Public Law 91–596). OSHA applies to nearly all employees and includes all of those working in nursing homes.

Federal Implementation

Two federal agencies have been set up to implement OSHA. The Act is administered by the Occupational Safety and Health Administration in the Department of Labor. The National Institute of Occupational Safety and Health (NIOSH) was established to conduct research and develop standards.

A major goal of the Act has been to turn workplace safety enforcement back to the states with a strengthened work-safety law. States have been encouraged to establish their own inspection programs and industrial safety laboratories.

In addition to meeting all standards set, OSHA imposes on employers a general duty to provide each employee a safe work place, free from recognized hazards causing or likely to cause death or serious physical harm. For example, pending the publication of final regulations regarding the control of infections (e.g., AIDS), OSHA invoked the "general duty" obligation when inspecting nursing facilities.

Three OSHA Impact Areas

OSHA directly affects the operations of nursing care facilities in at least three main areas:

1. Meeting the standards set by OSHA
2. Cooperating in OSHA inspections of the facility
3. Keeping the necessary records on job related accidents and illnesses

Sources of Standards

OSHA standards may originate from a variety of sources. The Secretary of Labor may issue and revise standards at will. This may be done on the Secretary's own initiative, on recommendation of the National Institute of Occupational Safety and Health, or at the urging of interested parties such as labor unions or groups of affected employees.

Adopting Standards of Other Organizations

OSHA has adopted several national consensus standards that were developed by other groups, including the National Fire Protection Association's *Life Safety Code*® and the *Standards for the Physically Handicapped* of the American National Standards Institute.

Definition of *Standard*

OSHA safety standards are "practices, means, operations or processes, reasonably necessary to provide safe . . . employment" (Ivancevich & Glueck, 1983, p. 595; Noe et al., 2000, p. 101). Each employer is responsible for knowing OSHA standards for their facility (either federal or a combination of federal and state).

The original standards ran to 350 pages of small print in the Federal Register. Subsequently, supplementary volumes of standards have been published. Some annual volumes have been over 700 pages in length. Even so, each manager is responsible for knowing applicable standards and is subject to both fines and imprisonment if found to be in violation of them.

Some OSHA Requirements

OSHA bulletins have listed the following as among OSHA's requirements.

Employers

Every employer must furnish a workplace free from recognized hazards that are causing or are likely to cause death or serious harm to employees and shall comply with OSHA standards, displaying the OSHA poster that informs employees of their rights and responsibilities, and compiling annual figures on work-related illnesses and accidents.

Employees

Each employee shall obey all OSHA requirements. However, the facility is held responsible for worker violation of OSHA standards. The employer has the choice of dismissing a worker who ignores OSHA requirements, but there are no punishments for the worker who willfully ignores them. Willful disregard of OSHA rules is, however, grounds for termination permitted under federal law.

Any employee may lodge a complaint with OSHA. The complaint must be in writing and signed with a description of the hazardous condition. The signed complaint is submitted to the OSHA regional director and to the employer, unsigned, if the employee wishes to remain anonymous.

Inspections

OSHA inspectors will visit at times of their own choosing, or at the invitation of any employer, union, or employee. Employees requesting an inspection need not be identified.

The employer and the employees must each designate a representative to accompany the OSHA inspector(s). If the employees do not do so, the OSHA compliance officer must consult several employees during the visit. This officer must hold an opening conference to discuss the scope and reason for the inspection and a concluding conference in which findings are presented to the employer.

Employers must not discriminate against any employee(s) who asks for an OSHA safety or health inspection. Any employee may file a complaint with the nearest OSHA office within 30 days for any such alleged discrimination.

OSHA inspectors examine *the premises* for compliance with regulations and *the records* of illnesses and injuries to employees.

Citations

Citations may be issued at the end of the inspection itself or later by mail. Any citation issued must be posted at or near the site of violation for 3 days or the duration of the violation, whichever is longer. One citation must be issued for each serious and nonserious violation found and a time limit specified for its correction.

OSHA compliance officers may categorize employer violations as

1. *imminent danger* (can close operations down)
2. *serious* (calls for a major fine)
3. *nonserious* (a violation in which a direct and immediate relationship exists between the condition and occupational health, but not such as to cause death or serious physical harm)
4. *de minimus* (small violation)—a notification is given, but no fine imposed; a violation of a standard that is not directly or immediately related to occupational safety or health.

In every case, a time period is specified within which the violation must be corrected. A fine of $7,000 per day per violation may be imposed after the time limit set for abatement (correction) of the violation.

Fines

Fines, some mandatory, under OBRA 1990, are to be imposed for the following:

1. *willful or repeated violations:* up to $7,000 per violation (mandatory); may double after first conviction
2. *serious violation:* mandatory penalty up to $7,000 for each violation
3. *nonserious violation:* optional penalties up to $7,000 each
4. *failure to correct* within proposed time period: up to $7,000 per day
5. *willful violation:* minimum fine: $5,000

Employers have the right to appeal fines or citations within the OSHA structure or in the courts. Notice of contest must be filed within 15 days.

Record Keeping

The area that most directly affects nursing home administrators on a daily basis is keeping standardized records of illnesses and injuries from which ratios must be calculated. This record is OSHA Form "Log and Summary of Occupational Injuries and Illnesses," which must be kept by each facility.

Accidents and illnesses that do not have to be reported are those that require only first aid and do not result in any work time lost. Accidents and illnesses that do have to be reported are those that result in death(s), disabilities that cause the employee to miss work, and injuries that require treatment by a physician. Reporting requirements were tightened on May 2, 1994. Fatal or serious multiple cases (three or more hospitalized) must be reported to the OSHA regional director orally by telephone within 8 hours, which begins as soon as any facility representatives becomes aware of the situation. Also, such incidents must be reported if death or hospitalization occur within 30 days of the incident. Other cases must be recorded within 6 days and reported on routine forms as requested by OSHA.

Occupational illness is a definition of special relevance to the nursing home setting. An occupational illness is any abnormal condition or disorder, other than one resulting from an occupational injury, caused by exposure to environmental factors associated with employment. It includes acute and chronic illnesses or diseases that may be caused by inhalation, absorption, ingestion, or direct contact (Chruden & Sherman, 1980, p. 524).

OSHA defines an occupational injury as any injury, such as a cut, fracture, sprain, or amputation, that results from a work accident or from an exposure involving a single accident in the work environment (Chruden & Sherman, 1980, p. 524).

Each time a recordable case is entered in the log mentioned previously, a "Supplementary Record of Occupational Injuries and Illnesses" must be completed, giving information on what the employee was doing, which part of the body was affected, and the identity of the employee.

An OSHA Form "Summary of Occupational Injuries and Illnesses" must be submitted annually and posted where employees can easily see it, for example, above the time clock, at least during January and February of every year.

In 2003, the number of occupational injuries and illnesses with days away from work, job transfer, or restriction in the health care industry was 3.1 cases per 100 full time workers (334,000 actual cases) making health care one of the more injury and illness prone industries (DHHS, 2005, p. 230).

The Current and Emerging Situation

Completing, submitting, and posting accident and illness forms as required will remain a continuing requirement for nursing home administrators, but the inspection issue is another matter. After years during which few, if any, nursing facilities were being inspected in the various states, OSHA inspectors have begun showing up to perform routine inspection of nursing facilities. In many locales OSHA inspectors will, at the invitation of the facility, perform "dry run" inspections for an employer, advising on any "violations" and providing an opportunity for correction before any official inspection.

Since OSHA was enacted, fatalities in the work force are estimated to have decreased by 10% and total injuries to have decreased by 15% (Ivancevich & Glueck, 1983, p. 601; Noe et al., 2000, p. 103).

In 2006, the nursing home injury incident rate was 13.9 injuries and illnesses per 100 full time workers. This was more than double the incident rate of 6.1% of industry as a whole.

OSHA Web Site

The OSHA Web site offers extensive nursing home specific downloads such as *Safety and Health Topics: Guidelines for Nursing Homes.* OSHA issued an ergonomics guideline for the nursing home industry March 13, 2003, which may be accessed on the OSHA Web site. OSHA estimates that nursing homes and personal care facilities employ approximately 1.8 million workers at 21,000 worksites (www.osha.gov, August, 2006).

4.6 Fire Safety: The *Life Safety Code®*

The National Fire Protection Association is a private, nonprofit organization with headquarters in Quincy, Massachusetts. It is not a government agency, nor does it write federal regulations. However, because the regulations for licensing nursing homes include adherence to the *Life Safety Code®* these fire safety standards have, in effect, the force of law for nursing homes.

The National Fire Protection Association has more than 150 committees, one of which, the Committee on Safety to Life, establishes and revises these standards. The committee has met since 1913 and currently has several standing subcommittees.

The Code has evolved over the years, benefiting from the hindsight gained from the experience of many tragic fires. This Code represents the collected wisdom on fire prevention and fire containment.

The regulations passed in the Federal Register in 1974 required nursing facilities to "meet such provisions of the *Life Safety Code®* of the National Fire Protection Association as are applicable to nursing homes" (405.1134A). These regulations have been revised regularly with new editions approximately every 3 years. The ones described in the following sections are from the 2000 *Life Safety Code®* edition. While the 2006 Life Safety Code wording is available the 2000 Life Safety Code is used here because the Director of the Office of the Federal Register has approved the NFPA 101 2000 edition issued January 14, 2000 for incorporation by reference into CFR (Code of Federal Regulations). Until the Director of the Office of the Federal Register designates a later year's Life Safety Code it is the Life Safety Code issued January 14, 2000, which the nursing facility is required to meet.

Generally, actual wording of the *Life Safety Code®* is not used in the following pages. The major concepts and a number of the essential features of the

---

Note: The materials on the Life Safety Code® in this section are from NFPA 101–2000, *Life Safety Code®*, Copyright © 2000, National Fire Protection Association, Quincy, MA 02269. This material is not the complete and official position of the National Fire Protection Association on the referenced subject, which is represented only by the standard in its entirety.

Code presented later in this section are summaries of the Code presented for study purposes. The Code itself is usually paraphrased. Under no circumstances, then, should the reader treat this material as a substitute for obtaining the actual *Life Safety Code®*.

The Eighth Edition, 2000 volume edited by Ron Cote, P.E., Editor, offers highly useful interpretations of the *Life Safety Code®* and the National Fire Protection Association's Health Care Facilities Handbook®, 8th Edition, (2000) Ron Cote, Editor, and copies of the Code itself may be ordered from National Fire Protection, Inc., Batterymarch Park, Quincy, MA 02269; telephone 1-800-344-3555, or by visiting the Web site, www.catalog.nfpa.org.

The material here is available in NFPA 101®, the eighth edition of the Life Safety Code Handbook, © 2000. National Fire Protection Association, Quincy, MA 02269. This material is neither the actual wording, nor the complete and official position of the NFPA on the referenced subjects, which are represented only by the standard in its entirety. This material is intended to apprise persons in the nursing home field of the general nature and functions within the facility of *The Life Safety Code®*.

Health Care Occupancies

Chapter 18 New Health Care Occupancies of the Life Safety Code

Life Safety Code® and 101® are registered trademarks of the National Fire Protection Association, Inc., Quincy, MA 02269.

Compromised Health. Due to the compromised health and mobility of residents a primary emphasis in placed on superior construction, quick discovery of fire, quick notification of the fire department, and early extinguishment.

18.1.3 Total Concept All health care facilities shall be designed, constructed, maintained, and operated to minimize the possibility of a fire emergency requiring the evacuation of occupants. Because the safety of health care occupants cannot be ensured adequately by dependence on evacuation of the building, their protection from fire shall be provided by appropriate arrangement of facilities; adequate, trained staff; and development of operating and maintenance procedures.

18.1.1.2 Goals and Objectives The goal is to close as many doors as possible to prevent smoke from spreading and, to the extent feasible, to confine the fire to the room of origin. Studies show that no or low loss of life occurs when staff close the doors. Closing the doors has the most significant effect on limiting the spread of fire and smoke and limiting or eliminating any loss of life. The goal is to be accomplished by limiting the development and spread of a fire emergency to the room of fire origin and deducing the need for occupant evacuation, except from the room of fire origin.

Emphases. Emphasis must be placed on removing patients from the room of fire origin and anyone directly exposed to the fire.

18.7.1 Evacuation and Relocation Plan and Fire Drills

18.7.1.1 The administration of every health care occupancy shall have, in effect and available to all supervisory personnel, written copies of a plan for the protection of all persons in the event of fire, for their evacuation to areas of refuge, and for their evacuation from the building when necessary. All employees shall be periodically instructed and kept informed with respect to their duties under the plan. A copy of the plan shall be readily available at all times in the telephone operator's position or at the security center.

18.7.1.2 Fire Drills shall include the transmission of a fire alarm signal and simulation emergency fire conditions. Drills shall be conducted quarterly on each shift to familiarize facility personnel (nurses, interns, maintenance engineers, and administrative staff) with the signals and emergency action required under varied conditions. When drills are conducted between 9:00 P.M. and 6:00 A.M. a coded announcement shall be permitted to be used instead of audible alarms. Exception: Infirm or bedridden patients shall not be required to be moved during drills to safe areas or to the exterior of the building.

18.7.1.3 Employees of health care occupancies shall be instructed in life safety procedures and devices.

18.7.2 Procedure in Case of Fire

The basic response required of staff shall include the removal of all occupants directly involved with the fire emergency, transmission of an appropriate fire alarm signal to warn other building occupants and summon staff, confinement of the effects of the fire by closing doors to isolate the fire area, and the relocation of patients as detailed in the health care occupancy's fire safety plan.

18.7.2.2 A written fire safety plan shall provide for the following:

- use of alarms
- transmitting of alarm to fire department
- response to alarms
- isolation of fire
- evacuation of immediate area

- evacuation of smoke compartment
- preparation of floors and building for evacuation
- extinguishment of fire

18.7.2.3 All personnel shall be instructed in the use of and response to fire alarms. In addition, they shall be instructed in the use of the code phrase to ensure transmission of an alarm under the following conditions:

- when the individual who discovers a fire must immediately go to the aid of an endangered person
- during a malfunction of the building fire alarm system

Personnel hearing the code announced shall first activate the building fire alarm using the nearest manual fire alarm box and then shall execute immediately their duties as outlined in the fire safety plan.

18.7.3 Maintenance of Exits

Health care occupancies that find it necessary to lock exits shall, at all times, maintain an adequate staff qualified to release locks and direct occupants from the immediate danger area to a place of safety in case of fire or other emergency.

18.7.4 Smoking

Smoking regulations shall be adopted and shall include no fewer than the following provisions:

- Smoking shall be prohibited in any room, ward, or compartment where flammable liquids, combustible gasses, or oxygen are used or stored and in any other hazardous location, and such areas shall be posted with signs that read NO SMOKING or shall be posted with the international symbol for no smoking.
- Smoking by patients classified as not responsible shall be prohibited.
- Ashtrays of noncombustible material and safe design shall be provided in all areas where smoking is permitted.
- Metal containers with self-closing cover devices into which ashtrays can be emptied shall be readily available to all areas where smoking is permitted.

18.7.5 *Furnishings, Bedding, and Decorations*

10.3.2 Upholstered furniture and mattresses shall be resistant to a cigarette ignition (that is smoldering) in accordance with NFPA 260 Standard Methods of Tests and Classification System for Cigarette Ignition Resistance of Components of Upholstered Furniture.

The peak rate of heat release for a single upholstered furniture item shall not exceed 250 kW (a heat release rate [HRR], that is, the rate at which heat energy is generated by burning).

The total energy released by the single upholstered furniture item during the first 5 minutes of the test shall not exceed 40 MJ (HRR).

The peak rate of heat release for the mattress shall not exceed 250 kW (HRR).

The total energy released by the mattress during the first 5 minutes of the test shall not exceed 40 mJ (HRR).

10.3.5 Furnishings or decorations of an explosive or highly flammable character shall not be used.

18.7.51 Draperies, curtains, including cubicle curtains, and other loosely hanging fabrics and films serving as furnishings or decorations in health care occupancies shall be in accordance with provisions of 10.3.1

Exception: Curtains at showers.

That is, contents and furnishings must be flame resistant as demonstrated by testing in accordance with NFPA 701, Standard Methods of Fire Tests for Flame Propagation of Textiles and Films

18.7.5.4 Combustible decorations shall be prohibited in any health care occupancy unless they are flame retardant. Exception: combustible decorations, such as photographs and paintings, in such limited quantities that a hazard of fire development spread is not present.

Note: Implication for administrator. There are NFPA tests for most objects in the nursing facility. It is important to learn from all vendors that the products being introduced into the facility have met NFPA or NFPA required tests.

18.7.5.5 Soiled linen and trash collection containers must be limited to a capacity of 32 gallons within any 64 square foot area. Mobile soiled linen and trash collection receptacles are limited to a maximum capactiy of 33 gallons. The average density of container capacity in a room or space shall not exceed .5 gal. A capacity of 32 gal. shall not be exceeded within any 64-foot area. Mobile soiled linen or Tran's collection receptacles with capacities greater than 32 gallons shall be located in a room protected as a hazardous area when not attended. Exception: Container size and density shall not be limited in hazardous areas.

18.7.7 New engineered smoke control systems must meet standards of NFPA 92A, Recommended Practice for Smoke-Control Systems and NFPA 92B, Guide for Smoke Management Systems in Malls, Atria, and Large Areas.

18.7.8 Portable Space Heating Devices are prohibited except for use in nonsleeping staff and employee areas where the heating elements do not exceed 212 degrees Fahrenheit.

18.1.1.4.1 Additions. Additions not meeting these standards must be separated by a fire barrier having at least a 2-hour fire resistance rating and of required construction materials.

18.1.1.4.2 Communicating openings. Shall be limited to corridors protected by approved self-closing fire doors. These doors, when necessary, may be held open by automatic release devices. These doors are normally kept closed.

18.1.2.3 Health care occupancies in buildings housing other occupancies shall be completely separated from them by construction having a fire resistance rating of not less than 2 hours.

A-12–1.1.4.5 Automatic sprinkler protection. Required of all new health care occupancies.

18.1.6.1 Construction requirements. The primary level of exit discharge of a building is the lowest story with a floor level at or above finished grade on the exterior wall with 50% or more of its perimeter. Figure 4.7 is a figure of a three-story building.

18.1.6.2 Construction and multistory buildings. Constructions types are specified for a variety of buildings. All multistory health care facilities must be constructed of noncombustible materials. In three- or more story buildings the major construction elements must be protected by a 2-hour fire resistance rating.

12–1.6.4 Openings for pipes, etc. All penetrations of walls must be protected with such means as metal plates, masonry fill, or similar approved product to prevent the spread of fire and smoke.

18.1.7 Occupant load. Means of egress must be provided for one person for each 120 square feet of gross floor area in health care sleeping areas and for one person each 240 square feet of gross floor area in inpatient treatment areas, for example, physical therapy. If the actual count of persons exceeds these numbers, the actual number of persons becomes the minimum occupant load for determining required egress.

18.2.2.2 Door locks are not permitted on patient sleeping room doors. An exception is permitted for using a device that locks a door so that staff can unlock it from the corridor and the patient can exit the room without use of any key. For example, such an approach would prevent patients from accidentally wandering into an isolation room, but the patient in the isolation room would be able to exit the room without use of a key or tool. Also, for

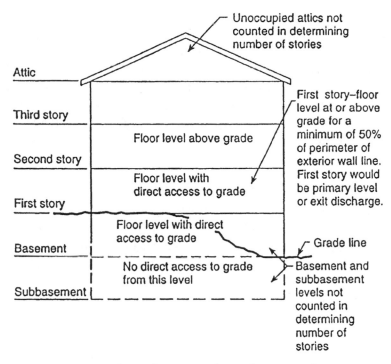

Determining number of stories for application of minimum construction requirements. Because of sloping grade, the primary level of exit discharge is not obvious. The 50% perimeter guideline of 12-1.6.1 clarifies that for the arrangement illustrated, the first story is the primary level of exit discharge. Number of stories includes primary level of exit discharge and all occupiable floors located above. This is an example of a three-story building.

FIGURE 4.7 Building section view illustrating grade line and story designation. Reprinted with permission from *NFPA Life Safety Code® Handbook*, 6th Ed., *Ron Cote, P.E., Editor*, 1994, p. 374.

patients that might endanger themselves, for example, Alzheimer patients, a lock may be installed provided staff carry keys at all times or other provision for remotely unlocking all such doors. Doors in a required means of egress may not be equipped with a latch or lock that requires the use of a tool or key from the egress side. At maximum, only one delayed egress device may be used along the length of any egress.

Means of Egress. Interior stairs, in general, must have a minimum clear width of 44 inches except for handrails not exceeding 3 1/2 inches at or below handrail height on each side. Riser maximum height is 7 inches, minimum height of risers is 4 inches. Minimum tread depth is 11 inches, minimum headroom is 6 feet 8 inches. Maximum height between landings is 12 feet.

Handrails are required on both sides, must be not less than 34 inches nor more than 38 inches above the surface of the tread measured vertically to the top of the rail from the leading edge of the tread. Handrail clearance must be at least 1 1/2 inches when smooth surfaces are used, more if rough surfaces. Handrails must be graspable firmly with a comfortable grip so the hand can slide along the rail without encountering any obstructions.

18.2.2.4 *Smokeproof Enclosures*

A smokeproof enclosure is a set(s) of enclosed stairs designed to limit the infiltration of heat, smoke, and fire gases from a fire in any part of a building, thereby limiting entry of the products of combustion into the stairway. Such stairwells must have a 2-hour fire resistance and a door with a 1 1/2 hour fire protection rating.

18.2.2.5 Horizontal Exits. A horizontal exit is a passage from one area of a building to another, separated by a fire barrier, space, or other protection enabling each area to be a fire compartment independent of the one in which a fire exists. It can be a bridge to another building. No stairs or ramps are normally involved. At least 30 square feet per patient must be provided within the aggregated area of corridors, patient rooms, treatment rooms, lounge dining area, and other low hazard areas on each side. A single door may be permitted provided the exit serves one direction only and is at least 41.5 inches wide. If separating two fire areas, two doors swinging opposite directions, each at least 41.5 inches are required.

18.2.2.5.4 A horizontal exit involving a corridor 8 feet or more in width serving as a means of egress from both sides of the doorway shall have the opening protected by a pair of swinging doors arranged to swing in opposite directions from each other, with each door having a clear width of not less than 41.5 inches or by a horizontal sliding door complying with 5 pounds of pressure to move that provides a clear width of not less than 83 inches.

18.2.2.6 Ramps. The usual definition is:

- 20 degrees to 50 degrees = a stairway.
- 7 degrees–20 degrees = a stairway and landings.
- under 7 degrees = a ramp.

Nearly horizontal landings are required at both ends of ramps. Ramps are to be slip resistant, and have a clear width of at least 44 inches, have a maximum slope of 1 inch in 12 inches and maximum cross slope of 1 inch in 48 inches. The maximum rise for a single ramp run is 30 inches.

18.2.3.3 Aisles, corridors, and ramps used for exit must be at least 8 feet in width clear and unobstructed.

18.2.4 Number of exits. At least two exits located remotely from each other must be provided for each floor and fire section of a building. At least one exit from each floor or fire section must lead directly outside, to a stair, a smokeproof enclosure, a ramp, or an exit passageway. At no time can an exit passageway require return through the compartment of origin.

18.2.5 Arrangement of means of egress. Every patient room must have an exit access door leading directly to an exit access corridor (some exceptions exist, e.g., a door opening directly to the outside).

18.2.6.2.1,2,3 Travel distance to exits. Travel distance between the door in any room and an exit access must not exceed 150 feet, and travel from within any patient room to same must not exceed 200 feet. Travel distance within a room to an exit must not exceed 50 feet.

18.2.7 Discharge from exits. Each required exit ramp or stair must lead directly outside at grade or be an enclosed passage meeting all fire-resistance regulations at grade.

18.2.8 Illumination of Means of Egress. Must be continuous with all exit floor surface illuminated at the level of 1-foot candle measured at the floor of the exit access, the exit, and the exit discharge. Failure of any single light source (electric bulb) must not leave any area in darkness, hence the need for overlapping light sources, separately wired.

18.2.9 Emergency lighting. Must have automatic transfer between normal power and an emergency source. Storage batteries are acceptable if they meet the candlelight requirements for a period of 1 1/2 hours. Automotive type batteries are not acceptable. An on-site generator normally is required as the second source of emergency lighting.

Exit marking. Exit signs must be readily visible from any direction of exit access. Tactile signage is required at each door into an exit stair enclosure. No point in the exit access route may be more than 100 feet. EXIT signs must have letters at least 6 inches high and not less than 3/4 inches wide and be of contrasting color.

18.2.10.2 Buildings equipped with or within which patients require the use of life-support systems shall have **emergency lighting equipment** supplied by the life safety branch of the electrical system.

Emergency power. Most facilities have an emergency electrical generator. This generator must go on within 10 seconds of a power failure. Such a generator is not required, however, in a freestanding building in which the management precludes the provision of care for any patient who may need to be sustained by electrical life-support equipment such as a respirator or suction apparatus, and in which battery-operated systems or equipment are provided to maintain power to exit lights and means of egress, stairways, medicinal preparation areas and the like for a minimum of 1 1/2 hours. Battery power is also required to operate all alarm systems. Separate power supplies controlled by separate switches that are protected from fire threat are required.

18.3 Protection

18.3.1 Vertical openings. Any stairway, ramp, elevator, hoist, or chute, for example, for laundry, between stories must be enclosed with protective construction, for example, fire resistance of 1 hour in buildings required to have 1-hour protection, 1-hour fire resistance for buildings of not more than three stories, and of 2 hours for enclosures in buildings of over three stories.

18.3.2 Protection from hazards. Hazardous areas are spaces with contents that are flammable or combustible and represent a higher than normal hazard.

Hazardous areas must be protected by fire barriers with a fire resistance rating of 1 hour or a completely automatic extinguishing system. Hazardous areas include

- mechanical equipment rooms
- laundry
- kitchens, repair shops
- handicraft shops
- employee locker areas
- gift shop

The following must have both 1-hour fire resistance and a complete extinguishment system: soiled linen rooms, paint ships, trash collection rooms, and rooms or spaces, including repair shops, used for the storage of combustible supplies and equipment in quantities deemed hazardous by the authority having jurisdiction.

18.3.2.5 Gift Shops Gift shops shall be protected as hazardous areas where used for storage or display of combustibles in quantities considered hazardous. Some exceptions apply if gift shop has separate storage.

18.2.3.6 Cooking facilities. Numerous regulations govern cooking facilities. A major focus is the requirement for a regularly serviced, fixed, automatic fire-extinguishing system for cook stoves. Small appliances such as equipment for food warming or limited cooking, protection such as a small microwave are exempted from cooking regulations for commercial cooking equipment.

18.3.3 Interior finish. A number of requirements specify the type of wall materials usable and the degree of flame spread, smoke development, and similar characteristics so as to assure that walls do not contribute to the spread of fire. No specific requirements pertain to interior floor finishes.

18.3.4 Detection, Alarm, and Communications Systems. This is an extensive section with numerous provisions and exceptions. The following are some of the more salient requirements.

A manually operated fire alarm system electrically monitored is required. This means that when any component part of the fire alarm system malfunctions, a continuous trouble alert indication is sent electronically to a continuously attended location.

The fire alarm system must be designed to notify all building occupants when any alarm station is activated. The local fire department (or its equivalent) must be automatically notified whenever any fire alarm station is activated. Codes for identifying fire zones are permitted.

Emergency control. Activating any fire alarm station must automatically activate all appropriate devices, for example, the sprinkler system, alarms, and door releases.

New nursing homes must have automatically operated smoke detection systems. Smoke detectors must be located no farther apart than 30 feet and not more than 15 feet from any wall.

The automatic smoke detection and fire detection systems must both be connected electrically. Manual pull stations should be located so no employee has to leave the fire area to activate the alarm. A distinct, supervisory signal must be provided to a constantly attended location in the event of any malfunction or action that would reduce sprinkler system performance. The main nursing station is often chosen for such a location.

18.3.4.5.3 Nursing Homes. An approved automatic smoke detection system shall be installed in corridors throughout smoke compartments containing patient sleeping rooms and in spaces open to corridors (some exceptions apply if each patient room is protected by an approved smoke detection system).

18.3.5 Extinguishment requirements. A supervised automatic sprinkler system must be installed. Quick response sprinklers must be used in the smoke compartment. Some exceptions may be made regarding sprinkler type.

Portable fire extinguishers meeting NFPA and local codes must be installed. Hand fire extinguishers are required on every floor and in every hazardous area. The travel distance to any extinguisher may be no more than 75 feet to a Class A extinguisher and 50 feet to a Class B or C extinguisher. Short persons must be able to reach the extinguisher.

Every extinguisher must be in operating condition at all items. Fire extinguishers must be checked quarterly by a qualified person and be serviced annually by a qualified examiner who must show the date that the inspection and servicing was accomplished on an attached tag.

18.3.6 Corridor doors. Doors protecting openings in corridor partitions must be able to resist the passage of smoke but need not have a fire protection rating. Doors must have a positive latch that cannot be held in the retracted position. Roller latches are not permitted. The latch must be able to hold the door in a closed position.

18.3.7 Subdivision of building spaces.

Smoke barriers are required

(a) to divide every story used by patients for sleeping or treatments into at least two smoke compartments;

(b) to divide every story having an occupant load of 50 or more persons, regardless of use, into at least two smoke compartments;

(c) to limit the size of each smoke compartment required above to no more than 22,500 square feet; and

(d) to limit the travel distance in the required smoke barrier to 200 feet.

Doors shall be 1 3/4 inches thick, solid bodied wood core or of construction of 20 minute resistance fire rating. Vision panels must be provided in swinging doors.

18.3.8 Outside window or door. Each patient sleeping room shall have an outside window or outside door. The maximum allowable sill height is 36 inches above the floor. The window does not have to be operable.

Concluding Observations

The administrator who is planning new construction must meet all state and local codes as well. Many areas covered by the *Life Safety Code*® have been left uncovered. There are, for example, additional sections on utilities, heating, ventilation, air conditioning, elevators, rubbish chutes, incinerators, laundry chutes, and so on that have not been discussed.

The reader realizes, of course, that this is an introduction to only a few of the more salient aspects of the Life Safety Code®. The reader is strongly urged to purchase the *Life Safety Code*® *Handbook* for the year containing the requirements that they must meet. For example, federal requirements may specify year 2000 Life Safety Code while the state may require a more current year's code.

The NFPA 101 Life Safety Code (annual edition) and its interpretative companion book *Life Safety Code*® *Handbook* are essential tools for administrators. It is the administrator's job to understand the Code and its basic requirements in order to assure that their facility is in basic conformity with regulations and to work intelligently with engineers, architects, and state building code officials in planning and pursuing any nursing facility construction project.

4.7 Americans With Disabilities Act of 1990 Accessibility Guidelines for Facilities

On Friday, July 26, 1991, the federal Department of Justice, Office of the Attorney General issued the following final rule Part III 28 CFR Part 36 for the purpose of achieving nondiscrimination on the basis of disability. These requirements apply to nursing facilities that are newly built or renovated and are available from the American with Disabilities Act's Architectural and Transportation Barriers Compliance Board, U.S. Department of Justice Civil Rights Division (Washington, DC) and are found in the *Federal Register* / Vol. 56, No. 144 / Friday, July 26, 1991, pages 35544–35691.

The following pages provide an overview of these requirements, most of which are based on the standards developed and approved by the Council of American Building Officials / American National Standards Institute, Inc., titled American National Standard Accessible and Usable Buildings and Facilities CABO/ANSI A117.1 1992, which, along with the federal final rule cited in the previous paragraph, must be obtained and utilized by any administrator planning, building, or renovating a nursing home. The following information, figures, and tables are reproduced here with the permission of the Council of American Building Officials, Executive Offices, 5203 Leesburg Pike, #708, Falls Church, VA 22041. As indicated in each figure and table, however, ordering address for copies of American National Standard Accessible and Usable Buildings and Facilities is located in Country Club Hill, IL. The information provided in this textbook is designed to provide only an introduction to the reader of the nature and importance of the directions of these requirements. Under no circumstances may the following pages be utilized in actual planning, construction, or renovating of a nursing facility (Maddox & Sussman, 2001, p. 81).

Obtain and Use Both the Following Documents:

American National Standard Accessible and Usable Buildings and Facilities CABO/ANSI A117.1–1992 from Buildings Officials and Code

Administrators International, 4051 West Flossmoor Road, Country Club Hill, IL, 60477

Americans With Disabilities Act of 1990, Accessibility Guidelines for Facilities, *Federal Register* / Vol. 56, No. 144, / Friday, July 26, 1991 / Final Rule Part III CFR 28, Part 36 from the Americans With Disabilities Act's Architectural and Transportation Barriers Compliance Board, 1331 F Street, N.W., Suite 1000, Washington, DC 20004–111.

Standards for Accessible Design (Appendix A to Part 36)

The following is an overview of the following standards.

1.   Purpose
2.   General
3.   Miscellaneous Instructions and Definitions
4.   Accessible Elements and Specifications of Sections
4.1 Minimum Requirements
4.2 Space Allowance and Reach Ranges
4.3 Accessible Route
4.4 Protruding Objects
4.5 Ground and Floor Surfaces
4.6 Parking and Passenger Loading Zones
4.7 Curb Ramps
4.8 Ramps
4.9 Stairs
4.10 Elevators
4.11 Wheelchair Lifts
4.12 Windows
4.13 Doors
4.14 Entrances
4.15 Drinking Fountains and Water Coolers
4.16 Water Closets
4.17 Toilet Stalls
4.18 Urinals
4.19 Lavatories and Mirrors
4.21 Shower Stalls
4.22 Toilet Rooms
4.23 Bathrooms, Bathing Facilities and Shower Rooms
4.24 Sinks
4.25 Storage
4.26 Handrails, Grab Bars, and Tub and Shower Seats

4.27 Controls and Operating Mechanisms
4.28 Alarms
4.29 Detectable Warnings
4.30 Signage
4.31 Telephones
4.32 Fixed or Built-in Seating and Tables
4.33 Assembly Areas
6.   Medical Care Facilities (included in 4 above).

1. Purpose

To set guidelines for accessibility for individuals with disabilities. Are to be applied during the design, construction, and alteration of facilities.

2. General

Departures from these guidelines are permitted where equivalent access is provided.

TABLE 4.8   Americans With Disabilities Act Graphic Conventions

Convention	Description
36 / 915	Typical dimension line showing U.S. customary units (in inches) above the line and SI units (in millimeters) below
9 / 230	Dimensions for short distances indicated on extended line
9 / 230 36 / 915	Dimension line showing alternate dimensions required
	Direction of approach
max	Maximum
min	Minimum
	Boundary of clear floor area
	Centerline

Americans with Disabilities Act of 1990, Accessibility Guidelines for Facilities. Federal, Register Vol, 56, No. 144 / Friday, July 26, 1991 / Rules and Regulations, p, 35622. Final Rule Part III CFR 2 & Part 36. A copy of the final federal rule should be obtained from American with Disabilities Act's Architectural and Transportation Barriers Compliance Bourd, U.S. Department of Justice, Civil Rights Division (Washington, DC). A copy of American National Standard Accessible and Usable Bu4#-CABO/ANSI A117.1-1992 should be obtained from American National Standards Institute, 25 West 43rd St., New York, NY, 10036.

3. Miscellaneous Instructions and Definitions

Graphic conventions. These are illustrated in Table 4.8.

Definitions: (selected)

Access aisle. An accessible pedestrian space between elements, such as parking spaces, seating, and desks that provides clearances appropriate for use of the elements.

Accessible. Describes a site, building, facility, or portion thereof that complies with these requirements.

Accessible element. An element specified by these requirements (e.g. telephone, controls, and the like).

Accessible route. A continuous unobstructed path connecting all accessible elements and spaces of a facility. Interior accessible routes may include corridors, floors, ramps, elevators, lists, and clear floor space at fixtures. Exterior accessible route may include parking access aisles, curb ramps, crosswalks at vehicular ways, walks, ramps, and lifts.

Accessible space. A space that complies with these requirements.

Addition. An expansion, extension, or increase in the gross floor area of a facility.

Area of rescue assistance. An area, which has direct access to an exit, where people who are unable to use stairs may remain temporarily in safety to await further instructions or assistance during emergency evacuation.

Assembly area. A room or space accommodating a group of individuals for recreational, educational, or amusement purposes or for consumption of food and drink.

Clear. Unobstructed.

Clear floor space. The minimum unobstructed floor or ground space required to accommodate a single, stationary wheelchair and occupant.

Egress, means of. A continuous and unobstructed way of exit travel from any point in a facility to a public way.

Element. An architectural or mechanical component of a facility, space or site, e.g. telephone, curb ramp, door, drinking fountain, seating, or toilet.

Signage. Displayed verbal, symbolic, tactile, and pictorial information.

Space. A definable area, e.g. room, toilet room, hall, assembly area, entrance, storage room, alcove, courtyard, or lobby.

Tactile. Describes an object that can be perceived using the sense of touch.

Walk. An exterior pathway with a prepared surface intended for pedestrian use.

4. Accessible Elements and Specifications of Section (6. Medical facilities)

(6)(3) Long-term care facilities, nursing homes—at least 50% of patient bedrooms and toilets, and all public use and common use areas are required to be designed and constructed to be accessible. (Author's observation: Given the nature of the patient mix in the typical nursing facility, it seems illogical to build any resident rooms and toilets that are not accessible to handicapped persons.)

4.1 Minimum Requirements

Accessible sites: must provide at least one accessible route that complies with 4.3 within the boundary of the site from public transportation stops, accessible parking spaces, passenger loading zones, if furnished, and public streets or sidewalks to an accessible building entrance.

Accessible routes: must have at least one complying with 4.3 connecting accessible buildings, accessible facilities, accessible elements, and accessible spaces that are on the same site.

Several other minimum requirements are stated, most of which are outlined in the following sections.

4.2 Space Allowance and Reach Ranges

Wheelchair passage width. 36 inches continuously, 32 inches at any one point (see Figure 4.8)

Width of wheelchair passing. 60 inches (see Figure 4.9).

Wheelchair turning space. (to make 180 degree turn) clear space of 60 inches or T-shaped space (see Figure 4.10).

Relationship of maneuvering clearances to wheelchair spaces. One unobstructed side adjoining an accessible route (see Figure 4.11).

High forward reach. Generally 48 inches. Demonstrated in Figure 4.12)

Side reach. Between 9 inches and 54 inches off the floor (see Figure 4.13).

4.3 Accessible Route

Must meet definition above; be at least 36 inches wide (32 at doors); allow for turns around objects (see Figure 4.14); have passing spaces 60 inches wide at least every 200 feet; 80-inch turn room; stable, firm, and slip-resistant surface texture; and meet change of level requirements.

FIGURE 4.8 Minimum clear width for single wheelchair.
Americans With Disabilities Act of 1990, Accessibility Guidelines for Facilities. *Federal Register* / Vol. 56, No. 144 / Friday, July 26, 1991 / Rules and Regulations, p. 35622. Final Rule Part III CFR 28 Part 36. A copy of the final federal rule should be obtained from Americans With Disabilities Act's Architectural and Transportation Barriers Compliance Board, U.S. Department of Justice, Civil Rights Division (Washington, DC). A copy of *American National Standard Accessible and Usable Buildings and Facilities,* CABO/ANSI A117.1–1992 should be obtained from American National Standards Institute, 25 West 43rd St. New York, NY 10036.

4.4 Protruding Objects

Objects located between 27 and 80 inches above the floor must protrude no more than 4 inches into any hall or passageway or walk. Objects with their leading edge 27 inches high or less may protrude any amount from the wall. Freestanding objects mounted on posts or pylons may overhang 12 inches when mounted between 27 and 80 inches above the floor, for example, a telephone booth. In no case may protruding objects reduce the clear width of an accessible route or maneuvering space (see Figure 4.15).

4.5 Ground and Floor Surfaces

General: Must be stable, firm, and slip-resistant.
Changes in level.
- Up to 1/4 inch may be vertical and without edge
- Between 1/4 and 1/2 inch beveled edge required
- Over 1/2 inch: ramp treatment required

FIGURE 4.9 Minimum clear width for two wheelchairs.
Americans with Disabilities Act of 1990, Accessibility Guidelines for Facilities. Federal Register / Vol. 56, No. 144 / Friday, July 26, 1991 / Rules and Regulations, p. 35622. Final Rule Part III CFR 28 Part 36. A copy of the final federal rule should be obtained from American with Disabilities Act's Architectural and Transportation Barriers Compliance Board, U.S. Department of Justice, Civil Rights Division (Washington, DC). A copy of American National Standard Accessible and Usable Buildings and Facilities, CABO/ ANSI A117.1–1992 should be obtained from American National Standards Institute, 25 West 43rd St., New York, NY 10036.

Carpet. Must be securely attached, firm or no pad, with maximum pile height of 1/2 inch, level cut, and trimmed along exposed edge that conforms to changes in level in previous paragraph (See Figure 4.16).

Gratings. Maximum width of openings: 1/2 inch. If in walkways, the 1/2 inch openings must be perpendicular to dominant direction of travel (See Figure 4.16).

4.6 Parking and Passenger Loading Zones

Space requirements

Parking spaces	Minimum Accessible Spaces
1–25	1
26–50	2
51–75	3

(a)
60-in (1525-mm)-Diameter Space

(b)
T-Shaped Space for 180° Turns

FIGURE 4.10 Wheelchair turning space.
Americans with Disabilities Act of 1990, Accessibility Guidelines for Facilities. Federal Register / Vol. 56, No. 144 / Friday, July 26, 1991 / Rules and Regulations, p. 35622. Final Rule Part III CFR 28 Part 36. A copy of the final federal rule should be obtained from American with Disabilities Act's Architectural and Transportation Barriers Compliance Board, U.S. Department of Justice, Civil Rights Division (Washington, DC). A copy of American National Standard Accessible and Usable Buildings and Facilities, CABO/ ANSI A117.1–1992 should be obtained from American National Standards Institute, 25 West 43rd St. New York, NY 10036.

76–100	4
101–150	5
151–200	6
201–300	7
301–400	8

Spaces shall be at least 96 inches wide with an accessible aisle at least 60 inches wide (two spaces may share one aisle). A van space must be provided and designated by signage (See Figures 4.17, 4.18).

The standard handicapped symbol must be placed so that it is not obscured by a parked vehicle. A passenger loading zone at least 60 inches wide and 20 feet long adjacent and parallel to the vehicle pull-up space must be provided.

4.7 Curb Ramps

Location. Wherever an accessible route crosses a curb (see Figures 4.19, 4.20).

(a)
Clear Floor Space

(b)
Forward Approach

(c)
Parallel Approach

NOTE: x ≤ 24 in (610 mm).

NOTE: x ≤ 15 in (380 mm).

(d)
Clear Floor Space in Alcoves

NOTE: If x > 24 in (610 mm), then an additional maneuvering clearance of 6 in (150 mm) shall be provided as shown.

NOTE: If x > 15 in (380 mm), then an additional maneuvering clearance of 12 in (305 mm) shall be provided as shown.

(e)
Additional Maneuvering Clearances for Alcoves

FIGURE 4.11 Minimum clear floor space for wheelchairs.
Americans with Disabilities Act of 1990, Accessibility Guidelines for Facilities. Federal Register / Vol. 56, No. 144 / Friday, July 26, 1991 / Rules and Regulations, p. 35622. Final Rule Part III CFR 28 Part 36. A copy of the final federal rule should be obtained from American with Disabilities Act's Architectural and Transportation Barriers Compliance Board, U.S. Department of Justice, Civil Rights Division (Washington, DC). A copy of American National Standard Accessible and Usable Buildings and Facilities, CABO/ ANSI A117.1–1992 should be obtained from American National Standards Institute, 25 West 43rd St., New York, NY 10036.

(a)
High Forward Reach Limit

(b)

NOTE: x shall be ≤ 25 in (635 mm); z shall be ≥ x. When x < 20 in (510 mm), then y shall be 48 in (1220 mm) maximum. When x is 20 to 25 in (510 to 635 mm), then y shall be 44 in (1120 mm) maximum.

FIGURE 4.12 Forward reach.
Americans with Disabilities Act of 1990, Accessibility Guidelines for Facilities. Federal Register / Vol. 56, No. 144 / Friday, July 26, 1991 / Rules and Regulations, p. 35622. Final Rule Part III CFR 28 Part 36. A copy of the final federal rule should be obtained from American with Disabilities Act's Architectural and Transportation Barriers Compliance Board, U.S. Department of Justice, Civil Rights Division (Washington, DC). A copy of American National Standard Accessible and Usable Buildings and Facilities, CABO/ ANSI A117.1–1992 should be obtained from American National Standards Institute, 25 West 43rd St., New York, NY 10036.

(a)
Clear Floor Space   Parallel Approach

(b)
High and Low   Side Reach Limits

(c)
Maximum Side Reach over Obstruction

FIGURE 4.13 Side reach.
Americans with Disabilities Act of 1990, Accessibility Guidelines for Facilities. Federal Register / Vol. 56, No. 144 / Friday, July 26, 1991 / Rules and Regulations, p. 35622. Final Rule Part III CFR 28 Part 36. A copy of the final federal rule should be obtained from American with Disabilities Act's Architectural and Transportation Barriers Compliance Board, U.S. Department of Justice, Civil Rights Division (Washington, DC). A copy of American National Standard Accessible and Usable Buildings and Facilities, CABO/ ANSI A117.1–1992 should be obtained from American National Standards Institute, 25 West 43rd St., New York, NY 10036.

4.8 Ramps

Ramp. Any part of an accessible route with a slope greater than 1:20.

Rise and slope. Least possible slope is to be used. Maximum slope is 1:12, maximum rise 30 inches.

Landings. Required at bottom and top of each run, as wide as widest ramp run leading to it (minimum of 60 inches). Minimum 60 inches x 60 inches if ramp changes direction at a landing.

FIGURE 4.14 Accessible route.
Americans with Disabilities Act of 1990, Accessibility Guidelines for Facilities. Federal Register / Vol. 56, No. 144 / Friday, July 26, 1991 / Rules and Regulations, p. 35622. Final Rule Part III CFR 28 Part 36. A copy of the final federal rule should be obtained from American with Disabilities Act's Architectural and Transportation Barriers Compliance Board, U.S. Department of Justice, Civil Rights Division (Washington, DC). A copy of American National Standard Accessible and Usable Buildings and Facilities, CABO/ ANSI A117.1–1992 should be obtained from American National Standards Institute, 25 West 43rd St., New York, NY 10036.

Handrails. If there is a rise of more than 6 inches or a horizontal projection of greater than 72 inches it must have handrails on both sides (see Figure 4.21).

Cross slopes. Maximum of 1:50.

4.9 Stairs

Treads and risers. On any given flight of stairs, riser heights and tread widths must be uniform. Treads must be no less than 11 inches apart, measured from one riser to another. Risers must be a maximum of 7

(b)
Walking Perpendicular to a Wall

FIGURE 4.15 Protruding objects: (a) Walking parallel to a wall; (b) walking perpendicular to a wall; (c) freestanding overhanging objects; (d) overhead hazards; (e) overhanging objects.

inches high. Open risers are never permitted on an accessible route. Nosing must project no more than 1 1/2 inches (see Figure 4.22).

Handrails. See "ramps" above. Also, at the bottom, the handrail shall continue to slope for the distance of one tread past the bottom riser, then extend parallel to the floor or ground surface for 12 inches. Gripping surfaces must be uninterrupted by newel posts, other construction elements, or obstructions. Top of handrail gripping surface shall be mounted between 34 and 38 inches above stair nosings. Ends of handrails shall be either rounded or returned smoothly to floor, wall, or post. Handrails must not rotate within their fittings. (See Figure 4.23)

FIGURE 4.15 (*Continued*)

FIGURE 4.16 Protruding objects: Carpet pile, gratings, and grating orientation.

4.10 Elevators

Numerous detailed requirements are set forth.

4.11 Wheelchair Lifts

Are permitted, must meet local requirements.

4.12 Windows

Reserved (i.e., no requirements set at this time)

4.13 Doors

Clear width. Must be 32 inches at openings which must be at an angle of 90 degrees to accessible route. Two doors in series must have at least 48 inches between them.

Thresholds at doorways. Shall not exceed 3/4 of an inch in height for exterior sliding doors or 1/2 inch for other types.

Hardware. Handles, pulls, latches, locks, and other operating devices on accessible doors must have a shape that is easy to grasp with one hand and does not require tight grasping, tight pinching, or twisting of the wrist to operate. Lever operated mechanisms, push type mechanisms, and shaped handles are acceptable designs, no more than 48 inches above the finished floor.

Door opening force. Five pounds maximum for interior and sliding or folding doors.

Automatic doors and power-assisted doors. Should be slow opening and low powered: not opening back to back faster than 3 seconds needing no more than 15 pounds to stop movement.

4.14 Entrances

Must be part of an accessible route and all accessible spaces and elements within a facility.

4.15 Drinking Fountains and Water Coolers

Spouts. Shall be no higher than 36 inches, located at the front of the fountain, flowing parallel with the front of the unit and at least 4 inches high (to allow for a cup or glass to be inserted under the stream of water; see Figure 4.24).

FIGURE 4.17 Dimensions of parking spaces.
Americans with Disabilities Act of 1990, Accessibility Guidelines for Facilities. Federal Register / Vol. 56, No. 144 / Friday, July 26, 1991 / Rules and Regulations, p. 35622. Final Rule Part III CFR 28 Part 36. A copy of the final federal rule should be obtained from American with Disabilities Act's Architectural and Transportation Barriers Compliance Board, U.S. Department of Justice, Civil Rights Division (Washington, DC). A copy of American National Standard Accessible and Usable Buildings and Facilities, CABO/ ANSI A117.1–1992 should be obtained from American National Standards Institute, 25 West 43rd St., New York, NY 10036.

Controls. Shall be located at or near the front edge of the fountain, be operable with one hand, easily grasped, needing no more than 5 pounds of pressure to operate

4.16 Water Closets

Toilets not in stalls must meet clear floor space requirements and may have either right-handled or left-handled approach. Height of 17–19 inches to top of toilet seat, with grab bars on walls mounted 33–36 inches off floor on side and rear walls. Flush control to require no more than 5 pounds of force to operate (see Figure 4.25).

4.17 Toilet Stalls

Toilet stalls must meet numerous dimension requirements (see Figure 4.26). They may be a specified standard or alternative size, must include grab bars, and if less than 60 inches in depth must provide 9 inches of toe clearance.

FIGURE 4.18 Access aisle at passenger loading zones.
Americans with Disabilities Act of 1990, Accessibility Guidelines for Facilities. Federal Register / Vol. 56, No. 144 / Friday, July 26, 1991 / Rules and Regulations, p. 35622. Final Rule Part III CFR 28 Part 36. A copy of the final federal rule should be obtained from American with Disabilities Act's Architectural and Transportation Barriers Compliance Board, U.S. Department of Justice, Civil Rights Division (Washington, DC). A copy of American National Standard Accessible and Usable Buildings and Facilities, CABO/ ANSI A117.1–1992 should be obtained from American National Standards Institute, 25 West 43rd St., New York, NY 10036.

4.18 Urinals

Urinals may be wall-hung or stall type with elongated rim a maximum of 17 inches above the finished floor; clear floor space of 30 inches by 48 inches is required; hand operated flush lever (5 pounds of force to operate at most) not more than 44 inches off floor.

4.19 Lavatories and Mirrors

Lavatories must be mounted with the rim or counter surface no higher than 24 inches above the finished floor, provide a clearance of at least 29 inches above the floor to the bottom or the apron (see Figure 4.27).

> **Hot water and drain pipes under lavatory.** Shall be wrapped and any sharp or abrasive surfaces protected.
> **Faucets:** Five pounds of pressure maximum to operate
> **Mirrors.** Mounted with bottom edge of reflecting surface no higher than 40 inches above the finished floor.

slope = Y:X
where X is a level plane

Adjoining slope shall
not exceed 1:20

walk   street

(a)

Measurement of Curb Ramp Slopes

Planting or other
nonwalking surface

flared side

1 10

(b1)
Flared Sides

(b2)
Returned Curb

If X is less than 48 in,
then the slope of the flared side
shall not exceed 1:12.

FIGURE 4.19 Measurement of curb ramp slopes.
Americans With Disabilities Act of 1990, Accessibility Guidelines for Facilities. *Federal Register* / Vol. 56, No. 144 / Friday, July 26, 1991 / Rules and Regulations, p. 35622. Final Rule Part III CFR 28 Part 36. A copy of the final federal rule should be obtained from Americans With Disabilities Act's Architectural and Transportation Barriers Compliance Board, U.S. Department of Justice, Civil Rights Division (Washington, DC). A copy of *American National Standard Accessible and Usable Buildings and Facilities,* CABO/ANSI A117.1–1992 should be obtained from American National Standards Institute, 25 West 43rd St. New York, NY 10036.

Must meet floor space requirements depending on arrangement of bathroom fixtures. They must have the following:

- an in-tub seat or a seat at the head of the tub
- grab bars and controls (5 pounds of pressure maximum pressure to operate) located on near side of tub enclosure
- a shower spray unit with hose at least 60 inches long usable as a handheld shower or fixed shower spray

4.21 Shower Stalls

Must meet size requirements; have grab bars, controls, and shower handheld sprayer unit as required for tubs and provide a seat.

FIGURE 4.20 Built-up curb ramp.
Americans with Disabilities Act of 1990, Accessibility Guidelines for Facilities. Federal Register / Vol. 56, No. 144 / Friday, July 26, 1991 / Rules and Regulations, p. 35622. Final Rule Part III CFR 28 Part 36. A copy of the final federal rule should be obtained from American with Disabilities Act's Architectural and Transportation Barriers Compliance Board, U.S. Department of Justice, Civil Rights Division (Washington, DC). A copy of American National Standard Accessible and Usable Buildings and Facilities, CABO/ ANSI A117.1–1992 should be obtained from American National Standards Institute, 25 West 43rd St., New York, NY 10036.

4.22 Toilet Rooms

These must meet requirements as outlined previously for doors, toilets, urinals, tubs, and so on. In addition, any medicine cabinet provided must be located so as to have a usable shelf no higher than 44 inches above the floor.

4.23 Bathrooms, Bathing Facilities and Shower Rooms

Must meet all the previous relevant requirements.

4.24 Sinks

Must be accessible and mounted with counter or rim no higher than 34 inches above the finish floor. Knee clearance at least 27 inches high, 30 inches wide, and 19 inches deep under sink. Water depth maximum is 6 1/2 inches. Clear floor space of at least 30 by 48 inches. All exposed pipes covered, faucets easily operated with maximum of 5 pounds of pressure to operate.

4.25 Storage

A clear floor space of 30 x 48 inches, within reach ranges of ADA Figures 5 and 6, clothes rods a maximum of 54 inches above the finish floor (see Figure 4.28).

elevation   section

FIGURE 4.21 Examples of edge protection and handrail extensions.
Americans with Disabilities Act of 1990, Accessibility Guidelines for Facilities. Federal Register / Vol. 56, No. 144 / Friday, July 26, 1991 / Rules and Regulations, p. 35622. Final Rule Part
III CFR 28 Part 36. A copy of the final federal rule should be obtained from American with Disabilities Act's Architectural and Transportation Barriers Compliance Board, U.S. Department of
Justice, Civil Rights Division (Washington, DC). A copy of American National Standard Accessible and Usable Buildings and Facilities, CABO/ ANSI A117.1–1992 should be obtained
from American National Standards Institute, 25 West 43rd St., New York, NY 10036.

4.26 Handrails, Grab Bars, and Tub and Shower Seats

Handrails and grab bars must be 1 1/4 to 1 1/2 inches or provide equivalent
gripping surface. If wall mounted, at least 1 1/2 inch space between the grab
bar and wall. Bending, sheer stress point: must be 250 pounds of pressure or
greater. Must not rotate within fittings and have no sharp edges (minimum
radius of edge = 1/8 inch) (see Figure 4.29)

(a)
Flush Riser

(b)
Angled Nosing

(c)
Rounded Nosing

FIGURE 4.22 Usable tread width and examples of acceptable nosings.
Americans with Disabilities Act of 1990, Accessibility Guidelines for Facilities. Federal Register / Vol. 56, No. 144 / Friday, July 26, 1991 / Rules and Regulations, p. 35622. Final Rule Part III CFR 28 Part 36. A copy of the final federal rule should be obtained from American with Disabilities Act's Architectural and Transportation Barriers Compliance Board, U.S. Department of Justice, Civil Rights Division (Washington, DC). A copy of American National Standard Accessible and Usable Buildings and Facilities, CABO/ ANSI A117.1–1992 should be obtained from American National Standards Institute, 25 West 43rd St. New York, NY 10036.

4.27 Controls and Operating Mechanisms

Electrical switches must be located at least 15 inches above the floor.

Clear floor space must allow a forward or parallel approach by a person in a wheelchair.

4.28 Alarms

At least, **visual signal appliances** shall be provided in facilities in each of the following areas: restrooms and any other general usage areas, (e.g., meeting rooms), hallways, lobbies, and any other area for common use.

> **Audible alarms.** If provided shall produce a sound that exceed the prevailing equivalent sound level in the room or space by at least 15 decibels or exceeds any maximum sound level with a duration of 60 seconds by 5 decibels, whichever is louder. Maximum decibel level is 120 decibels.
>
> **Visual alarms.** Must be provided, may be integrated into the facility alarm system. Must have following features:
>
> - a xenon strobe type lamp or equivalent
> - color clear or nominal white
> - .2 second maximum pulse duration
> - minimum 75 candle intensity
> - flash rate minimum of 1 Hz and maximum of 3 Hz

(a)
Plan

(b)
Elevation of Center Handrail

(c)
Extension at Bottom of Run

(d)
Extension at Top of Run

NOTE:

X is the 12 in minimum handrail extension required at each top riser.

Y is the minimum handrail extension of 12 in plus the width of one tread that is required at each bottom riser.

FIGURE 4.23 Stair handrails.

Americans with Disabilities Act of 1990, Accessibility Guidelines for Facilities. Federal Register / Vol. 56, No. 144 / Friday, July 26, 1991 / Rules and Regulations, p. 35622. Final Rule Part III CFR 28 Part 36. A copy of the final federal rule should be obtained from American with Disabilities Act's Architectural and Transportation Barriers Compliance Board, U.S. Department of Justice, Civil Rights Division (Washington, DC). A copy of American National Standard Accessible and Usable Buildings and Facilities, CABO/ ANSI A117.1–1992 should be obtained from American National Standards Institute, 25 West 43rd St., New York, NY 10036.

FIGURE 4.24 Drinking fountains and water coolers.
Americans with Disabilities Act of 1990, Accessibility Guidelines for Facilities. Federal Register
/ Vol. 56, No. 144 / Friday, July 26, 1991 / Rules and Regulations, p. 35622. Final Rule Part
III CFR 28 Part 36. A copy of the final federal rule should be obtained from American with Dis-
abilities Act's Architectural and Transportation Barriers Compliance Board, U.S. Department of
Justice, Civil Rights Division (Washington, DC). A copy of American National Standard Acces-
sible and Usable Buildings and Facilities, CABO/ ANSI A117.1–1992 should be obtained from
American National Standards Institute, 25 West 43rd St., New York, NY 10036.

- 80 inches above highest floor level or 6 inches below ceiling, whichever is lower
- no more than 50 feet from all space in a room, 100 feet in large spaces such as auditoriums
- maximum 50 feet apart in hallways and common corridors.

FIGURE 4.25 Grab bars at water closets.
Americans with Disabilities Act of 1990, Accessibility Guidelines for Facilities. Federal Register / Vol. 56, No. 144 / Friday, July 26, 1991 / Rules and Regulations, p. 35622. Final Rule Part III CFR 28 Part 36. A copy of the final federal rule should be obtained from American with Disabilities Act's Architectural and Transportation Barriers Compliance Board, U.S. Department of Justice, Civil Rights Division (Washington, DC). A copy of American National Standard Accessible and Usable Buildings and Facilities, CABO/ ANSI A117.1–1992 should be obtained from American National Standards Institute, 25 West 43rd St., New York, NY 10036.

Auxiliary alarms: required in sleeping accommodations and connected to the building emergency alarm system and visible to all areas of the room

4.29 Detectable Warnings

On walking surfaces shall be 0.9 inches in diameter and 0.2 inches in height with 2.35 inch spacing, contrast visually, and be of material similar to of that used on the surface. Shall be provided at hazardous vehicular areas that are without curbs and at edges of reflecting pools not having railings, walls, or curbs.

4.30 Signage

Letters must have a width to height ratio between 3:5 and 1:1 and a stroke-width-to-height ratio between 1:5 and 1:10.
Character height. Sized to viewing distance with a minimum of 3 feet.
Raised and Brailed Characters and Pictorial Symbol Signs. Must meet several size and type specifications.

FIGURE 4.26 Toilet stalls.
Americans with Disabilities Act of 1990, Accessibility Guidelines for Facilities. Federal Register / Vol. 56, No. 144 / Friday, July 26, 1991 / Rules and Regulations, p. 35622. Final Rule Part III CFR 28 Part 36. A copy of the final federal rule should be obtained from American with Disabilities Act's Architectural and Transportation Barriers Compliance Board, U.S. Department of Justice, Civil Rights Division (Washington, DC). A copy of American National Standard Accessible and Usable Buildings and Facilities, CABO/ ANSI A117.1–1992 should be obtained from American National Standards Institute, 25 West 43rd St., New York, NY 10036.

(a)

(b)

FIGURE 4.27 (a) Lavatory clearances; (b) clear floor space at lavatories.
Americans with Disabilities Act of 1990, Accessibility Guidelines for Facilities. Federal Register / Vol. 56, No. 144 / Friday, July 26, 1991 / Rules and Regulations, p. 35622. Final Rule Part III CFR 28 Part 36. A copy of the final federal rule should be obtained from American with Disabilities Act's Architectural and Transportation Barriers Compliance Board, U.S. Department of Justice, Civil Rights Division (Washington, DC). A copy of American National Standard Accessible and Usable Buildings and Facilities, CABO/ ANSI A117.1–1992 should be obtained from American National Standards Institute, 25 West 43rd St., New York, NY 10036.

(a) Shelves   (b) Closets

FIGURE 4.28 Storage shelves and closets.
Americans with Disabilities Act of 1990, Accessibility Guidelines for Facilities. Feder-
al Register / Vol. 56, No. 144 / Friday, July 26, 1991 / Rules and Regulations, p. 35622.
Final Rule Part III CFR 28 Part 36. A copy of the final federal rule should be obtained from
American with Disabilities Act's Architectural and Transportation Barriers Compliance Board,
U.S. Department of Justice, Civil Rights Division (Washington, DC). A copy of American
National Standard Accessible and Usable Buildings and Facilities, CABO/ ANSI A117.1–
1992 should be obtained from American National Standards Institute, 25 West 43rd St. New
York, NY 10036.

Symbols of accessibility. International symbols shall be used and displayed for areas required to be identified as accessible (see Figure
4.30).

4.31 Telephones

Seating/location. At least 30 inches by 48 inches of clear floor space.
Mounting heights. Highest part shall be within ranges of 15 to 48 inches
of forward reach and 54 inches to 9 inches above the floor for side
reach.
Hearing aid compatible and volume controllable. Both are required.
Volume capable of a minimum of 12 decibels and a maximum of 18

FIGURE 4.29 Sizes and spacing of handrails and grab bars.
Americans with Disabilities Act of 1990, Accessibility Guidelines for Facilities. Federal Register / Vol. 56, No. 144 / Friday, July 26, 1991 / Rules and Regulations, p. 35622. Final Rule Part III CFR 28 Part 36. A copy of the final federal rule should be obtained from American with Disabilities Act's Architectural and Transportation Barriers Compliance Board, U.S. Department of Justice, Civil Rights Division (Washington, DC). A copy of American National Standard Accessible and Usable Buildings and Facilities, CABO/ ANSI A117.1–1992 should be obtained from American National Standards Institute, 25 West 43rd St., New York, NY 10036.

(a)
Proportions
International Symbol of Accessibility

(d)
International Symbol of Access for Hearing Loss

(b)
Display Conditions
International Symbol of Accessibility

(c)
International TDD Symbol

FIGURE 4.30 International symbols. Americans with Disabilities Act of 1990, Accessibility Guidelines for Facilities. Federal Register / Vol. 56, No. 144 / Friday, July 26, 1991 / Rules and Regulations, p. 35622. Final Rule Part III CFR 28 Part 36. A copy of the final federal rule should be obtained from American with Disabilities Act's Architectural and Transportation Barriers Compliance Board, U.S. Department of Justice, Civil Rights Division (Washington, DC). A copy of American National Standard Accessible and Usable Buildings and Facilities, CABO/ ANSI A117.1–1992 should be obtained from American National Standards Institute, 25 West 43rd St., New York, NY 10036.

decibels above normal, directories provided within reach and a 29 inch or longer cord. A text telephone may be required.

4.32 Fixed or Built-In Seating and Tables

Knee space of 27 inches high, 30 inches wide, and 19 inches deep must be provided.

Height. Tops of accessible tables and counters shall be from 28 to 34 inches above the floor or ground (see Figure 4.31).

FIGURE 4.31 Minimum clearances for seating and tables.
Americans with Disabilities Act of 1990, Accessibility Guidelines for Facilities. Federal Register / Vol. 56, No. 144 / Friday, July 26, 1991 / Rules and Regulations, p. 35622. Final Rule Part III CFR 28 Part 36. A copy of the final federal rule should be obtained from American with Disabilities Act's Architectural and Transportation Barriers Compliance Board, U.S. Department of Justice, Civil Rights Division (Washington, DC). A copy of American National Standard Accessible and Usable Buildings and Facilities, CABO/ ANSI A117.1–1992 should be obtained from American National Standards Institute, 25 West 43rd St. New York, NY 10036.

FIGURE 4.32 Space requirements for wheelchair seating spaces in series.
Americans with Disabilities Act of 1990, Accessibility Guidelines for Facilities. Federal Register / Vol. 56, No. 144 / Friday, July 26, 1991 / Rules and Regulations, p. 35622. Final Rule Part III CFR 28 Part 36. A copy of the final federal rule should be obtained from American with Disabilities Act's Architectural and Transportation Barriers Compliance Board, U.S. Department of Justice, Civil Rights Division (Washington, DC). A copy of American National Standard Accessible and Usable Buildings and Facilities, CABO/ ANSI A117.1–1992 should be obtained from American National Standards Institute, 25 West 43rd St. New York, NY 10036. Private Voluntary Health Planning.

4.33 Assembly Areas

Floor space requirements are provided in Figure 4.32. Wheelchair seating areas must allow a choice of admission prices and lines of sight comparable to those for members of the general public and adjoin an accessible route that serves as a means of egress in case of emergency. At least one companion fixed seat shall be next to each wheelchair space. Readily removable seats may be installed in wheelchair areas when not occupied. Floor surfaces of wheelchair areas must be level. Wheelchair persons must have full access to performing areas. Views of the stage must be complete. Assisted-listening systems may be installed.

4.8 Expanding Facility Services: Health Planning Regulations

Health planning in 20th-century America has moved through three phases. During the first 50 years it was mainly the concern of voluntary private groups. In the 1960s and 1970s, health planning leadership was assumed by the federal agencies. Since 1980, any formal health planning is carried out by each state.

Phase 1: Private Voluntary Health Planning

The Local Health Council Movement

Consumers were the first to recognize a need for coordinating planning of health organizations in the public and private sectors. Dissatisfaction about overlapping and duplication of services, lack of data collection efforts and a desire to lobby for health legislation proposals brought a number of private citizens together in the early 1920s in the local health council movement. By the 1950s there were approximately 1,200 local health councils meeting in 32 of the 48 states.

Many professional health administrators equally deplored the lack of co-ordination and increasing costs in hospitals during those years, and this gave rise to a number of hospital planning associations.

The Hill Burton Act

A new phase in health planning began shortly after the passage in 1946 of the Hill Burton Act, which, over the next several decades, was to fund the building of hundreds of hospitals, long-term care facilities, and other related structures around the country.

Increasing Federal Involvement

During the 20 years following World War II, the federal government became actively involved for the first time in financial support of almost every aspect of health care, from sponsoring research, building hospitals, and actually providing health care to the poor and elderly to underwriting the education of nurses and physicians.

Phase 2: Federally Dominated Health Planning

Comprehensive Health Planning Act, 1966

In 1966, seeking to rationalize health planning and to give consumers a meaningful role in health care policy making, the federal government passed its first health planning law: Public Law 89–749, the Comprehensive Health Planning Act.

This legislation mandated that all participating states set up state and local health planning entities called Comprehensive Health Planning Agencies (CHPs). The hospital planning associations often served as the nuclei for these agencies. Consumers were to constitute 51% of the boards and have an active voice in program planning.

Within 5 years it became evident that the CHPs were all too often dominated by concerned health professionals. To counteract this trend, a new health planning law was passed in 1974, defining a "consumer" much more narrowly so as to assure that professionals were not over-represented on the local and state health planning agency boards.

The National Health Planning and Resources Development Act, 1974

Public Law 93–641, the National Health Planning and Resources Development Act of 1974, was intended to rationalize health planning in the United States. To accomplish this, 213 local offices, called Health Systems Agencies, were established. In many cases, the former Comprehensive Health Planning Agencies won the contracts to become the new Health Systems Agencies (HSAs).

Each local HSA was made responsible for estimating the health needs in its geographical area for the prospective 5 years. This included the need, or lack of need, for nursing home beds. Based on this plan, the Agency would attempt to determine whether the health care needs of its area were being met. It is this process that so directly affects nursing home operations in many states.

Certificate of Need

If the local health planning agency believed that there were insufficient nursing home beds in the area, it was willing to issue what is called a Certificate of Need, which is often referred to as a CON.

If the local health planning agency considered that there were enough or perhaps too many nursing home beds in the geographical area, it might refuse to issue a Certificate of Need. In effect, the agency could deny permission to build new long-term care beds in that geographical region.

Capital Project Review

A second area in which local HSAs could affect nursing home administrators and owners was through review of capital projects. Each HSA was responsible for reviews of requests by nursing homes and other health providers to make capital expenditures for building new facilities or renovating existing structures.

Phase 3: Health Planning as a State Level Activity

De-emphasis of the Federal Role

Under former President Ronald Reagan's leadership toward reducing federal government's role in health matters, Congress formally killed Public Law 93–641 as of October 1, 1986. Health planning then became a state activity.

Increased Reliance on States

Certificate of Need requirement is now an activity at the state level.

About half the states have dispensed with any "Certificate of Need" type of requirements, or are exempting all but the most expensive projects from requiring a Certificate of Need to build or renovate. In the several states that still retain some form of Certificate of Need, the rationale is that by controlling the number of new nursing home or hospital beds built or renovated, the state is able to exercise some control over health care costs.

4.9 Voluntary Operating Standards: Joint Commission on Accreditation of Healthcare Organizations

Long-term care facilities that meet certain requirements are eligible to apply for accreditation from the Joint Commission on Accreditation of Healthcare Organizations (JCAHO). Accreditation by JCAHO is voluntary, and currently, less than 10% of long-term care facilities have applied for it.

Some states are beginning to use JCAHO accreditation in lieu of state or federal inspections for meeting the federal or state requirements (Miller, 1982, p. 5039).

Origins of JCAHO

The JCAHO had its origins in a program for hospital evaluation established in 1918 by the American College of Surgeons (JCAHO, 1982, p. ix). Its 22-member board consists of representatives from the American College of Physicians, the American College of Surgeons, the American Dental Association, the American Hospital Association, and the American Medical Association (JCAHO, 1982).

JCAHO Membership

Slightly over 1,000 long-term care facilities are members of JCAHO. The Veterans Administration has traditionally required its long-term care facilities to be JCAHO accredited. As nursing home facilities seek to offer more medically complex care to the case managers of third-party payers, such as insurance companies and HMOs, these third-party payers frequently prefer the contracting nursing facilities have JCAHO accreditation, because that is the accreditation process with which they are familiar.

Nearly all U.S. hospitals seek accreditation by JCAHO, because the federal Medicare and Medicaid payers in effect "require" JCAHO accreditation to be eligible to receive Medicare and Medicaid payments. For nursing facilities to receive Medicare and Medicaid payments they must be certified by the federal Medicare and Medicaid officials and licensed by their individual state. Thus, JCAHO accreditation for hospitals has the same funding eligibility function as "Certification" for nursing facilities. For nursing facilities, then, JCAHO accreditation is an extra; for hospitals JCAHO accreditation is a must until Congress permits other agencies in addition to JCAHO to accredit hospitals.

Trend Toward Seeking JCAHO Accreditation

A number of managed care organizations, more acquainted with the hospital accreditation process than with Medicare/Medicaid inspection in nursing facilities, are demanding that those facilities seeking to offer subacute care, or negotiating similar contracts with third-party private reimburses, acquire JCAHO accreditation as a quality control measure (National Senior Citizens Law Center, 1995, p. 9).

Eligibility to Apply for JCAHO Accreditation

An eligible long-term care facility is one that is either hospital-based or free-standing and established "for inpatient care, that has an organized medical staff, or its equivalent, or a medical director, and that it provide continuous nursing service under professional nurse direction" (JCAHO, 1983b, p. 1).

The facility must also have been under the same ownership for at least 6 months, have a current unrestricted state license, and operate without restriction by reason of race, color, sex, or national origin. It must, in addition, submit a completed JCAHO application with all information requested.

JCAHO Accreditation Process

The JCAHO offers a concise manual summarizing all JCAHO accreditation requirements. After the application is accepted and processed, a survey team consisting of an administrator, a registered nurse, and a social worker visit the facility. The survey team report is evaluated by the JCAHO headquarters staff and a recommendation from the staff is forwarded to the Accreditation Committee of the JCAHO Board of Commissioners, who make the final decision. The entire process is normally completed in a total of 100 days and costs between $6,000 and $11,000, depending on the number of team members and the number of days they are at the facility. A recent base fee was $8,000+ (Morrissey, 1995, p. 21).

The JCAHO survey team examines the facility to discover if it is meeting the standards for the following (JCAHO, 1983b, p. v):

- building and grounds safety
- dental services
- dietetic services
- functional safety
- governing body and management
- infection/environment control
- laboratory, radiological, and other diagnostic services
- medical records, medical services, nursing services
- resident activities, care management, rights and responsibilities
- pharmaceutical services
- quality assurance
- rehabilitation services
- social services
- spiritual services
- transfer agreements

In concert with the federal thrust on outcomes, the JCAHO accreditation process is increasingly focused on the quality of care actually being received by residents. These JCAHO standards do not differ substantially from the Federal Requirements.

The Quality of Life

In general, the JCAHO requires that each accredited organization have the equivalent of a continuous quality improvement program in place and functioning (Quality Assurance in Long-Term Care, p. 11).

REFERENCES

Adams, E. K., Meiners, M. R., & Burwell, B. O. (1993). Asset spend-down in nursing homes. *Medical Care, 31*(1), 1–23.

Aetna Life Insurance Company. (1994). Covered level of care. *Medicare Bulletin.* Aetna Health Plans. All skilled nursing facilities 94–02 (Sept. 19), p. 1.

American Hospital Association. (1976). *Taft Hartley Amendments: Implications for the health care field.* Report of a symposium. Chicago: Author.

Argenti, P. A. (1994). *The portable MBA desk reference.* New York: Wiley.

Blake, J. B. (1959). *Public health in the town of Boston.* Cambridge, MA: Harvard University Press.

Boling, T. E., Vrooman, D. M., & Sommers, K. M. (1983). *Nursing home management*. Springfield, IL: Thomas.

Burda, D. (1995). Hospitals rank high as health hazard for employees. *Modern Healthcare, 25*(2), 24.

Carley, M. M. (1991). New medical devices. Reporting requirements. *Contemporary Long Term Care, 14,* 66.

Centers for Medicare and Medicaid Services (CMS). (1982). Conditions of participation for skilled nursing and intermediate care facilities (a proposed rule), 42 CFR Parts 405, 442, and 483, March 19, 1980. In D. B. Miller (Ed.), *Long term care administrators desk manual* (pp. 7042–7076). Greenvale, NY: Panel.

Cherry, R. L. (1993). Community presence and nursing home quality of care: The ombudsman as a complementary role. *Journal of Health & Social Behavior, 34,* 336–345.

Chruden, J. J., & Sherman, A. W., Jr. (1980). *Personnel management: The utilization of human resource* (6th ed.). Dallas, TX: South-Western.

Clement, P. F. (1985). History of U.S. aged poverty. *Perspectives on Aging, 9*(2), 4–7.

Committee on Nursing Home Regulation, Institute of Medicine. (1986). *Improving the Quality of Care in Nursing Homes*. Washington, DC: National Academy Press.

Council on Scientific Affairs. (1990). Home care in the 1990s. *Journal of the American Medical Association, 263,* 1241–1244.

Dainton, C. (1961). *The story of England's hospitals*. Springfield, IL: Charles C Thomas, p. 21.

Department of Health and Human Services. (2005). Centers for Disease Control and Prevention, National Center for Health Statistics. Hyattsville, MD: Author.

Department of Health and Human Services. (2003). Centers for Medicare and Medicaid Services, Oscar Form 671: F10–F39.

Department of Health and Human Services. (2006). Centers for Medicare and Medicaid Services, Oscar Form 672: F75–F139.

Department of Labor. (1976). *Brief history of the American labor movement* (Bulletin 1000). Washington, DC: U.S. Government Printing Office.

Duke University Medical Center. (1995, Summer). *Duke health*. Durham, NC: Author.

EEOC Notice 915.002. (1994, May 19). Enforcement guidance (revised EEOC form 106 (6–91)). Washington, DC: U.S. Government Printing Office.

Fact Sheet #17N: Nurses and the Part 541 July 2004 Exemptions Under the Fair Labor Standards Act.

Fair Labor Standards Act (FLSA). 29 United States Code ö201, et seq.

Federal Register, 39(12), Part 3, pp. 2238–2249.

Freymann, J. G. (1980). *The American health care system: Its genesis and trajectory*. Huntington, NY: Krieger.

Giacalone, J. A. (2001). *The U.S. nursing home industry*. Armonk, NY: M.E. Sharpe.

Greene, V. L., Lovely, M. E., & Ondrich, J. I. (1993). The cost-effectiveness of community services in a frail elderly population. *The Gerontologist, 33*(2), 177–187.

Harrington, C.H., Carrillo, M.S., Thollaug, S.C., Summers, P. R., & Wellin, V. (2000). *Nursing facilities, staffing, residents, and facility deficiencies, 1993 through 1999*. San Francisco: University of California at San Francisco, Department of Social & Behavioral Sciences.

Health care labor manual: Vol. 1. (1983). Rockville, MD: Aspen.

Hunter, R. J. (1955). *The origin of the Philadelphia General Hospital*. Philadelphia: Rittenhouse Press, p. 27.

Ivancevich, J. M., & Glueck, W. F. (1983). *Foundations of personnel: Human resource management* (Rev. ed.). Plano, TX: Business Publications.

Johns, G., & Saks, A. (2001). Organizational Behavior (5th ed.). Toronto: Addison Wesley Longman.

Joint Commission on Accreditation of Hospitals. (1982a). *Facts about JCAHO*. Chicago: Author.

Joint Commission on Accreditation of Hospitals. (1983b). *JCAHO eligibility criteria*. Chicago: Author.

Kaplan, B. (1985). Social Security: 50 years later. *Perspectives on Aging, 9*(2), 4–7.

Kart, C. S. (1981). *The realities of aging*. Boston: Allyn and Bacon.

Lagore, R. J. (1994). Adding nursing facility beds: Impact on hospital nonacute care. *Hospital and Health Services Administration, 39*(3), 327–340.

Landefeld, C. S., Palmer R. M., Johnson M. A., Johnston C. B., & Lyons W. L. (2004). *Current geriatric diagnosis & treatment*. New York: Lange Medical Books/McGraw-Hill.

Liu, F., Manton, K., & Allston, W. (1982). Demographic and epidemiological determinants of expenditures. In R. Vogel & H. Palmer (Eds.), *Long term care* (pp. 81–132). Washington, DC: Health Care Financing Administration.

Lutz, S. (1994). Hospitals' profit margins jump as costs are adjusted. *Modern Healthcare, 24*(43), 68.

Maddox, G. L., & Sussman, S. W. (2001). *The encyclopedia of aging* (3rd ed.). New York: Springer Publishing Company.

Manton, K. G., Stallard, E., & Woodbury, M. A. (1994). Home health and skilled nursing facility use: 1982–90. *Health Care Financing Review, 16*(1), 155–183.

McCarthy, M. J. (1994, November 8). Frayed lifeline: hunger among elderly surges: Meal programs just can't keep up. *Wall Street Journal*, p. 1 and 11.

Miller, D. B. (Ed.). (1982). *Long term care administrator's desk manual*. Greenvale, NY: Panel.

Miller, D. B., & Barry, J. T. (1979). *Nursing home organization and operation*. Boston: CBI.

Moore, J. D., Jr. (1995). Hillhaven nurses stage strike. *Modern Healthcare, 25*, p. 12.

Morrissey, J. (1995). JCAHO decides against survey fee hike. *Modern Healthcare, 25*, p. 21.

Muse, D. N., & Sawyer, D. (1982). *The Medicare and Medicaid Handbook*. Washington, DC: Health Care Financing Administration, p. 96.

National Center for Health Statistics. (1999). National Nursing Home Survey, Vital and Health Statistics, Series 13, Number 152.

National Fire Protection Association, Inc. (1985). *Life safety code 1985* (NFPA 101 ANSI-NFPA 101). Quincy, MA.

National Health Planning and Resources Development Act of 1974. Public Law 93–641.

National Senior Citizens Law Center. (1995). Quality assurance in nursing facilities. *Nursing Home Law Letter,* Issue No. 1, May 16, 16 pp.

Noe, R. A., Hollenbeck, J. R., Gerhart, B., & Wright, P. M. (2000). *Human resource management: Gaining a competitive advantage* (3rd ed.). Boston: McGraw-Hill Companies, Inc.

Occupational Safety and Health Act (OSHA). (1970). Public Law 91–596.

Perspectives. (1984, October 1). *Washington Report on Medicine and Health,* p. 3.

Pointer, D., & Metzger, N. (1975). *The National Labor Relations Act: A guidebook for health care facility administrators.* New York: Spectrum.

Prospective payment: DRG era dawns. (1983). *Medicine and Health,* p. 3.

Raskin, A. H. (1981, December). From sitdowns to solidarity: Passage in the life of American labor. *Across the Board,* pp. 12–32.

Robbins, S. P., & Coulter, M. (2007). *Management* (9th Ed.). New York: Pearson / Prentice Hall.

Robinson v. Jacksonville Shipyards, 790 F. Supp. 1486 (M.D. Fla. 1991).

Rosenfeld, L. S., Gaylord, S. A., & Allen, J. E. (1983). *Introduction to long-term care for the aging.* Chapel Hill, NC: The University of North Carolina Independent Study by Extension.

Rosmann, J. (1975). One year under Taft-Hartley. *Hospitals, 49*(24), 64–68.

Scott, L. (1994). NLRB order against Beverly voided. *Modern Healthcare, 24*(1), 8.

Service Employees International Union. (1995a, July). *Falling short.* Austin, TX: Author.

Service Employees International Union. (1995b). *National nurse survey.* Washington, DC: Author.

Service Employees International Union-AFL-CIO. (1995). *Caring till it hurts: How nursing home work is becoming the most dangerous job in America.* Washington, DC: Author.

Short, P. F., Kemper, P., Llewellyn, J. C., & Walden, D. C. (1992). Public and private responsibility for financing nursing home care: The effect of Medicaid asset spend down. *The Milbank Quarterly, 7*(2), 277–298.

Shriver, K. (1995). Union can't stop Vencor-Hillhaven deal. *Modern Healthcare, 25,* 18.

Simon-Rusinowitz, L., & Hofland, B. F. (1993). Adopting a disability approach to home care services for older adults. *The Gerontologist, 33*(2), 159–166.

Sloan, F. A., & Shayne, M. W. (1993). Long-term care, Medicaid, and impoverishment of the elderly. *The Milbank Quarterly, 71*(4), 575–599.

Smith, D. B. (1981). *Long-term care in transition: The regulation of nursing homes.* Washington, DC: Association of University Programs of Health Administration.

State of health planning. (1984, October 22). *Medicine and Health* (Insert).

Steinberg, R. M., & Carter, G. W. (1983). *Case management and the elderly.* Lexington, MA: Lexington Books, pp. 1–11.

Strahan, G. (1994). An overview of home health and hospice care patients. *Advance Data, 256,* Vital and Health Statistics, Centers for Disease Control, National Center for Health Statistics (July 22).

Wall Street Journal, January 21, 2006, p. A4.

Wall Street Journal, February 26, 2006, p. B1.

Weissert, W. G. (1989). Models of adult day care. *Gerontologist, 29,* 648.

Wilson, F. A., & Neuhauser, D. (1982). *Health services in the United States* (2nd ed.). Cambridge, MA: Ballinger.

PART V

Patient/Resident Care

5.1 The Aging Process

How many Americans die of old age each year? Depending on the definitions used, the answer could range from more than 1 million persons to no one. Our answer is, "no one." Old age is not a disease process.

It used to be customary to say that a person died of old age. But this is too imprecise an observation. It seems more functional to approach disease and disabilities and causes of death among older persons as one approaches these concerns in younger persons: to look for causes and seek either cure or relief.

Every older person, just as every younger one, dies of specific causes. Generally, one or more of the body systems (which are described later in this chapter) becomes overwhelmed for some specific reason, such as a disease or an injury to the person, and death results (Kane, Ouslander, & Abrass, 1989, p. 4; Kane et al., 2004). It is important to understand that age changes are not in themselves diseases, but rather are natural losses of function (Hayflick, 1995, p. 113–114; McCormick et al., 2006, pp. 152–154).

Research on Aging

The two groups who study aging individuals are identified by different titles. Physicians who specialize in treating the elderly are called geriatricians. Professionals who study the problems of the aging population in society, and usually are not physicians, are called gerontologists.

How much have the geriatricians and gerontologists learned about aging? With the development of clinical medicine over the past century, attention to diseases of aging persons and the aging process itself have become increasingly active areas of scientific investigation. Much has been learned, and some of this knowledge will be discussed later. However, a good deal of uncertainty remains. Much of the so-called knowledge about aging is still being tested and is not yet well established.

General Observations

One observation that seems safe to make is that aging is highly individual-ized. In the typical nursing home there are individuals whose chronological age is 90, yet their physiologic appearance and strong activity level are more characteristic of a 60-year-old person (Maddox & Sussman, 2001, p. 10). Similarly, there are those in their 60s and 70s in the same facility who appear to be more aged than the 90-year-old (Evans, Williams, Beattie, Michel, & Wilcock, 2000, p. 483).

The extent to which this is due to genetic inheritance, or is influenced by an individual's lifestyle and health behaviors remains a subject of lively debate.

A few additional general observations can be made about aging, none of them entirely safe, because for every such observation the reader may be able to produce valid exceptions.

Take, for example, observations of Alexander Leaf in *Scientific American* (1973, pp. 44–52). Leaf compared persons aged 75 with 30-year-olds and found that among those he studied, a person aged 75 has

92% of the former brain weight
84% of the former basal metabolism
70% of the former kidney filtration rate
43% of the former maximum breathing capacity

Those are impressive figures. What do they mean? Does the progressive loss of cortical neurons (brain cells) mean that older persons are that much less smart? Apparently not. There is little substantial clinical evidence that reduction of mental competence accompanies reduction in brain weight.

If Leaf's data are correct—that, on average, when a person reaches 75 the brain weighs about 10% less, the body is burning calories at a reduced rate, the kidneys are filtering about three-fourths as fast, and the lungs process oxygen more slowly, what is the significance? Certainly this may be important for the physician and the pharmacist concerned about drug tolerance and dosages, but these data do not make the 75-year-old individual any more or less of a person than the 30-year-old (Evans et al., 2000, p. 134).

The main import of Leaf's data may be to confirm that, in general, aging is a continuous process that may begin at birth, that it is a gradual decline of at least some systems of the body that proceed at different rates in dif-ferent individuals. Kane et al. (1989) suggest the 1% theory: that the ma-jority of body organs lose function at the rate of 1% per year after age 30 (p. 5). They caution, however, that newer findings suggest that functional decreases observed in some groups of persons and not others may point to disease patterns among some groups rather than normal aging in the general population.

5.1.1 OVERVIEW OF SOME APPEARANCE AND FUNCTIONAL CHANGES BELIEVED TO BE ASSOCIATED WITH AGING

The following observations are discussed at greater length under the headings of the 10 body systems described. By way of gaining an overall perspective, these phenomena can be observed.

Change in Collagen

Collagen is connective tissue that loses elasticity over time and appears to account for sagging of the skin often observed in the aging person. Sagging can occur around the eyes and jaws and can affect the general body tone of the muscles, especially in the arm (Balen & Vilenchik, 2006, pp. 259–262).

Reduced Reserve

Leaf's observation that the lungs' ability to process oxygen by age 75 to less than half their previous capacity tends to be true of several other body systems. One researcher believes that after age 20 the heart muscle, too, loses strength every year at the rate of 0.85% (Starr, 1964, p. 771). Another concludes that at-rest heart output at age 75 is no more than 70% of at-rest heart output at age 30 (Leaf, 1973, p. 44).

Gradual Changes in the Immune System

Usually, the body rejects foreign cells, but as the body ages, one theory holds that a progressive weakening of the immune response increases susceptibility to respiratory and other illnesses (Kane et al., 1989, p. 10; Kane et al., 2004; Maddox & Sussman, 2001, p. 527).

Temperature Response Changes

A reduction of capacity to maintain body temperature within a narrow range appears to lead to a diminished shivering and sweating response, allowing the body temperature of some older individuals to range dangerously. This can lead to the elderly dying in heat waves and cold waves that do not so adversely affect younger people. Ten percent of those over 65, or 2.5 million

Americans, are believed to be vulnerable to hypothermia (lowered body heat) due to reduced heat production by the body (Reichel, 1983, p. 8).

Postural Imbalances

The balancing mechanisms appear to function less well, resulting in some persons aged 65 and over being progressively at risk of tripping (Redford, 1989, p. 180).

Decalcification of the Bones

Many older persons are at increased risk of bones breaking, especially if they fall (Glowacki, 1989, p. 29).

Decreases in Bowel Function Control

As the central nervous system tends to function less and less well in some older persons, the ability to control the bowels lessens.

Frequent Anorexia

Anorexia (loss of appetite) among some elderly leads to skipping meals and a reduced level of nutrition (Gibbons & Levy, 1989, p. 197; Maddox & Sussman, 2001, p. 189).

Skin

With the loss of some subcutaneous fat, an older person may feel colder, and the skin may wrinkle. Some pigment (color) cells of the skin enlarge with age, resulting in the pigmented plaques often seen on the skin of aged persons.

Decreased Bone and Muscle Mass

This process among some elderly individuals can result in stooped posture, reduced height, loss of muscle power, misshapen joints, and limitations in mobility (DHHS, 2005, p. 340).

Renal System

The bladder of some persons appears to reduce to less than half its former capacity, and micturition, the desire to urinate, appears delayed until the bladder is at near capacity instead of triggering at one-half of capacity. One researcher (Lindeman, 1989, p. 248) estimates that the average 80-year-old resident has about one-half the glomerular filtration rate of a 30-year-old person.

Hearing and Vision

Both hearing and vision appear to become reduced among many aged persons.

Memory

Recall of names and information takes longer, learning new information is more difficult, and processing of information takes longer (Jones, 2004; Kline, 2006, pp. 1212–1214).

5.1.2 SOMATIC THEORIES OF AGING

Most investigators of the causes of aging agree that there is no one theory that currently explains the somatic aging phenomenon fully (Hayflick, 1995, pp. 113–118; Hefti, 1995, pp 686–687; Landfield, 1995, pp. 903–905; Meites & Quadri, 1995, pp. 677–681). Reichel, for example (1983, p. 8) defines aging as a progressive deterioration in functional capacity occurring after reproductive maturity.

Because no one really knows why people age, there are several theories instead of one generally accepted explanation. Hayflick thinks perhaps the question might more usefully be asked as why do we live so long (1995, p. 118). He observes that theorists are increasingly suspecting that the forces that produce age changes are different from those that drive longevity determination (p. 115).

There has been an explosion of biogerontologic theory about why we age. The main criticism of these theories is that changes such as reduced exercise capacity, may be indicative of certain more fundamental change processes (Hayflick, 1995, p. 114).

A Limit to the Number of Cell Divisions?

Some theories of aging relate to the genome or genetic apparatus, age-related changes in cell metabolism and function (Hayflick, 1995, p. 115). Leonard Hayflick, while doing research at Stanford University, found that normal human fibroblasts (embryonic cells that give rise to connective tissue), when cultured in vitro (in a test tube or other artificial environment), undergo only a limited number of divisions, usually about 50, before they die. His hypothesis is that the life span of a normal human cell is a programmed event under genetic control (1965, pp. 614–636). He obtained support for his theory by showing that cells from adult human tissue undergo about 20 divisions before they die. Kane et al. express their doubt about his theory, however (1989, pp. 8–9).

An Answer in Cancer Research?

Cancer cells appear to be able to continue reproducing indefinitely (Evans et al., 2000, p. 45; Rimer, 1995, p. 131). If this is so, what causes noncancerous cells to lose their ability to divide? Some researchers think that the answer to cancer cell divisions may hold information that will reveal the factor that limits the normal human cell's ability to continue dividing.

Somatic Mutation Theory

Some researchers have speculated that a sufficient level of accumulation of mutations in body cells produce the physiologic decrements we identify as aging (Hayflick, 1995, p. 116).

The Error Theory: A Loss in Genetic Programming?

At the University of California, Bernard Strehler hypothesized that age-related changes in cell metabolism are a programmed loss of the genetic material found in the DNA molecule (the molecule of heredity in most organisms). Essentially this is based on the theory that there is increasing inaccuracy in the protein synthesis. The idea is that the ends of linear chromosomes (the telemere length) decrease until encoded instructions for cell division disappear (Brown, 2006, pp. 445–446; Evans et al., 2000, p. 38; Hayflick, 1995, p. 116).

Random Mutations?

When he was working at the Boston University Medical School, Marott Sinex (1977) proposed that random mutations of cells may produce aging by causing damage to DNA molecules. His theory is that as mutations (changes) accumulate in the body cells, they progressively lose their ability to reproduce and perform their original functions.

Program Theory

Proponents of this approach contend that the events we associate with aging are programmed into the genome, that just as progressive maturation is programmed, progressive deterioration is programmed (Hayflick, 1995, p. 117).

An Autoimmune Explanation?

Several investigators (Evans et al., 2000, p. 49; Heidrick, 2006, pp. 95–96) suggest that a progressive failure of the body's immune system, which consists of white blood cells and various antibodies that are our first line of defense against diseases (discussed later), lead to autoimmune responses in older persons. Their idea is that "copying errors" in repeated cell divisions lead to cells that are progressively not recognized by the body, triggering the immune system to attack these cells, thinking foreign cells have invaded (Maddox & Sussman, 2001, p. 110).

This is similar to the wear and tear theory, which postulates that as mutations progress over time unrepaired changes of DNA and similar processes result in aging (Maddox & Sussman, 2001, p. 1053; Medevedev, 1995, p. 965).

Entropy and Aging

The Second Law of Thermodynamics postulates that ordered systems move toward disorder. In this theory, aging is an inevitable expression of the idea that closed systems, such as our bodies, tend to a state of equilibrium in which nothing more happens (Evans et al., 2000, p. 48).

Longevity Assurance Genes

In this approach aging is thought to be under the control of hormones and to be genetically based (Hayflick, 1995, p. 118; Meites & Quadri, 1995, p. 677).

Stress Theory of Aging: Wear and Tear

Some theorists have suggested that the body simply wears out, or that vital parts wear out, similar to what occurs in machines (Evans et al., 2000, p. 36; Landfield, 1995, p. 904; Maddox & Sussman, 2001, p. 979; Medvedev, 2006, pp. 964, 1224–1225). Hans Selye (cited in Landfield, 1995) suggests that the body's response to long-term stress resembles the normal life cycle, leading to the final stage of senescence. In this view, repeated experiences with stress are associated with a speeding up of the aging process (Landfield, 1995, p. 903). Some researchers have focused on the possible role of adrenal steroids or stress hormones that appear to accelerate aging of the brain (Landfield, 1995, p. 904; Medvedev, 2006, pp. 1224–1225).

Neuroendocrine Theory of Aging

Several theorists believe that the brain and the endocrine glands control aging. The concept is that as derangements in normal functioning occur tissues and organs are affected in ways we identify with "aging." Some of their thinking is based on the immune–neuroendocrine interactions. Basically, the brain and endocrine glands are believed to affect, for example, the immune system, which leads to impairment of antibody formation (Meites & Quadri, 1995, p. 681).

Some researchers have focused on caloric restriction being associated with delaying the maturing of the neuroendocrine functions, delaying body growth, puberty, lowering blood temperature, lowering cell division, decreasing body metabolism, and so on, thus delaying what we think of as the aging process (Maddox & Sussman, 2001, p. 736).

Neurotrophic Factors and Aging

Neurotrophic factors are observed to control the survival of neurons or nerves over time, and some theorists believe understanding this phenomenon will lead to greater understanding of what we identify with the aging process (Hefti, 1995, pp. 686–687).

Failure of Collagen?

Collagen is a protein fiber that is distributed in the walls of the blood vessels, the heart, and the connective tissue. Is age accompanied by a reduction in the elasticity of this protein, possibly leading to heart muscle inefficiency and, because of rigidity, to reduced cell permeability, making cell nutrition more difficult?

Regardless of which, if any, of these explanations of the aging process turns out to be correct, the nursing home administrator must deal with the effects of aging in planning the care of residents in the facility.

5.1.3 RESIDENT EXERCISE AND FITNESS

As we will see later, a degradation of function in the cardiovascular system usually interferes with the supply of nutrients and oxygen to the cells (Sullivan, 1995, p. 138). This, in turn, damages the tissues and organs in the body, leading to the decline of other major organs in the body and of other major processes. It is not surprising, then, that a consensus is emerging: Moderate exercise is important to the cardiovascular system of aged persons (Evans et al., 2000, p. 386 ff.; Landefeld, Palmer, Johnson, Johnston, & Lyons, 2004, p. 436; Maddox & Sussman, 2001, p. 145). Harris cites studies by deVries, Frankel, Kraus, Jokl, and others that demonstrate that physical conditioning can improve the cardiovascular system, the respiratory system, the musculature, and the body composition of older persons (Harris, 1989, p. 86). The Paffenbarger study of 16,920 Harvard male alumni attributed 1–2 years of increased longevity to 80-year-old men who had exercised moderately over the years (Paffenbarger, Wing, & Hsieh, 1986, p. 605).

This all makes sense (Landefeld et al., 2004, p. 437). The body systems we have mentioned and will describe in more detail later all depend on oxygen and nutrients from the blood (Evans et al., 2000, p. 326). Exercise increases the blood supplied to the body systems. Improved supplies of oxygen and nutrients lead to improved organ and cell status (Evans et al., 2000, p. 330; Landefeld et al., 2004, p. 2).

Claims for the benefits or exercise for the elderly are extensive. Beneficial effects on depression, in reducing the risk of developing heart disease, improved oxygenation and oxygen transport, greater protection against deterioration of glucose tolerance, and denser bone mass are some of the perceived benefits (Harris, 1989, p. 86; Landefeld et al., 2004, p. 1; Maddox & Sussman, 2001, p. 287).

Sedentary lifestyle and poor physical fitness are thought to be responsible for some of the typical nursing facility symptoms such as headaches, constipation, joint pain, back aches, insomnia, and fatigue (Harris, 1989, p. 86; Landefeld et al., 2004, p. 2).

Keeping the cardiovascular system at its peak through regular exercise, then, is seen to have beneficial effects upon many of the body's systems (Maddox & Sussman, 2001, p. 145).

There are many studies of dosages of exercise, particularly those suggesting maximal benefits from 30 minutes of moderate exercise 5 to 7 days per week. There is also literature on benefits of exercise at different ages, including very-advanced age. There is some literature on the promotion of exercise in the aged, including in residential settings. Promotion of exercise in the nursing home setting is complicated because each patient's condition is unique and varies over the stay in the facility. The physical therapists in the facility will be up to date on the changing world of exercise recommendations, but all "exercise" must be ordered by the physician and included in the patient's plan of care.

Inclusion of a level of aerobic exercise (i.e., exercise sustaining the heart rate at an elevated level, delivering increased oxygen for specified minimum period of time each week) matched to each resident's capabilities in the plan of care seems appropriate as facility policy (Evans et al., 2000, p. 968, 1140 ff.; Landefeld et al., 2004, p. 1; Maddox & Sussman, 2001, p. 372).

In the following sections we further explore some of the possible important relationships between diseases and aging found in the typical nursing facility population. Before turning to an exploration of these relationships, however, the following section, which presents and defines a number of medical and related terms, is offered. The section is divided into four vocabulary-building topics: (a) a list of medical and related specialists, (b) therapeutic action of some drugs, (c) abbreviations commonly used in patient charting, and (d) a series of the more common prefixes and suffixes.

5.2 Medical and Related Terms

5.2.1 MEDICAL SPECIALIZATIONS

"Specialization" is typically a 3-year training program taken beyond medical school curriculum, which itself is usually 4 years. By professional custom, physicians usually place only "MD" after their names, omitting any reference to certification they may hold as a "specialist." The following is not a list of all the prominent specialists—rather, it is a list of those more commonly seen in or consulted by residents in the nursing facility.

Cardiologist—a physician who specializes in the diagnosis and treatment of heart diseases.

Chiropodist—see Podiatrist.

Dermatologist—a physician who diagnoses and treats diseases of the skin.

Endocrinologist—a physician who specializes in disorders affecting the endocrine (ductless gland) system. This system includes the pituitary, thyroid, pancreas, and adrenal glands, which secrete hormones into the blood stream.

Family medicine specialist or practitioner—In 1879, 80% of physicians were general practitioners (GPs), 20% were specialists. With the proliferation of medical knowledge the reverse is true today: 80% of physicians are specialists, 20% are general practitioners. The general practitioner of yesteryear, since the late 1980s, has gone full circle and is itself a specialty requiring 3 years of internship beyond medical school. In this sense, nearly all physicians are now specialists. They specialize in diagnosing diseases and making referrals to specialists when appropriate and still provide the bulk of care in nursing facilities.

Gastroenterologist—a physician who treats and diagnoses diseases of the digestive tract.

General surgeon—a physician who specializes in operative procedures to treat illnesses or various injuries.

Geriatrician—a physician who concentrates on the treatment of elderly persons. Gerontology became a specialization only in 1987.

Note: There are currently a number of physicians who, during the grandfather period in the late 1980s, by taking the written exam only, became certified gerontologists without doing the required 3-year specialization. Still at issue, and an important question for the nursing home industry, is whether gerontology will be a small subspecialty or see "all" of the elderly. Current expert opinion is that gerontology will move toward being a small subspecialty because the typical needs of older persons, especially perhaps nursing home residents, will best be met by other specialists, regardless of age. Persons with hip fracture, prostate problems, cardiac problems, and so forth, will require the care of a specialist (Maddox & Sussman, 2001, p. 441).

(A **gerontologist** is a professional who studies the problem of the aging population in society and usually is not a medical doctor.)

Internist—a physician who specializes in diagnostic procedures and treatment of nonsurgical cases.

Neurologist—a physician who diagnoses and treats diseases of the brain, nervous system, and spinal cord.

Ophthalmologist—a physician who diagnoses and treats eye diseases and disorders, performs eye surgery, refracts the eyes, and prescribes corrective eye glasses and lenses.

Optician—a technician, not a physician, trained to grind lenses and to fit eye glasses.

Orthopedist—a physician who specializes in diseases and injuries to bones, muscles, joints, and tendons. An orthopedic surgeon is a physician who specializes in surgical procedures relating to the bones, muscles, joints, and tendons.

Osteopath—a doctor of osteopathy, not an allopathic trained medical doctor, who uses methods of diagnosis and treatment that are similar to those of a medical doctor, but who places special emphasis on the interrelationship of the musculoskeletal to the other body systems.

Physiatrist—a physician who specializes in physical medicine, body movements, and conditioning much like the focus of a physical therapist, often associated with sports medicine.

Podiatrist—a trained professional, who is not a medical doctor, concerned with care of the feet, including clipping of toenails for diabetics, and who treats ailments such as corns and bunions.

Proctologist—a physician specializing in the diagnosis and treatment of the large intestine, particularly the rectum and anus.

Psychiatrist—a physician who specializes in the diagnosis and treatment of mental disorders.

Psychoanalyst—a psychiatrist who specializes in the use of psychoanalytic technique of therapy.

Psychologist—one who studies the function of the mind and behavioral patterns and administers psychological tests; not a physician.

Pulmonologist—a physician specializing in treatment of the lungs.

Radiologist—a physician specializing in the use of "X-ray" and similar medical diagnostic machines such as magnetic resonance imaging (MRI), computer automated tomography (CAT) scans, and other medical techniques or modalities.

Rheumatologist—a physician who specializes in the treatment of rheumatic and arthritic diseases.

Urologist—a physician specializing in the diagnosis and treatment of diseases of the kidney, bladder, and reproductive organs.

5.2.2 MEDICATIONS / THERAPEUTIC ACTIONS OF DRUGS

Note: The nature and uses of several of the drugs and concepts mentioned, but not defined in this section, are discussed later in the context of individual body systems.

Extent of Drug Prescriptions in the Nursing Facility

Medications are among the most common types of treatment prescribed by physicians for the nursing home resident (Jones, 1989, p. 41). According to one National Nursing Home Survey, 95.5% of nursing home residents receive at least one or more medications (Evans et al., 2000, pp. 127 –130; Hing, 1977, p. 23; Maddox & Sussman, 2001, p. 17). This is not surprising, because admission usually depends on being ill and in need of continuing treatment. However, another study revealed that more than half of nursing home residents receive 3 to 7 different medications a day (USDHEW, 1976, p. 13).

Routes Used in Drug Administration

Drugs typically function in the body after being absorbed, usually through the digestive tract, into the bloodstream, following a pathway similar to that traveled by nutrients from food.

Drugs may be administered several ways: orally (by mouth); intramuscularly (IM) by an injection; directly on skin (topically); on membranes or other tissue, such as being held under the tongue (sublingually); or as suppositories. Usually medications eventually become inactive in the liver and are removed from the body by the kidney.

Injections and Intravenous Therapy

Injections are provided by facilities for a variety of reasons. Injections rates remained essentially level from 1993 through 1999. In 1993, 11.5% of residents in facilities were receiving injections compared with 12.6% in 1999 (Harrington, Carrillo, Thollaug, Summers, & Wellin, 2000, p. 51).

Intravenous therapy rates, on the other hand, rose. Intravenous therapy and blood transfusions are used to provide fluid, medications, nutritional substances, and blood products for residents. The percent of residents reported receiving these therapies in nursing facilities rose from 1.5% in 1993 to 2.7% in 1999, possibly reflecting an increasingly higher acuity level of residents (Harrington et al., 2000, p. 51).

In 2006, 17.85% of nursing home residents were receiving injections (DHHS, 2006, F78, F124–F128).

Five Basic Drug Actions

The following are the five basic types of actions drugs will produce (Poe & Holloway, 1980, pp. 14–15):

- blocking nerve impulses
- stimulating nerve impulses
- working directly on living cells
- working to replace body deficiencies
- any combination of the above

Every person is affected by drugs differently because of individual body chemistries, so every resident must be monitored to determine the appropriateness of different dosages (Evans et al., 2000, p. 129; Jones, 2004, p. 58).

As a result of age-related changes in the liver, kidney, and other organs throughout the body that alter the normal utilization of drugs, the elderly are at much greater risk of suffering from drug reactions, which are often the result of a buildup or excess amount of drugs in the body. In addition there may also be an increase in the occurrence of side effects that are commonly associated with most medications (Jones, 1989, pp. 42–44).

Policy Implications

Because nursing home residents are more likely to suffer from multiple diseases and use multiple medications, these drug combinations can produce dangerous drug interactions (Maddox & Sussman, 2001, p. 311; Roberts & Snyder, 1995, p. 289). The same residents are also at a much greater risk of suffering from an adverse drug reaction, many of which are the result of chemical incompatibilities among the different medications.

For these reasons, the nursing home administrator must assure that drug regimens in the facility are appropriately monitored by the consulting pharmacist with properly in-depth periodic reports to the facility management. Special precautions can be mounted to prevent the consequences of illness or disability from drug reactions.

Nursing facilities are increasingly moving to a system in which the nursing home staff use bedside handheld devices linked to an encrypted wireless network to scan bar codes on patient bracelets or enter information at workstations. The patient's identification is matched with records stored in off-site databases (*Wall Street Journal*, August 1, 2006, p. B3). A national electronic system is being built that allows authorized caregivers to access a patient's medical file from anywhere at any time. This both cuts down on medical mistakes and makes conforming to the HIPAA privacy regulations a complex process.

Use of P.R.N.

Often physicians rely on what is commonly referred to as p.r.n. (*pro re nata,* literally meaning "as the thing is necessary") approach. These "prescribe as needed" orders allow licensed nurses to determine when to administer a particular medication. A study of nursing home medication practices by Segal, Thompson, and Floyd revealed that approximately 46% of medications were prescribed on a p.r.n. basis. These practices, while functional and probably desirable, nevertheless need to be monitored closely.

A policy involving the facility pharmacy consultant and medical director, along with the nursing staff, in a constant monitoring of drug reactions is a major step. Increasing concern has been generated concerning polypharmacy (too many drugs) being given to the elderly patient (Evans et al., 2000, p. 1185; Landefeld et al., 2004, p. 421). However, closer and more active monitoring seems appropriate, inasmuch as undesirable drug interactions are a major ongoing concern in nursing facility administration.

The five rights of medication administration include identifying

1. the right medication
2. the right dose
3. the right time for administration
4. the right route (oral, shot, etc.)
5. the right patient (a picture with the Medication Administration Record [MAR] is always a good idea)

Generic and Brand Names

Familiarity with some of the more commonly prescribed medications by both the generic (chemical) names and brand (manufacturing) names can be useful. In the following discussion the generic names are mentioned first, with the brand names following in parentheses. Brand names are often used among health professionals unless a particular medication, for example, aspirin, is produced by a number of companies. Some of the more frequently prescribed medications are discussed later.

Antianxiety and Antipsychotic (Psychoactive) Medications

Antianxiety and antipsychotic medications act on the central nervous system to enable residents to deal with changes in their own behavior or stressful and anxiety-provoking changes in their environment. The two major classes of this type of drug are tranquilizers and sedatives/hypnotic.

These medications act directly on the major control center—the brain—and should be administered very cautiously. Many of the drug-related fatalities among the elderly are associated with these medications (Basen, 1977, p. 44; Maddox & Sussman, 2001, p. 83).

Some of the most commonly prescribed tranquilizers and sedatives/hypnotics used in the nursing home are thioridazine and chlordiazepoxide. Thioridazine (Mellaril®) is a major tranquilizer and antipsychotic drug prescribed for mild to moderate anxiety relief. This medication has been used for long-term alcoholics to control their illness. Chlordiazepoxide hydrochloride (Librium®) is a minor tranquilizer prescribed for relief of anxiety.

The side effects associated with these medications include drowsiness, dizziness, disorientation, and allergic reactions (Evans et al., 2000, p. 950).

An extensive and apparently successful effort has been made over the past few years to reduce the number of antipsychotic drugs used in the typical nursing facility (Ray, 1993, p. 713; Selma, Palla, Padding, & Brauner, 1994, p. 648).

Vitamins and Minerals

Vitamins and minerals are the most common classes of medications prescribed for the elderly nursing home resident, according to the National Nursing Home Survey (Evans et al., 2000, p. 131; Johnson, 2006, pp. 854–859). Ferrous sulfate, which is an iron supplement, and multivitamins are among the most popular in this category.

A common side effect of iron supplements is irritation of the gastrointestinal tract, which may cause some stomach upset. Too much iron is suspected to contribute to heart attacks. Other frequently prescribed minerals include calcium and potassium supplement.

Analgesics

Nonsteroidal Anti-Inflammatory Drugs (NSAIDs)

NSAIDs (e.g., Ibuprofen) are widely used for treating arthritis and chronic pain. NSAIDs provide fast and effective pain relief. However, adverse effects are experienced in elderly nursing home patients. NSAIDs inhibit cyclooxygenase (COX) enzymes, which catalyze the conversion of prostaglandins from arachidonic acid, which has adverse health effects on the body. Prostaglandins are vasodilators and help maintain blood flow and glomerular filtration through the kidneys, especially when blood volume is decreased (Landefeld et al., 2004, p. 424).

Analgesics are often administered for pain relief (Sengstaken & King, 1993, p. 541). Acetylsalicylic acid, or aspirin, may be relatively safe, except for nursing home residents with kidney problems and ulcers. Aspirin may also act as an anti-inflammatory agent for arthritic patients. Such medications serve to reduce the amount of damage to the joints and to lessen the painful side effects associated with the inflammatory process.

Some of the side effects associated with aspirin include stomach upset, ringing in the ears, deafness, dizziness, confusion, and irritability.

Acetaminophen (Tylenol®) is an analgesic similar to aspirin, but without anti-inflammatory properties, and hence it may serve only as a pain reliever (Weiner, 2006). Some side effects associated with acetaminophen are redness and itching of the skin and possible liver damage.

Another group of much stronger analgesics is the narcotics. Federal regulations require that they be kept under lock and key in a safe place because of their potential for abuse. A dangerous side effect with these drugs is the potential to depress breathing and respiratory functions that are controlled by the central nervous system. Alterations in consciousness or blood pressure may also occur. Some of the more commonly prescribed narcotic analgesics include codeine (Methylmorphine®), meperidine (Demerol®), morphine sulfate, and oxycodone terephthalate (Percodan®).

Laxatives and Gastrointestinal Agents

Gastrointestinal agents are among some of the more commonly prescribed medications for nursing home residents. Laxatives are also referred to as cathartics. This category includes suppositories, such as bisacodyl (Dulcolax), bulk laxatives like plantago seed (Metamucil®) and stool softeners such as milk of magnesia.

Often these agents are prescribed with other medications to neutralize their irritating effects on the gastrointestinal tract. Antacids, one of the most commonly indicated for this purpose, unfortunately may also cause side effects such as diarrhea. Milk of magnesia is frequently prescribed for gastrointestinal problems.

Cardiovascular Agents

Various groups of cardiovascular agents work to reduce blood pressure by different actions (this and similar topics are explored at length later in this section).

Methyldopa (Aldomet®) is an antihypertensive that works directly on the central nervous system to lower blood pressure. Orthostatic hypotension, or decreased blood pressure on standing, may be associated with this medication and increases the likelihood of residents falling.

Diuretics work by forcing the body to excrete excess fluids. Furosemide (Lasix®) and hydrochlorothiazide (Esidrix®) are commonly prescribed. But they cause the body to excrete potassium, and this may result in muscle weakness, lethargy, and muscle cramping (White & Sullivan, 2006, pp. 163–168).

Other medications act directly on heart muscle. Digoxin (Lanoxin®) acts to slow down the heart rate by decreasing the speed of impulses traveling along muscle fibers. Propranolol hydrochloride (Inderal®) is another medication that works to block chemicals from increasing the heart rate. Some side effects from these medications include a loss of appetite, nausea, vomiting, confusion, blurred vision, and arrhythmias (irregular heart beats).

Antianginal medications work to alleviate the pain associated with a decreased oxygen supply to the heart muscle. Nitroglycerin (NTG) works as a vasodilator to increase the size of blood vessels so they will carry more oxygen. This medication is administered sublingually (under the tongue).

Amitriptyline hydrochloride (Elavil®) is one of the most commonly prescribed drugs for elderly residents in a nursing facility (Cooper, 1978, p. 25). This medication also acts as a tranquilizer. The extent of its use is not surprising, considering that depression is one of the most common forms of illness (see Jones, 2004, pp. 55–56). Depression is also common among residents suffering from other chronic ailments, especially Alzheimer's and Parkinson's diseases (Blazer, 2006, pp. 303–306; Evans et al., 2000, p. 987 ff.; Kaszniak, 1995, p. 729; Maddox & Sussman, 2001, p. 287).

Some of the side effects associated with antidepressant medications such as Elavil® include confusion, drowsiness, decreased blood pressure, constipation, dry mouth, heart flutter, rashes, and retention of urine.

Anti-Infectives

Anti-infectives kill or decrease the growth of infectious organisms, complementing the natural body defense mechanisms.

Antibiotics are one of the more notable groups of medications within this class. Among the different types are the penicillins, cephalosporins, and tetracyclines. One of the most important side effects associated with these medications are allergic reactions, which are often identified by skin rashes.

Some antibiotics may be used to combat fungal and viral infections. Intravenous (IV) therapy is introduced when dealing with the more resistant organisms.

Miscellaneous Medications

Respiratory Agents

Expectorants, including ammonium chloride (Robitussin®), terpin hydrate, and acetylcysteine (Mucomyst®), are used to break up and expel mucus from the respiratory tract. The first two medications are taken orally; the third is usually administered by inhaling it in the form of a vapor. Tetracycline and ampicillin can be effective antibiotics for residents with respiratory tract infections due to chronic bronchitis (Evans et al., 2000, p. 57).

Optical Medications

Mydriatics are often used for residents with glaucoma. Pilocarpine and physo-stigmine are two often prescribed medications. They act to decrease the fluid buildup in the eye resulting from glaucoma. These medications are administered as eye drops. Some of their more common side effects are headaches, diarrhea, and sweating.

Controlled Drug Schedules

Federal regulations require all drugs to be stored in locked compartments. Separately locked, permanently affixed compartments are required for Schedule II drugs listed in the Comprehensive Drug Abuse Prevention and Control Act of 1970.

Formerly, drugs were regulated under the 1914 Harrison Narcotic Act, which placed them into classes A, B, X, and M narcotics. Subsequently, each state passed drug acts. Today, pharmacists and nursing facilities must meet the individual state drug laws and the federal drug laws. Most states have passed a State Uniform Controlled Substances Act, some with six instead of five drug group classifications.

The federal government has classified drugs into the following five schedules.

Schedule I Drugs: Drugs with a high abuse potential and no accepted medical use in the United States, for example, heroin, marijuana, LSD, peyote, mescaline, and certain other opiates and hallucinogenic substances.

Schedule II Drugs: Drugs with accepted medical use in the United States, having high abuse and dependency potential, for example, opium, morphine, codeine, methodone, cocaine, amphetamine, seco-barbital, methaqualone (Quaalude), and phencyclidine ("angel dust"). These were formerly Class A narcotics.

Schedule III Drugs: Drugs with less abuse potential than schedules I and II drugs. Several compounds are included, for example, Empirin compound with codeine, Tylenol® with codeine, and Phenaphen® with codeine. These were formerly Class B drugs.

Schedule IV Drugs: Drugs with less abuse potential than Schedule III drugs, for example, barbital, Librium®, diazepam, Valium®, and Dalmane®.

Schedule V Drugs: Drugs with less abuse potential than Schedule IV drugs. These typically are compounds containing limited qualities of narcotic drugs for antitussive (anticough) and antidiarrheal purposes.

Examples are Lomotil®, Phenergan® expectorant with codeine, and Robitussin® A-C syrup. These were formerly Class X (exempt narcotics) under the Harrison Act.

Therapeutic Actions of Drugs

Analgesic—reduces pain, e.g., aspirin

Antacid—neutralizes the acid in the stomach, e.g., Maalox®

Antianemic—used in treatment of anemia, e.g., liver extract

Antibiotic—destroys microorganisms in the body, e.g., penicillin

Anticoagulant—depresses (slows) the clotting of blood

Antidote—used to counteract poisons

Antiseptic—slows down growth of bacteria, but does not kill all of the bacteria, e.g., hydrogen peroxide

Antispasmodic—relieves smooth muscle spasm, e.g., Valium® (diazepam)

Antitoxin—neutralizes bacterial toxins in infections, e.g., tetanus antitoxin

Astringent—used to constrict skin and mucous membranes by withdrawing water, e.g., alum

Carminative—an agent that reduces flatulence (gas) in the stomach or intestinal tract

Cathartic—laxative, purgative, inducing bowel movements, e.g., cascara sagrada

Caustic—destroys tissue by local application, e.g., silver nitrate

Chemotherapeutics—chemicals used to treat illness, e.g., sulfanilamide for streptococcal infection

Coagulant—stimulates clotting of the blood

Diaphoretic—used to induce perspiration

Disinfectant—destroys pathogenic organisms, e.g., Zephiran® chloride

Diuretic—stimulates elimination of urine, often used with medications prescribed to reduce hypertension, e.g., diazide

Emetic—induces vomiting, e.g., warm salt water

Emollient—used to soften and soothe tissue, e.g., cold cream, petroleum jelly

Expectorant—used to induce coughing, an agent that increases bronchial secretion and facilitates its expulsion (coughing), e.g., Robitussin®

Hypertensive—helps raise blood pressure

Hypnotic—assists patients/residents to fall asleep, e.g., Nembutal

Miotic—constricts the pupil of the eye

Mydriatic—dilates the pupils of the eye

Sedative—relieves anxiety and emotional tensions, e.g., Seconal®

Tonic, or stimulant—used to stimulate body activity, e.g., Eldertonic® or Ritalin®

Vasoconstrictor—causes blood vessels to narrow or constrict

Vasodilator—expands or dilates blood vessels

Vitamins—used in replacement therapy, e.g., vitamin C

5.2.3 ABBREVIATIONS

aa	of each
Abd	abdomen
ac	before meals
Ad lib	as much as desired, at pleasure
A/G	albumin/globulin ratio
AIDS	acquired immune deficiency syndrome
amp	ampule
amt	amount
aq	water
aq dist	distilled water
ASH.D.	arteriosclerotic heart disease
BE	barium enema
bId	twice a day
BMR	basal metabolic rate
BP, or B/P	blood pressure
BRP	bathroom privileges
c	with
Ca	carcinoma
CAD	coronary artery disease (Evans et al., 2000, p. 194)
caps	capsules
cath	catheter
CBC	complete blood count
c c	cubic centimeter
cf	compare
CNS	central nervous system
COLD	chronic obstructive lung disease; same as COPD
comp	compound
COPD	chronic obstructive pulmonary disease
CVA	cerebral vascular accident
d/c	discontinued
decub	lying down
Diab	diabetic

Diag, or **Dx**	diagnosis
Diff	differential blood count
Dil	dilute
Disc	discontinue
Disch, or **D/C**	discharge
dx	diagnosis
EEG	electroencephalogram
EKG, or **ECG**	electrocardiogram
exam	examination
fl, or **fld**	fluid
FUO	fever of unknown origin
Fx	fracture
GII	gastrointestinal
gm	gram
gr	grain
gtt, or **gtts**	drop (s)
H, or **hr**	hour
hs	at bedtime
hypo	hypodermically
IDDM	insulin dependent diabetes mellitus
IM	intramuscular
inf	infusion
IV	intravenous
KUB	kidney–ureter–bladder
l	liter
lab	laboratory
Lat	lateral
lb	pound
liq	liquid
mg	milligram
min	minute
ml	milliliter
mm	millimeter
MN	midnight
MRSA	methicillin-resistant Staphylococcus aureus
N	noon
NIDDM	noninsulin dependent diabetes mellitus
no	number
noct.	at night
NPO	nothing by mouth
NV	nausea and vomiting

od	right eye
os	left eye
OT	occupational therapy
ou	each eye
oz	ounce
p	pulse
pc	after meal
PEARL	pupils equal and reactive to light
po	by mouth
prn	as needed
prog	prognosis
PROM	passive range of motion
pt	pint
PT	physical therapy
PX	physical examination
qd	every day
qh	every hour
qhs	each bedtime
qid	four times a day
qn	every night
qod	every other day
qs	sufficient quantity
ROM	range of motion
Rx	prescription
s	without
SOB	shortness of breath
sol	solution
sos	one dose, if necessary
spec	specimen
SS	soap solution
ss	half
stat	immediately
surg	surgery
T	temperature
tab	tablet
TB	tuberculosis
tId	three times a day
tinct, or tr	tincture
TO	telephone order
TPR	temperature, pulse, and respiration
u	unit

ung	ointment
URI	upper respiratory infection
UTI	urinary tract infection
VO	verbal order
vol	volume
vs	vital signs
WBC	white blood cells
W/C	wheelchair
wt	weight

5.2.4 PREFIXES

a-, an-	*without,* e.g., anorexia (loss of appetite; Evans et al., 2000, p. 158).
ab-	*from, off, away,* e.g., abnormal (not normal)
ad-	*toward, to, at*
an-	*without,* e.g., anoxia—absence of oxygen supply to the tissues despite adequate perfusion of the tissue by blood, sometimes used to mean hypoxia or reduced oxygen supply, e.g., anoxic encephalopathy (any degenerative brain disease, meaning a degenerative brain disease characterized by insufficient supply of oxygen)
adeno-	*gland,* e.g., adenoma, a benign (noncancerous) epithelial (surface-covering) tumor in which the cells form recognizable glandular structures
ambi-	*both,* e.g., ambilateral (relating to both sides)
ana-	*up, toward,* e.g., anabolism (building up metabolism)
angio-	*relating to a vessel,* e.g., angiofibrosis (hardening of a vessel wall)
ante-	*in front of, before,* e.g., ante cibum (before a meal)
arthro-	*pertaining to the joints,* e.g., arthropathy (any disease affecting the joints)
auto-	*self, same,* e.g., autoanalysis (analysis by a person of their own disorder)
bact	*relating to bacteria,* e.g., bacteuria—the presence of bacteria in the urine.
bi-	*two,* e.g., bilateral (relating to both sides)
bio-	*relation to life,* e.g., biopsy (the process of removing tissue from living residents for a diagnostic examination)

brady-	*slow*, e.g., bradycardia (a slow heart)
broncho-	*relating to the trachea or windpipe*, e.g., bronchoedema (swelling of the mucosa of the bronchial tube)
carcino-	*pertaining to cancer*, e.g., carcinogen (any cancer producing substance) or carcinoma (a malignant neoplasm or cancer)
cardio-	*pertaining to the heart*, e.g., cardioplegia (paralysis of the heart), cardiomyopathy (a generalized term denoting heart disease)
cata-	*downward, against*, e.g., catabolism (the breaking down in the body of complex chemical compounds into simpler ones, often accompanied by the liberation of energy
celio-	*pertaining to the abdomen*, e.g., celiectomy (excision of the stomach) or celiocentesis (puncture of the abdominal cavity)
cephalo-	*head*, e.g., cephalogram (an X-ray image of the structures of the head)
cervico-	*neck or cervix*, e.g., cervicovesical (pertaining to the urinary bladder and the cervix)
chiro-	*pertaining to the hand*, e.g., chiroplasty (plastic surgery on the hand)
chole-	*pertaining to bile*, e.g., cholecystotomy (incision into the gall bladder)
circum-	*around*, e.g., circumcorneal (around or about the cornea of the eye)
com-, con-	*with, together*, e.g., complication (a disease or adverse condition associated with another disease or adverse condition)
contra-	*against, opposite*, e.g., contraindicated (not recommended, advised against)
counter-	*against, opposite*, e.g., counteraction (action of a drug or agent opposed to that of some other drug or agent)
cranio-	*pertaining to the head*, e.g., cranioplasty (any plastic operation on the skull)
cysto-	*pertaining to the bladder*, e.g., cystitis (inflammation of the urinary bladder) or cystocele (hernia of the bladder)
cyto-	*relation to a cell*, e.g., cytolysis (the dissolution of a cell)

de-	*down, away from,* e.g., defibrillation, the arrest of fibrillation, that is, irregular or rapid randomized contractions of the cardiac muscle restored to normal rhythm; e.g., debridement, [Evans et al., 2000, p. 108] removal of foreign material and contaminated or devitalized tissue from adjacent to a traumatic or infected lesion until healthy tissue is exposed, for example, to debride a pressure sore; e.g., detrusor, a general term for a body part; or a muscle, that pushes down).
derm-	*pertaining to the skin,* e.g., dermatitis (inflammation of the skin)
dextro-	*toward or on the right side,* e.g., dextrocardiogram (the part of the electrocardiogram that is derived from the right ventricle of the heart)
di-	*double, twice,* e.g., diarthric (relating to two joints)
dia-	*through, apart,* e.g., diagastric (through the stomach)
dys-	*painful, difficult,* e.g., dysphasia (difficulty in talking) or dyspnea (difficulty in breathing)
ecto-	*out, away from,* e.g., ectoderm (the outermost layer of the skin)
em-, en-	*in,* e.g., embolic (pushing or growing in)
encephalo-	*condition in the brain or head,* e.g., encephalomyolitis (an acute inflammation of the brain and spinal cord) or encephalosclerosis (a hardening of the brain)
endo-	*within, inner,* e.g., endocarditis (inflammation of the endocardium or lining membrane of the heart; Evans et al., 2000, pp. 61, 428); or endoscope (an instrument for the examination of the interior of a body canal or hollow area)
entero-	*relating to the intestines,* e.g., enterocolitis (inflammation of the mucous membrane of both small and large intestines)
epi-	*above, upon, over,* e.g., epidermititis (inflammation of the epidermis or the superficial layer of the skin)
eu-	*good,* e.g., euphoria (a feeling of well-being, commonly exaggerated and not necessarily well founded) or eupnea (easy, free respiration)

fibro-   *pertaining to fiber,* e.g., fibromyalgia (a condition char-
                  acterized by fatigue, stiffness, and chronic pain of the
                  muscles, tendons, and ligaments)

gastro-   *stomach,* e.g., gastrostomy (the establishment of an
                  artificial opening into the stomach, usually for feeding
                  purposes)

glyco-   *relationship to sweetness* (sugar), e.g., glycogen, the
                  chief carbohydrate storage material in animals formed
                  by and largely stored in the liver and, to a lesser extent,
                  in the muscles

gyneco-, gyno- *pertaining to a female,* e.g., gynecology (the science
                  of diseases of women, especially those of the genital
                  tract)

hemato-, hema- *pertaining to the blood,* e.g., hemorrhage (bleeding, a
                  flow of blood) or hematuria (blood in the urine)

hemi-   *half,* e.g., hemialgia (pain affecting one entire half of
                  the body) or hemiplegia (paralysis of one side of the
                  body)

hepato-   *liver,* e.g., hepatitis (inflammation of the liver)

histo-   *relationship to tissue,* e.g., histolysis (disintegration of
                  the tissue)

hydro-   *pertaining to water,* e.g., hydrocyst (a cyst or sore with
                  clear, watery contents)

hyper-   *excessive,* e.g., hyperesthesia (abnormal acuteness of
                  sensitivity to touch, pain, or other stimuli)

hypno(a)-   *relating to sleep,* e.g., hypnotherapy (the treatment of
                  disease by inducing prolonged sleep)

hypo-   *deficiency, lack of,* e.g., hypochondria (a false belief
                  that one is suffering from some disease); hypoten-
                  sion

hystero-   *relating to the uterus,* e.g., hysterogram (an X-ray of the
                  uterus)

ileo-   *relating to the ileum* (remote end of the small intestine),
                  e.g., ileocolitis (inflammation of the mucous mem-
                  brane of both ileum and colon)

infra-   *below, beneath,* e.g., infracardiac (beneath the heart,
                  below the level of the heart)

inter-   *between,* e.g., intercostal (between the ribs)

intro-   *in, into,* e.g., introgastric (leading or passed into the
                  stomach, e.g., a nasogastric tube for feeding)

kerato-	*relating to the cornea, or horny tissue,* e.g., keratoconjunctivitis (inflammation of the conjunctiva at the border of the cornea of the eye)
labio-	*relating to the lip,* e.g., labiocervical (pertaining to the lip and to the neck)
macro-	*large, long,* e.g., macrocyte (a giant red cell)
mast-	*relating to the breast,* e.g., mastectomy (amputation of the breast)
mega-	*large, oversize,* e.g., megacardia (enlargement of the heart)
meta-	*after, beyond, transformation,* e.g., metastasis (the shifting of a disease)
micro-	*small,* e.g., microinfarct (a very small infarct, i.e., death of tissue due to lack of blood supply, due to obstruction of circulation in capillaries or small arteries)
multi-	*many,* e.g., multicellular (composed of many cells)
myel-	*pertaining to the spinal cord,* e.g., myeloplegia (spinal paralysis)
myo-	*relating to muscle,* e.g., myotrophy (muscular atrophy) or myocardial infarction (death of some heart muscle due to lack of blood supply, a heart attack)
necro-	*relating to death,* e.g., necrocytosis (death of cells)
neuro-	*relating to the nerves,* e.g., a neurogenic bladder is one that is controlled by the nervous system rather than by voluntary control by the person; or neuroleptic, an antipsychotic agent
nephro-	*pertaining to the kidney,* e.g., nephritis (inflammation of the kidney)
odont-	*relating to the teeth,* e.g., odontalgia (a toothache)
omo-	*pertaining to the shoulder,* e.g., omodynia (pain in the shoulder joint)
opthalmo-	*relating to the eye,* e.g., opthalmoplegia (paralysis of the motor nerves of the eye)
opto-	*relating to vision,* e.g., optometer (an instrument for determining the refraction of the eye)
ortho-	*straight,* e.g., orthostatic (standing upright from a sitting or reclining position)
osteo-	*pertaining to the bones,* e.g., osteoporosis (reduction in the quantity of bone or atrophy of skeletal tissue)

oxy-	*sharp, acute,* e.g., oxyesthesia (a condition of increased acuity of sensation)
pachy-	*thick,* e.g., pachylosis (a condition of roughness, dryness, and thickening of the skin)
pan-	*all,* e.g., pancarditis (diffuse inflammation of the heart)
patho-	*disease,* e.g., pathogenesis (the origin or development of a disease)
per-	*through,* e.g., perfusion (the act of pouring over or through, especially the passage of a fluid through the vessels of a specific organ)
peri-	*around,* e.g., peribronchitis (inflammation of the tissues surrounding the bronchial tubes)
phlebo-	*relating to a vein,* e.g., phlebitis (inflammation of a vein)
pneumo-	*lung,* e.g., pneumonia (inflammation of the lung)
poly-	*many, much,* e.g., polyarthritis (inflammation of several joints)
procto-	relating to the anus, e.g., proctoscope, a short tubular instrument with illumination for inspecting the rectum. A sigmoidoscope, a foot-long tube, is used to examine the sigmoid (shaped like the letter M) colon, i.e., left colon from the descending colon to the rectum. A colonoscope, which is the longest, is used to examine the entire colon.
pseudo-	*false,* e.g., pseudo dementia (a condition of indifference to one's surroundings without actual mental impairment)
psycho-	*pertaining to the mind,* e.g., psychotherapy (counseling help)
pyo-	*signifying pus,* e.g., pyoderma (any infection of or on the skin that contains pus, that is, a collection of white blood cells and other materials generated by the immune response)
rachi-	*spine,* e.g., rachiocampsis (curvature of the spine)
rhino-	*nose,* e.g., rhinoplasty (a repair of the nose)
sub-	*under,* e.g., subcutaneous (under the skin)
syn-	*loss,* e.g., syncope (to faint, a temporary loss of consciousness due to generalized cerebral ischemia, that is, too little blood getting to the brain; Evans et al., 2000, p. 111; Landefeld et al., 2004, p. 138). Syncope

itself is not a diagnosis but rather a symptom of an underlying disorder.

tachy-	*rapid,* e.g., tachycardia (rapid beating of the heart)
thermo-	*heat,* e.g., thermophobia (morbid fear of heat)
uni-	*one,* e.g., unicellular (composed of one cell)
uro-	*relating to the urine,* e.g., urosepsis (septic poisoning from retained and absorbed urinary substances)
vaso-	*vessel,* e.g., vasoconstriction (narrowing of the blood vessels) or vasodilation (widening of the blood vessels)

5.2.5 SUFFIXES

-ac	*pertaining to,* e.g., cardiac (pertaining to the heart)
-algia	*pain,* e.g., neuralgia (nerve pain)
-cele	*hernia,* e.g., protrusion of a portion of an organ or tissue through the wall that normally contains it
-centesis	*surgical puncture,* e.g., paracentesis (a puncture of the body cavity for removing fluid)
-clasis	*breaking,* e.g., thromboclasis (the breaking up of a blood clot)
-clysis	*washing, irrigation,* e.g., enteroclysis (enema of the intestines)
-cyte	*cell,* e.g., hematocyte (any blood cell)
-ectasia	*dilation, stretching,* e.g., gastrectasia (dilation of the stomach)
-emesis	*vomiting,* e.g., hyperemesis (excessive vomiting)
-emia	*denoting a condition of the blood,* e.g., glycemia (sugar in the blood)
-ectomy	*excision (cutting out) of,* e.g., tonsillectomy (cutting out of the tonsils)
-genesis	condition of producing, e.g., carcinogenesis (the origin or production of cancer)
-itis	*inflammation,* e.g., dermatitis (inflammation of the skin)
-lith	*stone,* e.g., nephrolith (kidney stone)
-lysis	*breakdown,* e.g., hemolysis (the destruction of red blood cells)
-malasia	*softening,* e.g., osteomalasia (a disease characterized by gradual softening and bending of the bones)
-megaly	*enlargement,* e.g., cardiomegaly (enlargement of the heart)

-odynia	*painful condition,* e.g., cardiodynia (pain in the heart)
-oma	*tumor,* e.g., carcinoma (a malignant tumor)
-opsy	*vision,* e.g., biopsy (excision of a small piece of living tissue from a patient for microscopic examination)
-orexia	*appetite, desire,* e.g., anorexia (loss of appetite)
-orrhaphy	*suture,* e.g., gastrorrhaphy (the suture of a perforation of the stomach
-orrhea	*flow, discharge,* e.g., gastrorrhea (excessive secretion of gastric juice or mucus by the stomach)
-ostomy	*to make a new opening,* e.g., colostomy (the establishment of an artificial anus by an opening into the colon)
-otomy	*incision, to cut into,* e.g., nephrotomy (an incision into the kidney)
-path	*morbid or diseased,* e.g., a sociopath (a person who feels no remorse or guilt about behaving in socially unaccepted ways, e.g., physically beating a roommate and feeling no guilt or remorse)
-pathy	*disease,* e.g., neuropathy (any nerve disease), or angiocardiopathy (disease of the heart or blood vessels), or cardiomyopathy a disease of the heart; diabetic neruropathy is a common term in the nursing facility
-penia	*deficiency,* e.g., leukopenia (any situation in which the total number of leukocytes (white blood cells) in the circulating blood is less than normal)
-pepsia	*digestion,* e.g., dyspepsia (indigestion or upset stomach)
-pexy	*fixation, to put into place,* e.g., nephropexy (surgical attachment of a floating kidney)
-phobia	*fear,* e.g., claustrophobia (fear of being closed in a small space)
-plasty	surgical repair, e.g., thoracoplasty (reparative or plastic surgery to the chest)
-pnea	*breath,* e.g., polypnea (very rapid breathing)
-rhythmia	*rhythmical,* e.g., arrhythmia (any variation from the normal rhythm of the heart)
-sclerosis	*hardening,* e.g., arteriosclerosis (hardening of the arteries)
-spasm	*sudden violent involuntary contraction of muscles,* e.g., myospasm (spasm of a muscle)

-stasis	*arrest, control,* e.g., cholestasia (an arrest in the flow of bile from the liver)
-taxis	*order, arrangement,* e.g., thermotaxis (regulation of the temperature of the body
-tripsy	*crushing,* e.g., lithotripsy (the crushing of a stone in the kidney by a machine, called a lithotripter, that uses sound waves to break stones into minute particles, which can then be passed in the urine)
-trophy	*development, nourishment,* e.g., hypertrophy (an overgrowth or increase in the bulk of a body part or organ)
-uria	*urine,* e.g., albuminuria (the presence of protein in urine, chiefly albumin; albumin is any protein that is soluble in water)

5.3 The Aging Process As It Relates to Diseases Common to the Nursing Home Population

It is useful for the administrator to be familiar with the rudiments of biological processes and human anatomy and to be able to recognize the parts of the body that are most affected by the aging process. In this way the administrator will be better able to appreciate the special problems with which the facility must cope.

All physical processes in the body may undergo some changes as a result of aging, including a slowing down, a decrease in the overall energy reserve, breakdown of some of the body functions, and an alteration of some individual cell structures, which ultimately affects the functioning of some body tissues and organs as well.

The systems referred to are groups of structures that perform a specialized function for the body. Following is a list of 10 systems of the body processes and structures as they are most commonly categorized. They are presented to reflect also the prevalence of diseases affecting them in the nursing home population.

It is important to remember that these systems are highly interrelated and that most nursing home residents typically suffer from multiple chronic diseases that may affect combinations of body systems (Kane et al., 1989, p. 29).

1. **Blood circulation**—the basic processes and structures that enable the body to transport oxygen to the cells and tissues.
2. **Breathing**—the process by which the body obtains oxygen from the environment and distributes it throughout the body.
3. **Nervous system**—responsible for controlling all of the body functions and assuring that they are functioning properly; these are the regulatory activities.
4. **Digestion**—the process by which the body breaks down food into a form in which the nutrients may be used by the individual cells.

5. **Nutritional needs**—needs of the body for nutrients (Evans et al., 2000, p. 140 ff.).

6. **External and internal defense mechanisms**—the skin and an internal immune system, which play important roles in protecting the body from any harmful invasions.

7. **Musculoskeletal system**—the bones, muscles, tendons, and joints used in movement (Tonna, 1995c, p. 147).

8. **Excretory system**—the way in which the body relieves itself of fluid and chemical waste products.

9. **Reproductive system**—sexuality in the elderly.

10. **Emotional and mental well-being**—the psychological status.

Chronic vs. Acute

The nursing facility administrator typically focuses on caring for persons with chronic illnesses. Chronic illnesses are conditions that are persistent and last over an extended period of time. Usually these are diseases of slow progression and long duration. Chronic illness is thought of as long-term or permanent illnesses that often result in disabilities that may require help with various activities. Acute illness, on the other hand, is an illness characterized by an abrupt or rapid onset and usually of short duration. The typical acutely ill person in the hospital is said to be in an unstable condition, that is, in need of constant monitoring by physicians and nurses. In contrast, the typical nursing home resident exhibits one or more chronic illnesses that are thought to be in a stabilized state. The hospital focuses on acutely ill persons; the nursing facility focuses on chronically ill persons. As hospitals have discharged patients quicker and sicker, the acuity level of the nursing home patient has increased thus requiring increasing nursing care skills more and more often resembling the care needs of persons experiencing acute illness.

5.3.1 BLOOD CIRCULATION

The circulatory system, also called the cardiovascular system, may be thought of as an elaborate pumping mechanism. It is powered by the heart, which pumps the blood throughout the body within a network of blood vessels (arteries and veins).

Arteries

Arteries are the vessels that carry blood rich in nutrients away from the heart to the remainder of the body cells.

Nutrients combined oxy produced energy

Nutrients obtained from the food are processed in the digestive tract. Combined with oxygen, nutrients permit individual cells to perform the chemical reactions that produce energy.

Oxygen is a colorless, odorless, gaseous chemical element that is found in the air. Oxygen is most plentiful in the arteries, which divide into smaller and smaller branches until they become capillaries. These capillaries are the smallest blood vessels and form a network connecting the smallest arteries to the smallest veins (see Figure 5.1). It is here at the capillaries that the function of oxygenation occurs.

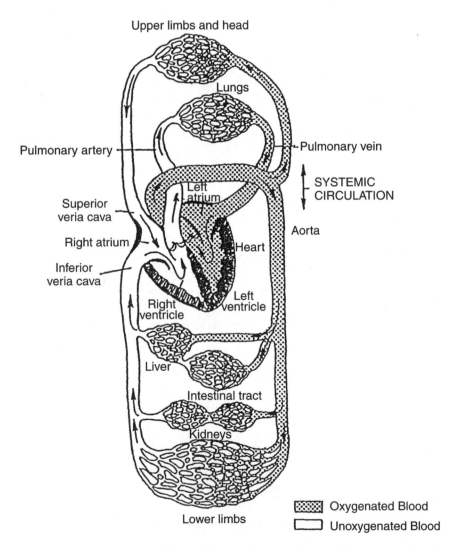

FIGURE 5.1 Representation of the circulatory and oxygenation process.

Oxygenation is the transfer of oxygen from the blood cells at the capillary level into the necessary tissues in exchange for carbon dioxide. Carbon dioxide is also a gas. It is produced as a waste product of the chemical reactions in the cells.

Veins

The blood cells carry carbon dioxide through the vein network and back to the heart. Veins return blood that is carrying carbon dioxide back to the heart through the superior (from upper body) and inferior (lower body) vena cava (see Figure 5.1).

The blood then enters the right side of the heart. When a sufficient amount of blood has collected, the right ventricle of the heart contracts, actually squeezing its contents into the artery that leads to the lungs (pulmonary artery).

Lungs

Within the lungs the carbon dioxide that has been collected by the veins is discarded and exchanged for oxygen. The carbon dioxide is then exhaled into the air as the breath is expelled. It has followed the reverse of the oxygen pathway until it is removed from the body. This is a simplification of the respiratory process (breathing), which will be discussed further in the next section.

The newly oxygenated blood returns to the heart through the pulmonary vein. The blood is then channeled into the left side of the heart. When enough blood has collected, this blood is then pumped forcefully out of the heart into the aorta. The aorta is the largest artery from which all the smaller arteries branch off, carrying blood that is rich in oxygen throughout the rest of the body again. This process occurs with every heartbeat (Pierce, 1995, p. 784; see Figure 5.1).

In 2006, under 2% (1.62%) of nursing home residents were receiving IV therapy (nutritional or blood; DHHS, 2006, F78–F93).

The Heart

The heart itself is a complex organ. It is a muscle composed of various types of cells to facilitate the pumping process. The heart requires oxygen to function and is supplied by a network of coronary arteries that stem from the aorta (see Figure 5.2).

The inner structure of the heart is also very complex, with four distinct changes and a valve network that regulates blood flow.

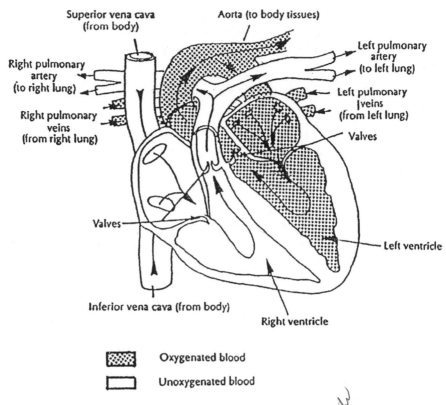

FIGURE 5.2 Schematic representation of blood flow through the heart.

Cell Changes

Any substantial change in these structures or the circulatory process itself can eventually affect all the body cells. The significance, then, of the oxygenation process is that when the health of cells has deteriorated, it is usually due to a change in the cardiovascular system that interferes with the supply of nutrients to the cells and with the supply of oxygen. This in turn damages the tissues and organs in the body, leading to the decline of other major processes.

Aging Effects

The extent to which the aging process plays a role in this deterioration is still being argued. It is known that the cardiovascular system (heart and blood vessels) is not designed to last indefinitely. Many of the cells are not capable of dividing and remain part of the system for long periods of time (Cohen & Rao, 2006, pp. 139–142).

Decreased Elasticity

A specific age-related change in the heart may include a lessening of the force of contraction (pumping) due to the decreased elasticity of muscle. Elasticity is the ability of the heart muscle to stretch and return to normal size spontaneously. When this property has been decreased in the heart muscle, the heart becomes stretched. This loss of elasticity reduces the force of contractions by the heart (pumping), which ultimately diminishes the amount of blood pumped by the heart (also termed cardiac output).

Decreased Cardiac Output

The reduced cardiac output is also due to an increased resistance to blood flow within the blood vessels and a loss in the heart's ability to compensate by beating faster. This added resistance to blood flow within the blood vessels may be a direct result of arteriosclerosis (hardening of the arteries) or more specifically atherosclerosis (one type of arteriosclerosis; Maddox & Sussman, 2001, p. 102).

A change in any one of these components will affect the other two. If the amount of blood circulated is reduced, the organs and tissues will receive fewer nutrients and less oxygen, resulting in some cells dying (if deprived for more than 3 to 5 minutes).

It is estimated that in the elderly the blood flow to the kidneys is reduced by as much as 50% and to the brain by as much as 20%, due to these same processes (Kenney, 1982, p. 51). These changes can explain changes in other systems associated with age.

Blood Pressure Changes

There is much debate among scientists about the role of the aging process and its effect on blood pressure. In many elderly persons the blood pressure does increase (O'Brien & Bulpitt, 1995). This increased pressure may be attributed to the stiffness of the large arteries (arteriosclerosis) and *peripheral vascular resistance* (the resistance in the blood vessels throughout the body) that are commonly associated with the aging process. Other studies of individuals in isolated areas reveal no changes in blood pressure levels for the elderly. Some investigators feel there is a strong association of social and environmental factors contributing to the presence of high because of their higher risk of infection (*hypertension*) (Kane et al., 2004, pp. 384–386; The Johns Hopkins Medical Letter, June, 1995, p. 1).

Blood vessel changes due to this progressive stiffening have suggested that they become like rigid tubes. This promotes the resistance to blood flow throughout the body (peripheral vascular resistance) and may exacerbate an already adversely affected heart function and increased blood pressure.

The vein walls tend to weaken with increased deposits of fats, cholesterol, fibrin, platelets, cellular debris, and calcium over time. The capillary walls become thickened, thus decreasing their ability to exchange oxygen with the cells. This thickening also contributes to the overall decrease in perfusion of (flow or nutrients into) the tissues and organs.

In 2003, diseases of the heart were the leading causes of death among persons 65 years of age and older: 563,000. This differs little from 1980 when 595,000 persons 65 years of age and older died of this number one cause of death (DHHS, 2005, Table 32, p. 183).

Six Common Cardiovascular Diseases

Cardiovascular disease is the major cause of death in the elderly population. The primary diagnosis of approximately 40% of long-term nursing home residents is some problem associated with heart disease (Landefeld et al., 2004, p. 156). The distinction between changes related to the aging process and those related to disease is a fine one. This dilemma becomes clear with the discussion of arteriosclerosis.

Arteriosclerosis

Usually, arteries are smooth inside and can stretch to permit the passage of more blood and oxygen when needed. With arteriosclerosis, the blood vessels are not as responsive as they previously were. Everyone has arteriosclerosis to some degree. Almost half of all long-term nursing home residents manifest disease changes due to chronic arteriosclerosis. Two forms of this condition (atherosclerosis and aortic stenosis) account for much of the heart disease in the elderly.

Aortic Stenosis

The term describes a narrowing of the aorta, which is the major artery leading from the heart and channeling the oxygenated blood supply to the rest of the body. This stenosis, or narrowing of the vessel, increases the workload specifically for the left ventricle of the heart, because it now has to pump harder to overcome the obstructive resistance to blood flow.

The increased workload eventually is felt by the entire heart, and when combined with the normal changes attributed to the aging process, this disease places considerable stress on the cardiovascular system. It can result in congestive heart failure, which will be discussed at the end of this section.

For many elderly residents, the cause of the disease is either the result of scarring from a childhood outbreak or rheumatic fever or calcified deposits found lining the blood vessels.

Some of the **symptoms** of aortic stenosis are difficulty in breathing, dizziness, high blood pressure, chest pain, and symptoms associated with congestive heart failure.

Treatment can consist of surgical correction, rest to decrease the workload on the heart, and medication therapy.

Atherosclerosis

In this, the most common form of arteriosclerosis, there is a progressive buildup of fat deposits on the inner lining of blood vessel walls. The disease does not usually manifest itself until the blood vessel becomes completely obstructed or shows a markedly decreased ability to facilitate blood flow. The symptoms can be found affecting the body anywhere that an initial pathology (a disease-related change in a tissue or organ) may be present; this usually includes the main arteries. In 1980, atherosclerosis caused twice the number of deaths as cancer in older groups.

Cerebrovascular Disease

This disease manifests itself through restricted blood flow to the brain, caused by occlusions within the carotid arteries that supply blood to the brain. One of the most important causes of strokes is atherosclerosis (Landefeld et al., 2004, p. 147; Maddox & Sussman, 2001, pp. 191, 982).

Long-term nursing home residents who may be predisposed to cardiovascular disease are those with high blood pressure, previous history of heart disease, and overweight. The specific symptoms of the disease depend on the affected location in the brain. *Transient ischemic attacks* (also termed "mini-strokes") are caused by a temporarily diminished blood supply to the brain.

Signs of cerebrovascular disease can be slurred speech, blurred vision, dizziness, numb hands and fingers, and mental confusion. Some of these symptoms could be easily attributed to the "aging process" rather than this underlying disease pathology.

A much more severe consequence of cerebrovascular disease is a *stroke,* or cerebrovascular accident (CVA). This occurs when the lack of oxygen for a much larger area of the brain causes permanent damage. Again, the resulting damage will depend on the area of the brain affected and may range from temporary loss of taste or smell to paralysis of many of the body parts.

Diagnosis

- Stroke presents as a neurological deficit or headache of abrupt onset.
- Hemorrhagic strokes can be intracerebral or subarachnoid.
- Urgent neuroimaging studies are essential (get the patient to the hospital as soon as possible).
- Diagnosis must exclude nonvascular causes.
  (Landefeld et al., 2004, p. 147).

For relevant Web sites see: American Stroke Association, www.strokeasso ciation.org; and National Stroke Association, www.stroke.org.

Peripheral Vascular Disease

PVD

This actually describes a group of diseases that affect the veins, arteries, and other blood vessels of the extremities. The symptoms are a result of decreased blood flow to the affected area. The most frequent symptom is *intermittent claudication,* which is a complex of **symptoms** (Evans et al., 2000, p. 345) including the following:

- pain on movement of an extremity
- pain that is chronic in a localized area
- cold, numb feet
- changes in skin integrity, such as ulcers or infections that are slow to heal Poor circulation

Coronary Artery Disease — CAD

Also known as chronic ischemic heart disease, here the heart muscle itself suffers from a lack of oxygen due to blockages in the coronary arteries that usually supply it (Aronow, 2006, pp. 533–536; Evans et al., 2000, p. 332).

The current popular coronary artery bypass graft surgery is a common treatment for persons with severe blockages who do not respond to medical therapy. Because this is major surgery, some nursing facility residents would not be considered good surgical risks for such treatment. This may be increasingly true inasmuch as a growing number of researchers are coming to believe that medical treatment may be as effective as surgery.

Symptoms can include chest pain—commonly called angina—which results from a lack of oxygen to certain areas of the heart muscle. Pain may be located anywhere in the chest, especially in the left arm or neck. This symptom is commonly found in residents over 60 years of age.

Myocardial infarction (MI; literally meaning heart muscle death) results when a large enough area of the heart muscle does not receive oxygen for a period of time (Evans et al., 2000, p. 394; Landefeld et al., 2004, p. 172; White & Sullivan, 2006, pp. 163–168). With a massive myocardial infarction, the heart can no longer continue to act as a pump and may completely stop beating. There is a greater chance that residents over 60 years old will die from a heart attack than will younger patients (Evans et al., 2000, p. 335).

The phases in coronary artery disease range from diffuse, incomplete blockages throughout the arteries, to one or more large blockages that occlude more of the blood flow.

Symptoms can range from none at all to various types of angina or, most serious, to a complete cessation of heart activity that occurs after MI or complete heart block (Aronow, 2006, pp. 533–536; Evans et al., 2000, p. 402). Symptoms include shortness of breath on exertion, effort intolerance, fatigue, cough, dizziness on standing, swelling of the feet and ankles. Also, lethargy, anorexia, abdominal discomfort, and gastrointestinal disturbances are common symptoms among nursing facility patients (Landefeld et al., 2004, p. 172).

Treatments vary. Initially, patients without severe manifestations of the disease can be treated conservatively with restrictions on sodium and fat from their diet. Medications commonly used in the nursing facility are nitroglycerin and propranolol.

Nitroglycerin, the most common medication prescribed for persons with angina, is administered sublingually, the resident holding the pill under the tongue. This drug lowers the blood pressure by dilating the blood vessels, including the coronary arteries, to decrease resistance to blood flow.

Propranolol hydrochloride (Inderol®) is referred to as a beta blocker because of its action in blocking body chemicals that act to increase the heart rate. This acts to slow the heart down, thereby decreasing blood pressure and lowering the amount of oxygen required by the heart muscle.

There are also a variety of antiarrhythmic medications available, which are prescribed in accordance with the particular type of arrhythmia diagnosed (White & Sullivan, 2006, pp. 166–167).

A common result of prolonged or diffuse coronary artery disease is the inability of the heart to initiate contractions independently. When this occurs, another type of treatment is often prescribed: permanent pacemaker. The pacemaker is a mechanical device implanted under the skin with its wires attached to the heart muscle to provide a continuous flow of electrical impulses that stimulate the heart to contract with a steady rhythm (Aronow, 2006, pp. 533–536).

High Blood Pressure

High blood pressure is usually considered to be present when the blood pressure measurement is consistently greater than 140/90 (Landefeld et al., 2004, p. 183).

The numbers 140/90 are a measurement of the amount of pressure the blood exerts on the walls of the arteries. The first number (140) measures the maximum pressure (systolic) exerted when the heart is fully contracted near the end of the stroke output of the left ventricle. The second number (here 90) measures the minimum or diastolic pressure occurring when the heart ventricles are in the period of dilation or fully relaxed. This must be monitored for each individual to account for height and weight variations (Evans et al., 2000, p. 359).

There are two types of this disease: (a) essential hypertension and (b) secondary hypertension. The cause of essential hypertension is unknown, and therefore the disease is without a complete cure, but it can be successfully controlled by medication. Secondary hypertension in the elderly results from other underlying diseases, including anemia, fever, endocrine disease or hormonal disruption, arteriosclerosis, or kidney disease (Evans et al., 2000, pp. 204–205; Landefeld et al., 2004, p. 185; Rubin, p. 309). These diseases place a greater demand on the heart and may cause the blood pressure to increase during the disease episode or permanently.

The effects of continued high blood pressure, regardless of the cause, may be harmful to various organs within the body, especially the heart, brain, kidney, and eyes. When a person has high blood pressure, the heart must automatically pump harder to circulate the blood throughout the body. As the heart works harder and harder to compensate, eventually it begins to fail after being overworked for such long periods of time. This in turn reduces the blood flow to the vital organs, damaging their functioning as well.

Some **signs** of hypertension are prolonged, elevated blood pressure greater than 140/90, or the individual's norm, and prolonged presence of risk factors such as overweight, smoking, and high salt intake. Using the 140/90 definition, 40 to 50% of individuals over age 65 are hypertensive and should be actively treated (Kane et al., 1989, p. 249; Kane et al., 2004).

Treatments typically used include prescribing weight loss and diet therapy, including restricted salt intake (Landefeld et al., 2004, p. 42). The goal of medication therapy is to use as few drugs as possible. Some of the most common medications used in a nursing facility include diuretics, nitroglycerin, and propranolol.

Diuretics are frequently used to get rid of the excess fluids in the body to decrease the workload of the heart by decreasing the blood volume that it must pump. Vasodilators such as nitroglycerin are used to dilate blood vessels and therefore decrease the amount of resistance against which the heart must work. Cardiac drugs such as propranolol may also be used to relieve the workload of the heart by decreasing its rate of contractions or pumping.

Congestive Heart Failure

This is not a disease, but is actually a complex set of many symptoms associated with an impaired performance of the heart (Evans et al., 2000, p. 417; Landefeld et al., 2004, p. 163; White & Sullivan, 2006, pp. 163–168). A progressively weakening heart results in an increasing inability of the heart to pump enough oxygen to the various tissues of the body. This failure results in a congestion of blood being backed up in the circulatory system. This backup causes fluids to leak out of the bloodstream into the various tissues and organs, most notably the lungs. Taken together, these constitute the disease process called congestive heart failure (CHF; Evans et al., 2000, p. 336; White & Sullivan, 2006, pp. 163–168). See Figure 5.3 (The Johns Hopkins Medical Letter, p. 4). The most common symptom is central chest discomfort, often descried as pressure, tightness, or heaviness typically brought on by physical exertion or emotional stress and relieved by rest or nitroglycerin (Landefeld et al., 2004, p. 163).

The cause of congestive heart failure may be a variety of diseases or conditions, most notably arteriosclerosis, uncontrolled high blood pressure or a problem with one of the heart valves, heart attack, alcoholism, or chronic exposure to agents harmful to the body tissues (Evans et al., 2000, p. 1012). The lifetime prevalence of alcoholism of older hospitalized persons has been reported to be 20.4% for those aged 60–69, declining to 13.7% among patients aged 70–79, and to 0% for those aged 80 and older (Maddox & Sussman, 2001, p. 57).

Congested Heart

Congestive heart failure occurs when a healthy heart (*right, top*) loses its ability to contract fully. As a result, too much blood remains in the heart after each pump cycle, and the heart cannot supply the body with an adequate amount of oxygenated blood (*bottom*).

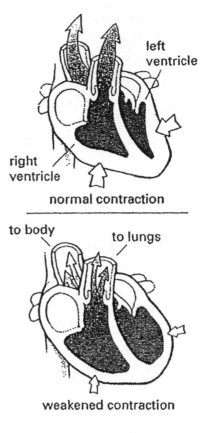

left ventricle

right ventricle

normal contraction

to body

to lungs

weakened contraction

FIGURE 5.3 Congested heart.

The symptoms usually are seen in other organs and can be classified according to whether the heart failure primarily affects the left or right side of the heart.

Right-Sided Failure of the Heart

- edema (a build-up of fluids outside of the blood vessels that forces fluid into the tissues; occurs mostly in the ankles; gradual loss of energy)
- anorexia (loss of appetite for food)
- constipation
- weight gain (because kidneys cause the body to keep too much sodium and water)
- grayish or blue color of the skin due to decreased blood flow

Left-Sided Failure of the Heart

- frequent coughing or wheezing
- shortness of breath (dyspnea), a result of the blood backing up into the lungs thus decreasing the amount of space in the lungs available to hold air. This is one of the definitive signs of CHF and usually occurs after exercise (Anderson, 1976, p. 136; Evans et al., 2000, p. 1013).
- confusion and loss of memory are severe symptoms that suggest the disease has progressed far enough to damage the brain tissue

Treatment generally consists of rest; monitoring weight to guard against sudden changes; diet therapy, including reducing salt intake and encouraging potassium intake with foods like bananas and oranges; and oxygen therapy to improve the oxygen content of red blood cells, because there is less and less exchange area available in the lungs (Moss, 1989, p. 65).

Technologic advances are being made in providing oxygen to residents. Machines called oxygen concentrators are available, obviating the constant need for oxygen tanks. The advantage is an ability to use ambient air in the resident's room to produce the required oxygen. The potential disadvantage is that, unlike the bulky and unsightly tanks, the oxygen concentrator must have a continuous supply of electricity.

Medications can include Digoxin (Lanoxin®), which acts directly on the heart muscle to increase the force of contraction. This is an extremely powerful medication that may cause severe side effects in the elderly when the level of the medication becomes too high in the blood. Confusion or severe behavioral changes may indicate this is occurring (Landefeld et al., 2001, p. 159).

To avoid fluid buildup, *diuretics* are also often prescribed to aid the body in eliminating toxic wastes and fluids that have accumulated (Crow, 1984, p. 45; White & Sullivan, 2006, pp. 163–168). Some of the more powerful diuretics deplete the body's supply of important electrolytes, such as sodium and potassium. Low levels of potassium can be particularly dangerous for the elderly resident, who is especially vulnerable to such imbalances. Potassium supplements are frequently prescribed, in addition to dietary supplements, to increase the blood level of this naturally occurring mineral.

5.3.2 RESPIRATORY SYSTEM

The chief function of the respiratory process is providing the body with oxygen while removing excess carbon dioxide. These processes occur during breathing, when air enters and exits the body through the nose and mouth. The air that enters the body is rich in oxygen, the gas necessary for many of the cells' basic chemical functions. The respiratory and circulatory systems are very closely related, because both are involved with the oxygenation process.

The Oxygenation Process

The circulatory system can be envisioned as a train carrying the oxygen in each car or blood cell. The lungs, then, are the depot terminals where the blood cells pick up oxygen and deposit carbon dioxide. The structures in the body that help the respiratory system do its work include the mouth, nose pharynx, trachea, bronchi, bronchioles, lungs, alveoli, diaphragm, and various respiratory muscles. The respiratory process involves all of these structures to promote the inhalation and exhalation of air that transports gases to the blood cells and diffuses oxygen into the body.

After the air is inhaled through either the nose or mouth, it travels through the trachea, which leads to the bronchi of the lungs. There, the two bronchi, the main airways into the lungs, divide and subdivide numerous times before ultimately forming the bronchioles (see Figure 5.4 The respiratory tract). The bronchioles are the smallest airways in the lungs and eventually terminate in the numerous alveoli that are the basic respiratory units (see Figure 5.5).

Alveoli are the many air-filled sacs that are the site of the actual oxygen–carbon dioxide exchange. In this transaction oxygen is absorbed by the blood, and carbon dioxide is released into the air as the breath is exhaled. Much of the volume within the lungs is taken up by blood undergoing this stage of the oxygenation process.

Because the respiratory and cardiovascular systems are closely related, any damage to one of these systems is likely to directly affect the other. A number of other structures are essential for breathing, including the diaphragm and associated respiratory muscles of the chest. These structures aid the lungs in expanding and contracting with each inhalation and exhalation.

Age-Associated Changes

Changes associated with the aging process do occur. However, in the elderly person without any significant disease, the overall result of these changes should not be incapacitating or prevent them from carrying on the activities of daily living (Kart, Metress, & Metress, 1978, p. 129).

One of the reasons for this is that the lung, unlike the heart, has a remarkable ability to repair itself after infection or damage. These repairs usually

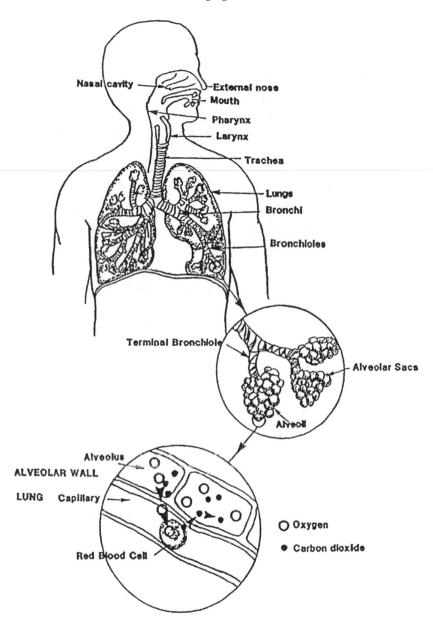

FIGURE 5.4 The respiratory tract. Oxygen–carbon dioxide exchange at alveolar wall where permeation of oxygen and carbon dioxide cells occurs.

FIGURE 5.5   Diagram of events occurring simultaneously during respiration.

leave only minor traces that could later be mistaken for degenerative changes. A list of changes due to aging that do affect the respiratory system includes the following:

- decreasing size (and therefore capacity) of the alveoli
- loss of elasticity of lung tissue
- stiffening of the ribs (requiring muscles to work harder to pump air in and out of the lungs)
- changes in the shape of the chest
- decreased resistance to infection

The decreased capacity of the alveoli is not in itself enough to cause any dramatic changes in the breathing process. However, this does reduce the efficiency of the breathing mechanism and may lead to disability and respiratory problems over time.

The elderly are more prone to infections than the rest of the population. When these additional factors are coupled with the fact that the lungs receive foreign materials continuously from the outside air, it is not surprising that many elderly persons suffer from some form of lung disease.

Influence of the Environment on the Lungs

Because the lungs are in almost direct contact with the air outside, the environment may play a more important role in the development of lung disease than in any other body system. Environmental exposure to a lung irritant over a prolonged period of time often produces the type of changes that result in respiratory disease. Some examples are miners' exposure to coal dust, welder's to asbestos, and chronic cigarette smokers' to tar and nicotine. Lung infection is one of the more common causes of death among older persons.

Chronic Respiratory Disease

Approximately 6% of long-term nursing home residents suffer from some type of chronic respiratory disease. The most common classification of lung disease is chronic obstructive lung disease (COLD), or chronic obstructive pulmonary disease (COPD). The COPD diagnosis includes chronic bronchitis, asthma, and emphysema (Landefeld et al., 2004, p. 205). There is no cure for these diseases, but there are a variety of treatments available (The Johns Hopkins Medical Letter, December, 1994, p. 6). New diagnostic instruments are becoming available such as a pulse oximeter, which uses infrared light through the finger to read the oxygen level within 30 seconds. Spirometers are used to detect the amount of lung volume the individual can exhale then results are compared with predicted curves. Death rates from chronic lower respiratory diseases among the general population increase dramatically with age rising from 165 deaths per 100,000 resident population among persons aged 65–74 to 635 deaths per 100,000 resident population among persons 85 years and over (DHHS, 2005, Table 41, p. 208).

The main complication brought on by COPD is that the body is unable to rid itself of the air containing carbon dioxide (Landefeld et al., 2004, p. 205). This may be because of a disruption of the alveoli or because the bronchial tubes are not expanding and permitting the gases to escape during respiration.

Chronic bronchitis and emphysema are two diseases of this type that are most commonly seen in the long-term nursing facility resident. The signs, symptoms, and treatment of the respiratory diseases mentioned are very similar, because they all affect the lungs. The symptoms listed following the discussion of the next two diseases will apply to all the diseases in the remainder of this section.

Chronic Bronchitis

As the name suggests, chronic bronchitis is caused by a continuing irritation of the bronchi (the two airways into the lungs). The inside of these airways swell and become clogged with mucus secretions, making it more difficult to breathe. This may be due to something irritating from the environment or a recurrent infection. Chronic smokers are the ones most likely to develop bronchitis. This disease is the most common respiratory condition found in the elderly and is defined as a chronic productive cough in more than 3 months of 2 successive years, unexplained by another diagnosis (Shashaty, 1989, p. 101).

Asthma is characterized by bronchial reactions to internal or external stimulants. It is generalized reversible airways obstruction. Usually a bronchodilator is administered orally, by inhalation, or both.

Emphysema

Emphysema results in a loss of elasticity in all of the lung tissue. As a consequence, the lung is less able to hold as much air, but the alveoli tend to have air trapped inside causing carbon dioxide to build up. The increasing amount of carbon dioxide only worsens the respiratory condition because the body is triggered to obtain more and more oxygen to compensate for this imbalance. Continuous oxygen therapy may be supplied from large oxygen tanks, liquid oxygen reservoirs, or an oxygen concentrator. Oxygen therapy reduces lung hypertension and promotes oxygenation of the other body systems.

The causes of emphysema are similar to those of bronchitis, the most common one being a recurrent infection or chronic irritant to the lung. Emphysema is much more serious than bronchitis, and usually residents with this disease die from heart failure as a result of prolonged stress on the cardiovascular system.

Symptoms common for most lung diseases are chronic cough, increased production of thick white mucus, and some shortness of breath. These symptoms are a result of the body attempting to rid itself of whatever is irritating the respiratory tract. Irritation of the inner lining of the respiratory tract results in the increased production of mucus, which is intended to coat the cause of the irritation and assist its excretion from the body.

A cough is another way the body has of rejecting whatever is causing the irritation. When this irritation is chronic, these mechanisms are continually being triggered.

These lung disease symptoms can be found in more severe forms:

- stress on the entire cardiovascular system with related symptoms
- enlarged heart
- heart failure (with emphysema)
- thick mucus plugs blocking the smaller airways within the lung
- alveoli that have become over inflated and eventually burst, decreasing the amount of space available for oxygen exchange

- barrel-shaped chest
- poor appetite
- weight loss
- dizziness

Treatments include medications to minimize airway irritation and obstruction, such as bronchodilators—to relax the breathing tubes, widening them, and thus improving air flow—and expectorants, to thin the mucus so that coughing is more successful.

Pneumonia

Pneumonia is an infection in the lungs caused by either a virus or bacteria. Residents with chronic obstructive lung disease are much more susceptible to this infection because bacteria grow in stagnant areas like those where the mucus is collecting. This infection further complicates the elderly person's ability to breathe and causes disruptions in other systems.

The signs and symptoms are very similar to those already described and may include a fever or very weak condition resulting from the infection. Treatment generally includes some type of antibiotic therapy when bacteria are the cause of this infection. A study of 124 nursing home patients with nursing home acquired pneumonia, some of whom were treated in the nursing home and some in the hospital, revealed that the majority of episodes were successfully treated with oral antibiotics (Evans et al., 2000, p. 57; McNeil, 2006, pp. 569–572).

Symptoms of pneumonia usually include fever and cough with sputum production. Sputum cultures are generally obtained for diagnosis.

Most studies in the elderly identify pneumococcus as the most prevalent pathogen. Other pathogens include H. influenza, S. aureus, enteric gram-negative organisms, Legionella species, and Chlamydia. The most serious infections are due to S. pneumoniae and Legionella (Landefeld et al., 2004, p. 353).

In recent years emphasis has been placed on giving nursing home residents annual pneumococcal vaccine. In 2006, 40.28% of residents received or had received this vaccine (which need not be given yearly; DHHS, 2006, F78, F143–F145). Beginning September 1, 2006, CMS included pneumococcal (and influenza) vaccination assessment as part of the MDS (Minimum Data Set) for nursing homes.

Nevertheless, pneumonia deaths among persons aged 65 and over in the United States remained a concern in 2003 when it was the 6th leading cause of death among older persons causing 57,000 deaths (DHHS, 2005, Table 32,

p. 183). Average length of stay of all males in U.S. hospitals was cut nearly in half between 1990 (10.2 days) and 2003 (6.2 days) likely shifting more days of pneumonia care to nursing facilities (DHHS, 2005, p. 333).

Treatment

For patients treated in the facility, the most common treatment is Levofloxacin plus clindamycin or moxifloxacin or levofloxacin or ceftriaxone.

Pneumonia is the most common reason for transferring nursing home residents to the hospital. Nursing home residents represent 10–18% of all patients hospitalized with pneumonia. The decision to transfer a patient with pneumonia from a nursing home to the hospital may be aided by published guidelines for predicting pneumonia mortality.

Independent Variables Associated With Mortality Within 30 Days in Nursing Home Acquired Pneumonia

- Respiratory rate > 30 breaths/minute
- Pulse > 125 beats/minute
- Altered mental status
- History of dementia

When 2 or more of these findings are present, mortality is 30%. Factors that have been associated with treatment failure in the nursing home include respiratory rate > 30, pulse > 90, temperature >38.1 degrees Centigrade, oxygen saturation < 92%, use of a mechanically altered diet, feeding tube dependence, and altered level of consciousness (Landefeld et al., 2004, pp. 353–354).

Chronic Tuberculosis

Tuberculosis is an infectious disease more commonly found among nursing home residents because of their higher risk of infection, resulting from multiple chronic diseases (Cohen, 1995b, p. 946; Lashley, 2006a, pp. 1196–1198; Maddox & Sussman, 2001, p. 1032).

Tuberculosis may infect a person while they are young, but often times a healthy immune system wards off the disease, which goes into a dormant state. As a person ages, this immunity may break down with an infection, and the dormant disease may become active (Evans et al., 2000, p. 59).

Signs and symptoms are similar to those listed for COLD, except that the secretions contain the tuberculosis bacteria. The disease is termed infectious because it may easily be transmitted through the secretions or when a patient coughs.

One of the most important treatments then, is to isolate the person as long as they are coughing and producing sputum. To prevent the spread of infection, staff and visitors generally are required to wear masks and gloves when in contact with the resident or in their room.

Lung Cancer

Lung cancer is a chronic lung disease and is among the leading causes of death for American men. It is also the most prevalent form of cancer found among nursing facility residents. Because the disease affects the lung, symptoms are similar to those of COLD.

Generally, the nursing home resident is receiving palliative treatment (just enough therapy to make them comfortable; Balducci, 2006, pp. 155–158; Evans et al., 2000, p. 1113; Landefeld et al., 2004, pp. 210, 307; Maddox & Sussman, 2001, p. 140). Other types of treatment include radiation, chemotherapy, or surgery, depending on the size and location of the tumor (Evans et al., 2000, p. 440). With improved understanding of this disease process, new drug regimens, and improved radiation treatments, lung cancer is becoming treatable (Johns Hopkins Medical Letter, August, 1995, p. 1; Evans et al., 2000, p. 74).

Respiratory Therapy Rates

Respiratory treatment is provided by respirators/ventilators, oxygen, inhalation therapy, and other treatment. In 1993, 6% of facility residents received treatment compared to 9% in 1999. Harrington et al., 2000, p.53). By 2006, nearly 12% of residents (11.96%) were receiving some type of respiratory therapy (DHHS, 2006, F78, F124–F128). An additional 1% were receiving tracheotomy (DHHS, 2006, F78, F124–F128).

5.3.3 NERVOUS SYSTEM

One of the body's most important mechanisms is the nervous system, which acts as its control center by coordinating functions and maintaining order. The brain can be thought of as a computer system with the nerves and spinal cord transferring input and output messages to and from each part of the body (Brody, 1995a, p. 674).

Some specific nervous systems functions for control of the body include responding to events outside the body through the five senses, performing voluntary activities such as walking, and storing memories, ideas, and emotions so they may be used at a later time for various thought processes. The nervous system also performs automatic responses such as breathing, maintaining heart rate, and controlling temperature.

Components of the Central Nervous System

The central nervous is composed of the brain, spinal cord, and nerves (Brody, 1995b, p. 171). The brain is considered by some to be the most important organ in the body because it is accorded a high level of priority among body functions. When the body is undergoing a great deal of stress, other organs will reduce nutrient intake so that more nutrients can be directed to the brain.

The brain is protected by the skull and surrounded inside by a protective layer of cerebrospinal fluid. This organ is very specialized, with different areas responsible for different body functions.

The cranial nerves connect the brain with the areas of the body responsible for sensory perception (identifying what is outside the body through the senses, including taste, smell, and hearing). The base of the brain is called the medulla. It is primarily responsible for controlling motor activity or movement. It is this area that connects the brain to the spinal cord.

The spinal cord looks like a tree trunk, with the nerves representing the branches of the tree and eventually leading to the blood vessels, muscles, and organs throughout the body.

The brain itself is made up of many specialized cells that are unique to the individual areas of the brain in which they are found. Because the brain cells perform complex processes, they need large amounts of oxygen to function continually. A lack of oxygen to the brain causes the cells and their tissues to die within minutes.

The nerves are composed of many individual fibers that are encased in a fatty substance called myelin for the same reason that electrical wires are covered with a plastic coating: to prevent them from "shorting out." These individual fibers are composed of neurons, which are the nerve cells. Unlike the heart cells, nerve cells can be replaced or regenerate themselves, although at a very slow rate.

The nerve fibers form an intricate network that is responsible for carrying a variety of messages to the brain. These messages are carried in the form of electrical impulses that stimulate the appropriate area of the brain, triggering either an involuntary response reaction (reflex) or a thought (cognitive) process.

The nerve fibers form a complex series of pathways that impulses travel along to reach the brain. It is important to remember that the left side of the brain controls the functions on the right side of the body, and the right side of the brain controls functions on the left side of the body.

Possible Effects of Aging

The effects of aging on the nervous system are most commonly believed to be the result of a change in the system that reduces the oxygen supply to the brain cells. This can lead to permanent alterations to those cells that are so sensitive to the level of the oxygen supply.

Apparently the weight of the brain, as mentioned previously, decreases with age possibly because of some loss of brain cells and nerve fibers. Researchers, using refined instruments, have been able to detect changes in the neurological system of the elderly when observing the speed with which impulses are transmitted to the brain. But this change is not directly associated with a slowing down of functioning in the thought process. It is probably a myth that older people's thought or cognitive process is much slower than other age groups.

Perceptual Changes

One of the perceptual changes commonly attributed to the aging process is a decreased sensitivity to touch.

Some of the visual changes associated with age include loss of range of vision for near objects, decreased flexibility of the lens of the eye, and reduced clarity of vision, or the "dusty windshield" effect of the lens of the eye, accompanied by a loss in ability to distinguish pastels (Evans et al., 2000, p. 869).

There may be a change in the central processing of sound in the inner ear. This has not been proven as yet, so residents who are hard of hearing are not necessarily that way just because of age. Among the general population an average of 7% of persons aged 65–74 report a lot of trouble hearing. This increases to 15% of persons aged 75 and over (DHHS, 2005, Table 59, p. 246). There does appear to be a loss of ability to hear high-pitched sounds; speaking to residents in deep tones can help compensate for this loss.

In many elderly individuals the taste buds appear to have degenerated, and the amount of saliva produced also appears to be diminished, producing a change in the capacity to taste different flavors (Evans et al., 2000, p. 904; Schiffman, 2006, pp. 1168–1170). Abuse of salt may result from patient efforts to "improve" or increase taste sensations. Ability to taste sweets is apparently unaffected, which may explain the preference of many elderly residents for eating dessert first.

There may also be an age-related decrease in neurons responsible for smell, resulting in the loss of smell for different odors.

Some of the elderly also appear to dream less and have increased periods of wakefulness throughout the night.

Diseases associated with the nervous system include those that affect sensory components, impair mobility and communication processes, and affect the ability to distinguish reality from fantasy.

The Eye

The eye is a complicated structure, with muscles holding it in place. The retina is the innermost layer of the eye and contains receptor cells that actually generate electrical nerve impulses when hit by light. These impulses are carried to the brain on the nerve fibers that leave the retina and form the optic nerve. This nerve leads to the area of the brain responsible for vision. The retina is protected by the lens covering the eye.

The lens can be thought of as a layer of skin, except that all of the old cells on the lens cannot be discarded like old layers of skin, and they are continually compacted within the eye. The aqueous humor is a substance that bathes the eye and protects it as well.

Presence of Eye Problems

Approximately 33% of all long-term nursing home residents experience some form of visual impairment, and 5.5% of these patients are blind. About 61% were found to wear some type of eyeglasses to correct their vision.

Among the general population 13% of persons aged 65–74 report trouble seeing even with glasses, and 21% of persons aged 75 and over report vision problems (DHHS, 2005, Table 59, p. 246).

The aging process may result in an overproduction of aqueous humor, resulting in a large amount within the eye. When this happens, glaucoma may result.

Glaucoma ↑ pressure from liquid

Glaucoma is a chronic condition that is actually a complex of many different symptoms. This condition is not a direct result of the aging process, but the incidence of the disease is definitely greater among older individuals

(Kane et al., 2004; Landefeld et al., 2004, p. 127; Rafuse & Kelly, 2006, pp. 405–410).

There are four different types of glaucoma: (a) chronic, (b) acute, (c) secondary, and (d) congenital. In each of these, the primary problem is that fluids within the eye undergo increasing pressure changes. These fluids are continually being formed, but not draining from the eye chamber because of some disruption in the drainage system (Landefeld et al., 2004, p. 128). As a result, the eyeball itself becomes very hard. This also causes an extremely painful pressure in the eye, which can lead to a range of other conditions.

Symptoms of glaucoma can induce acute pain in the eye, elevated blood pressure, blurred vision, and halos seen around lights. Untreated glaucoma can lead to blindness.

Treatment usually varies with the form or state of disease, but initially medical therapy is used to promote the drainage of excess fluids from the eye (Rafuse & Kelly, 2006, pp. 405–410). As a rule, medications are the critical variable in preventing blindness from glaucoma.

Mydriatics are a kind of medication that usually comes in the form of eye drops that act to dilate the pupil of the eye, helping to drain off some of the excess fluid.

Cataracts   Cloudy Lens

A cataract is a cloudiness that affects the transparency of the lens to the extent that light cannot get through to the retina of the eye. The retina is the area of the eye that transforms light into the objects seen. Usually cataracts form in both eyes (Landefeld et al., 2004, p. 122).

The major symptom of cataracts is increasingly blurred vision, with perceptions of shadows. Treatment usually consists of eyeglasses or contact lenses. The lens can be surgically removed and replaced with a new manufactured one (lens implant).

Importance of Vision Among Residents

When older persons with visual impairments are assisted to see better through intervention, they adapt better to the area around them. Interventions do not need to be complex. They can include provision of large-type books, magazines, and newspapers; painting color-coded boundaries and walkways throughout the facility for easy identification (e.g., a painted baseboard in the hallway helps distinguish spatial location for the resident); and using large letters and numbers in all visual displays such as doors, elevators, and clocks.

Hearing

The structures of the outer ear include those portions of the ear external to the eardrum (tympanic membrane). The middle ear contains three small bones that conduct the sound waves; they are called the incus (the anvil), the malleus (hammer), and the stapes (stirrup).

The inner ear contains the cochlea, which transmits sound waves to nerve impulses that travel down the auditory nerve (the eighth cranial nerve) to the auditory center of the brain.

Hearing Impairments

presby = Old

Presbycusis is the term used to describe any hearing impairment in old age (Kane et al., 2004; Landefeld et al., 2004, p. 136; Massoud, 2006, pp. 508–512). Approximately 26% of long-term nursing home residents suffer some hearing impairment, and it has been estimated that 5% of the residents are deaf. However, only 6% of them use hearing aids (which, in any case, are not invariably helpful).

Hearing impairments can also be due to a buildup of wax in the ear or to what is known as a conductive or sensorineural hearing loss. Conductive disorders and ear wax are the only ones that may be treated effectively. Usually surgery or hearing aids are prescribed for those with a conductive loss. The sensorineural disturbances result from a disruption in the structure of the inner ear or the nerve pathway to the brain stem.

Symptoms of hearing impairment can include tinnitus (an intermittent, sometimes constant, ringing in the ears), progressive hearing loss, and increased inability to hear high-frequency sounds, including shouting, warning bells, or buzzers (Landefeld et al., 2004, p. 133).

Treatment can include a hearing aid when appropriate; sign language; lip-reading; speech reading; slow, well-enunciated communication; always facing the resident when speaking to them; and providing appropriate warning signals to communicate the presence of fires or other dangerous occurrences within the facility. New technologies are being applied to hearing aids. Digital hearing aids in which sound is converted to digital computer code, which undergoes processing via a digital signal processor, are available that are small, barely visible, and programmable to the individual (Landefeld et al., 2004, p. 136). A relevant Web site is www.nidcd.nig.gov/ (National Institute on Deafness and Other Communication Disorders).

Mobility and Communication

A cerebrovascular accident (CVA), also known as a stroke, can be one of the most debilitating conditions that an elderly person faces (Evans et al., 2000, p. 452). It is believed that 16% of long-term nursing home residents have suffered from some form of stroke.

The cause of stroke is lack of oxygen to the brain. For treatment purposes, it is important to distinguish among the three types and causes of stroke. Cerebral thrombosis is blockage by a thrombus (clot) that has built up on the wall of a brain artery and accounts for about 40% to 50% of strokes. Cerebral embolism is blockage by an embolus (usually a clot) swept from below up into an artery in the brain and accounts for 30% to 35% of strokes. The third mechanism of stroke occurs when there is rupture of a blood vessel and bleeding within or over the surface of the brain and accounts for 20% to 25% of cases. New evidence suggests that getting a stroke victim to the hospital as rapidly as possible may permit minimizing damage by quick treatment once it is learned whether the stroke is due to a clot that can be dissolved by a blood thinner or to hemorrhage (a burst artery), which requires different treatment.

Warning signs can include headache, dizziness or confusion, visual disturbance, slurred speech or loss of speech, or difficulty swallowing.

Degrees of Disability

The degree of disability resulting from a stroke may range from only a slight impairment to complete immobility and loss of voluntary muscle control (Van Vilet, 1995b, p. 200). Signs following a stroke are usually specifically related to the area of the brain affected. These symptoms may include the following:

- muscle weakness on one side of the body (hemiplegia)
- difficulty standing or walking
- poor balance
- pain in arms and legs
- fatigue
- poor vision
- confusion
- difficulty in spatial judgment, distortion
- complete loss of muscle control (quadriplegia)
- paralysis of the body below the upper extremities (paraplegia)
- difficulty speaking (aphasia)

Para-half

Some of the results of decreased functioning of the nervous and muscular system is evidenced by the following. In 2006, residents suffered disabilities in the following percentages:

Bedfast	4%
Chair bound	57%
Physically restrained	7%
Contractures	29%

(DHHS, 2006, F78, F100–F106)

Aphasia *c̄ an't interpret*

Aphasia is the term used to describe an inability to interpret and formulate language (Maddox & Sussman, 2001, p. 84; Thompkins & Scharp, 2006, pp. 71–74, Van Vilet, 1995a, p. 76). Specifically, such problems may be seen as a slowdown in ability to retrieve vocabulary and inappropriate use of grammar or words, as well as problems in understanding what is being said.

Usually this occurs because the area of the brain responsible for speech is damaged during the stroke. There are many different types of aphasia with the most severe resulting in an individual being unable to understand what others are saying to them (receptive aphasia; Tompkins & Scharp, 2006, pp. 71–74).

Other types of aphasia result in an inability to express in words what the individual really wants to communicate (expressive aphasia). Other times, inappropriate words or vulgar language is uttered as if the individual has no control of what they say.

Dysarthria *Can't Speak*

Dysarthria (literally, imperfect articulation of speech) is a speech rather than a language abnormality that may accompany paralysis, weakness, or lack of coordination. This deficit can be a frustrating experience for the resident who has all other mental capacities intact. This frustration often leads to emotional upset. The most important need that residents have at this time is the ability to communicate. The incidence of these disorders may exceed 50% of the long-term population in a nursing facility (Corso, 1981, p. 211; Thompkins, Scharp, & Meigh, 2006, pp. 234–236).

Individually designed rehabilitative therapy is the most usual form of treatment. The ability of a person to recover from a stroke is best correlated with the cause. Lower brain stem damage from a stroke has a more favorable prognosis than an assault on the upper part of the brain.

Rehabilitation therapy usually focuses on standing, ambulating, taking initial steps, and walking with a cane or other appliance. Physical and occupational therapists are integral members of the rehabilitation team for these residents.

In 2006, about 3.83% of nursing facility residents required the use of nonoral communication devices, and 2.89% of residents were non-English speaking (DHHS, 2006, F76–F81). Another 1.38% of nursing facility residents required suctioning of the throat area (DHHS, 2006, F78, F124–F128).

Parkinson's Disease

Parkinson's disease is actually a group of symptoms that can progressively lead to complete disability in those severely affected. Scientists believe that selected groups of neurons (nerve cells) in the brain are lost as a result of this disease, but the cause of this loss remains a mystery (Maddox & Sussman, 2001, p. 789).

Symptoms of Parkinson's disease can include tremor, or trembling, of any of the limbs while at rest, rigidity or muscle stiffness, and bradykinesia (a slowness in body movements). Additional symptoms may include the following:

- stooped posture while standing
- walking with short, shuffling steps
- garbled speech
- illegible handwriting
- sad, lifeless facial expression
- facial droop
- mood swings
- dementia (an impairment in intellectual ability)

There is no cure for Parkinson's disease, so the treatment is determined by the specific symptoms and degree of physical impairment in functioning.

Often residents with Parkinson's disease suffer from mental disturbances similar to those seen in patients with Alzheimer's disease (Rogaevea & George-Hyslop, 2006), and physicians are finding it difficult to distinguish one from the other. Alzheimer's patients have the additional diagnosis of dementia (Evans et al., 2000, p. 922; Ripich, Wykle, & Niles, 1995, p. 16).

Drugs most often prescribed are Primidone (most effective for hand tremors) and propranolol (for general symptomatic relief; Landefeld et al., 2004, p. 99).

See: National Parkinson Foundation www.parkinson.org

Dementia

Dementia is a broad, nonspecific term denoting cognitive loss (Reichel & Rabins, 1989). The diagnosis and understanding of mental deterioration among some elderly is still in its early stages.

Riechel and Rabins identify three major causes of senile dementia. About 60% is due to Alzheimer's type, 25% to infraction of brain tissue due to cerebrovascular disease, and 15% to several other diseases such as paresis, Huntington chorea, Pick's disease, Parkinsonism, acquired immune deficiency syndrome (AIDS; Cohen, 1995a, p. 5; Lashley, 2006a), Wilson's disease, and several others (Evans et al., 2000, p. 923; Maddox & Sussman, 2001, p. 907).

More than one-half of long-term nursing home residents may have some form of dementing illness (Gwyther, 1983, p. 435). Persons intimately acquainted with the nursing facility population believe 80% to 90% of residents have some form of dementia (DePorter, 2006). Dementia is usually thought of as senility in an elderly person and may include behavior such as forgetfulness, a deterioration in personality, and a decrease in intellectual functioning (Reisberg, 1995, p. 846).

A common misperception is that these behaviors are all a normal result of the aging process. But none of these senile behaviors are considered to be normal aging effects and are instead due to some type of disease or disruption (Kane et al., 2004; Landefeld et al., 2004, p. 53).

Hardening of the arteries due to arteriosclerosis is a disease that may lead to dementia in the elderly person. In this situation, the arteries do not allow enough oxygen to pass through to the brain, with the result that areas of the brain die. This condition is also refereed to as multi-infarct dementia and may affect 25% of elderly nursing home residents (Chui, 1995b, p. 954; Howlett, 2006). The only way physicians currently have of distinguishing between multi-infarct dementia and Alzheimer's disease (Albert, 1995, p. 7; Rogaevea & George-Hyslop, 2006), is to perform a computer automated tomograph (CAT scan). The treatment, however, is no different for either diagnosis.

Figure 5.6, shows a slight increase in average percent of residents reported with dementia, rising from 37% in 1993 to 41% in 1999. The percent varied from 32% in Illinois to 55% in Maine in 1999.

Frontotemporal Dementia

Frontotemporal dementia is a heterogeneous syndrome that includes progressive aphasia and corticobasal degeneration syndrome. It is characterized by early changes in personality and behavior with relative sparing of memory. It is often associated with loss of social awareness, compulsive or repetitive

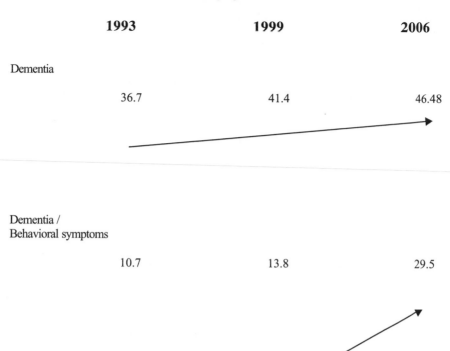

| **1993** | **1999** | **2006** |

Dementia

36.7   41.4   46.48

Dementia /
Behavioral symptoms

10.7   13.8   29.5

FIGURE 5.6 Trends in percent of U.S. residents in nursing facilities with dementia (other behavioral symptoms), 1993,1999, and 2006.

behaviors, reduction in speech, and marked changes in food preferences (Landefeld et al., 2004, p. 63).

Facility interventions can include

- maintain familiarity and routines as much as possible
- decrease number of choices
- tell, don't ask
- understand why they *can't*, rather than why they *won't*
- always keep goals in mind
  (Landefeld et al., 2004, p. 71).

Drugs used to treat behavioral and psychological symptoms of dementia include Halperidol, Risperidone, Olanzapine, Trazonone, and Carbamazepine (Landefeld et al., 2004, p. 72).

Delirium	Dementia
acute, sudden illness	chronic, slowly developing illness
often reversible	generally irreversible
fluctuates over time or worsens as medical problem worsens	often slowly worsens with time

POSSIBLE CONTRIBUTORS TO DELIRIUM

- urinary tract infection
- respiratory infection
- influenza
- pneumonia
- undiagnosed pain
- congestive heart failure
- COPD hypoxia
- renal insufficiency
- anemia
- hypoperfusion states (dehydration, low blood pressure)
- recent surgery
- sensory impairment (cataract, hearing loss)
- trauma: from a fall, accident, head injury (blood clot in brain), internal bleeding

Other causes of delirium

- silent heart attack
- stroke or mini-stroke
- diabetes not regulated
- thyroid problems not being treated
- not enough fluids taken in
- poor nutritional patterns

(Jones, 2004; Landefeld et al., 2004, p. 54)

When to be concerned about a resident: when there are any sudden changes in the 5As, such as:

- alertness vs. sleepiness
- ability to pay attention to you and others
- appetite/eating patterns
- aggression

- activities of daily living

(Jones, 2004; Landefeld et al., 2004, p. 62.)

When to call the physician:

- think "different"
- think "unusual"
- think "agitation": new pattern of hitting, punching, screaming, yell-ing out
- think "behavioral change of recent onset"
- think "pain unable to be expressed"
- if notice changes in baseline behaviors/activity level
- if you have a question about the care plan

(Landefeld et al., 2004, p. 54).

In 2006, the Food and Drug Administration approved Exelon (rivastigmine tartrate), the first drug for treatment of mild to moderate Parkinson's disease dementia, the same drug that had been approved in April, 2000 for treating mild to moderate Alzheimer's disease (www.fda.gov. Approved August, 20, 2006).

The percent of residents with other psychiatric conditions (other than or-ganic mental syndromes) such as schizophrenia, mood disorders, and other problems is reported in Figure 5.6. Other psychiatric conditions varied from 11% of residents in 1993 to 14% of residents in 1999. The percentage of con-ditions varied from 4% in Hawaii to 21% in Louisiana and Ohio in 1999.

Psychosis	Agitation
delusions (including paranoia)	aggression
hallucinations	combativeness
	hyperactivity (including wandering)
	hypervocalization
	disinhibition

Jones, 2004, ; Landefeld et al., 2004, pp. 56, 59.

Alzheimer's Disease

Alzheimer's disease is the most common form of dementia seen in persons over 60 years old; its incidence increased dramatically after that age (Maddox & Sussman, 2001, p. 62). The Alzheimer's patient displays an intellectual impair-ment that is irreversible. The disease progression varies from one resident to another and can extend from 1 year to over a decade. Alzheimer's type of dementia is also known as primary degenerative dementia, a disorder that involves alteration in the structure, number, and functions of neurons in some areas of the brain's cerebral cortex (Evans et al., 2000, p. 925; Kane et al., 2004; Maddox & Sussman, 2001, p. 63). Aging is the greatest risk factor (Jones, 2004).

Three distinct phases of Alzheimer's disease have been identified as: Stage I—forgetfulness or early stage, Stage II—confusion or mild stage, and Stage III—dementia or terminal stage.

The signs and symptoms of the disease vary with each state, but some, including memory loss and behavioral changes, progress in severity until they become profound in the final stage. The following list of signs and symptoms reveals the progressive nature of the disease.

Stage I

- memory loss
- time disorientation
- anxiety
- irritability
- behavior and personality change
- agitation
- inability to concentrate for long periods of time

Stage II

- excessive hunger
- aphasia
- temper tantrums
- restlessness
- muscle twitching
- aimless wandering, sometimes getting lost
- inability to read, write, or do arithmetic calculations
- obsession behavior (e.g., constant washing and rewashing of hands)
- repetitive movements (e.g., tapping, chewing, lip smacking)

Stage III (usually the shortest stage) bedridden

- unable to perform purposeful movement (i.e., walk)
- poor appetite
- poor articulation
- incontinence
- emaciation
- frequent seizures

The goal of treatment is to achieve the highest quality of life while maintaining physical function (Evans et al., 2000, p. 1148). Several nursing home chains as well as individual facilities have installed special Alzheimer's units, usually characterized by enclosed outdoor areas and indoor gates of various types to control wandering (e.g., coded key pads on doors). Typically, it is the Stage II resident who is the primary type of resident in these units due to the special management needs created by this stage of the disease process. A major recent trend is for assisted-living facilities to offer stand-alone Alzheimer's units. It is estimated that 30 to 50% of assisted-living facility residents have dementia. About 18% of assisted-living facilities offered Alzheimer's special care units in 1999 (Maddox & Sussman, 2001, p. 67). This is an area of special concern because staff in these assisted-living units have less training than staff in a nursing facility and nearly all such units are locked units, raising serious restraint issues for the United States.

Medications are palliative, often being tranquilizers to relax the resident and relieve any agitation or violence. Antidepressants are also used to improve the overall mood.

- Delusional thought content (e.g., paranoia) is common (studies suggest 34% to 50% incidence among Alzheimer's disease). Some common delusions are
  - marital infidelity
  - patients, staff are trying to hurt me
  - staff, family members are stealing my things
  - people on TV are real (Jones, 2001)

The high level of dependency among the nursing facility population is illustrated by the statistic that: 22.45% can move from bed to chair or bed to bath without assistance. Half (52.21%) require assistance while one-fourth (25.34%) are wholly dependent on staff.

Similarly, in the simple act of bathing over 95% of nursing home residents needed partial (60%) or total (36%) assistance (DHHS, 2006, F78–F81).

Breaking New Ground

Research into treatments appears promising, but no breakthroughs have been achieved. It seems likely that as more is learned, new disease patterns will be identified within the current broad categories of (1) Alzheimer's type, or (2) infarction of the brain tissue due to cerebrovascular disease, or (3) other. Researchers at Harvard Medical School studied 3,623 elderly Bostonians and found Alzheimer's present in 3% of those aged 65 to 74, 19% of the 75–84 year olds and 47% of those 85 or older.

Cognitive losses are being identified more successfully and, it is hoped, will become more treatable. Persons 85 and older make up the fastest growing segment of the U.S. population. The nursing facility is usually the institution of choice to care for persons of that age diagnosed as having dementia.

Articles and research reports concerning Alzheimer's disease abound (see, for example, Bennett & Knopman, 1994, p. 20; Herdman, 1992, p. 7; The Johns Hopkins Medical Letter, May, 1995, p. 3; Karcher, 1993, p. 34; McCaddon & Kelly, 1994, p. 334; Sterritt & Pokorny, 1994, p. 155; Swanson, Maas, & Buckwalter, 1993, p. 292; Zinn & Mor, 1994, p. 371).

5.3.4 DIGESTIVE SYSTEM

Digestion is the process by which the body breaks down food into needed nutrients. These nutrients are further broken down into particles small enough to pass through tissues and enter the bloodstream for delivery to the appropriate tissues and organs. After absorbing necessary nutrients, the leftover materials or waste products are discarded from the body.

The digestive system is commonly referred to as the gastrointestinal or alimentary tract in reference to the various organs that participate in the digestive process (see Figure 5.7; Bruns, 1995, p. 392).

A diagrammatic representation of the path of food through the digestive system is presented in Figure 5.8.

Mouth

Digestion begins when food enters the mouth. Chewing the food is an important step in preparing it for digestion. Saliva, produced by salivary glands in the mouth, contains enzymes that begin breaking down food substances while they are still in the mouth.

Esophagus

After food is swallowed, it enters the esophagus. The esophagus is the tube (made of smooth muscle) connecting the mouth to the stomach. When food is swallowed, the gastric (stomach) sphincter relaxes to allow food into the stomach. Swallowing initiates a wave like movement of the esophagus (called peristalsis) that propels food toward the stomach.

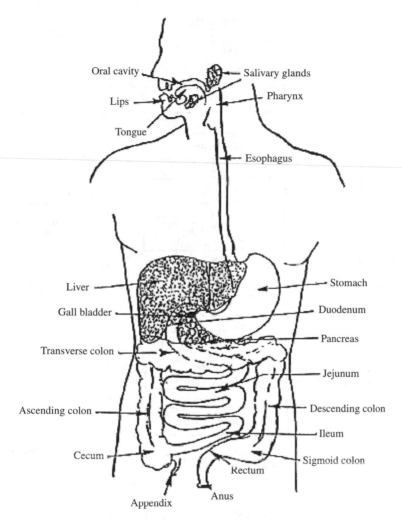

FIGURE 5.7 Organs involved in the digestive processes.

Stomach

The next phase of digestion begins in the stomach. The stomach has sphincters (muscles) at both ends that close when the stomach is full, enabling the stomach acids to have sufficient time to break down the food.

The digestive process in the stomach is controlled by the brain through the nerves, which constantly carry impulses directing the digestion process. In 2006, 4.52% of nursing facility residents were receiving ostomy care (an incision into the stomach through which the resident is fed; DHHS, 2006, F24, F128).

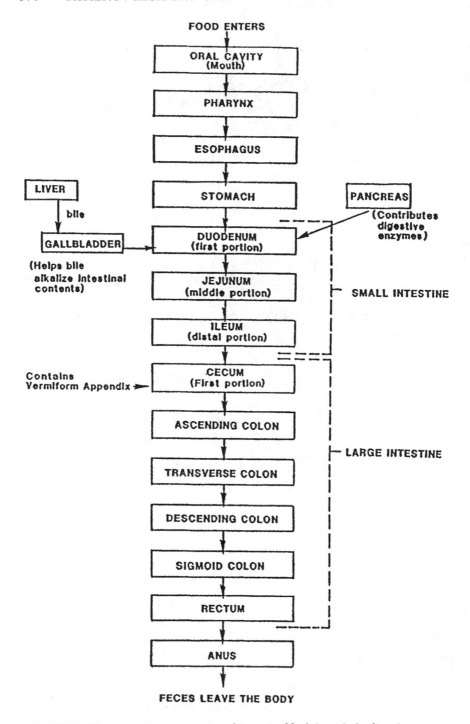

FIGURE 5.8 Diagrammatic representation of the path of food through the digestive system.

Intestines

The intestines may be thought of as a long tube. The intestines are also referred to as the bowels or lower gastrointestinal tract (lower GI). Despite its name, the small intestine is actually much longer than the large intestine.

When the digestive contents enter the small intestine (duodenum), further chemical digestive actions occur. The food is in liquid form at this stage and contains powerful enzymes that break down certain substances. The intestines are also filled with a supply of bacteria that help to digest some of the food substances. These same bacteria are very harmful to any other part of the body if allowed to escape.

Like the stomach, the intestines also have nerves carrying impulses to and from the brain. These nerves are especially important in stimulating the bowel to move the waste materials along the intestinal tract. As in the esophagus, the intestines contract in snakelike movements (peristalsis), propelling the food along the digestive tract.

If, for some reason, the brain does not send the appropriate impulses to the intestines, the waste moves much more slowly through these organs. Unlike the esophagus, the intestines do not have the added force of gravity to assist in this process.

Large Intestine

The large intestine is a continuation of the small intestine and plays its own role in the digestive process. One function of the large intestine is to store the waste so that the body can absorb excess fluids and nutrients before elimination.

By the time waste materials are excreted from the body, they are in a solid form, often referred to as feces or stool. It is important to note that usually patients have voluntary control over when they choose to eliminate these waste materials because the sphincters at the very end of the digestive tract are within the realm of voluntary control.

Possible Effects of Aging

Mouth

The amount of saliva secreted by the salivary glands may decrease. The saliva also may become thicker, until it is almost like mucus (MacHudis, 1983, p. 400). The loss of teeth may also cause digestive complications (Libow, 1981, p. 314). Increasingly, it is suspected that gum disease (periodontal disease) and tooth disease are entry points for germs to enter the body cavity causing various systemic diseases. In light of this, oral hygiene in the nursing facility is a major aspect of maintaining the resident's health state.

Esophagus

In some elderly persons food may not travel as quickly through the esophagus. Causes for this appear to be (a) a reduction in the effectiveness of the swallowing mechanism helping foods move toward the stomach, and (b) the gastric sphincter failing to travel as quickly as before.

Stomach

The lining of the stomach can decrease in thickness with age. This decreased thickness of the lining may allow the size of the stomach to increase. The amount of acid produced by the stomach may decrease.

Digestive Diseases

The digestive tract is an area of the body about which elderly nursing home residents often complain. Physicians use the general diagnosis "gastro-intestinal distress" to describe a range of diseases affecting this system.

Esophagus

The esophagus may be a common site of discomfort for the elderly resident. Esophagi (inflammation or irritation of the esophagus) is another name for heartburn, a frequent problem for elderly individuals. Often this sharp, burning pain may be confused with chest pain and may become worse when the person lies flat, allowing stomach contents to reenter the esophagus.

Dysphagia is difficulty in swallowing or transferring food from the mouth to the esophagus (Evans et al., 2000, p. 244; Lee, 2006, pp. 430–432). Persons with neurological damage may be subject to this problem. Persons who have recently suffered a stroke can be at increased risk because without this function they may aspirate (inhale particles of) food into their lungs.

Stomach

Peptic ulcers may occur anywhere in the gastrointestinal tract. Two of the most common types are gastric ulcers that affect the mid-stomach and duodenal ulcers that involve the lower stomach (Evans et al., 2000, pp. 270–273).

An ulcer is a wearing away of the inner lining of the stomach wall and is due to a chronic buildup of excessive levels of acid. Excessive stress, inactivity, prolonged bed rest, severe trauma, and irritating drugs may all serve to cause or irritate this condition. On examination at death 35% of persons under 50 years of age had gastric ulcers whereas 80% of those over 80 years of age (i.e., typical nursing facility resident) had gastric ulcers.

Medical views on what causes stomach ulcers and their treatment has changed in recent years. Currently, *H. pylori,* a Gram-negative spiral bacterium that colonizes the mucus layer overlaying the gastric mucosa, has become known as a transmitted disease, which causes stomach ulcers, contrary to earlier beliefs (Evans et al., 2000, p. 271). Standard treatment is a triple-antibiotic regimen for 14 days in conjunction with a 6-week course of acid suppression therapy (Evans et al., 2000, p. 271; Landefeld et al., 2004, p. 224).

Ulcer symptoms can include sharp burning abdominal pain 1 to 4 hours after eating, nausea, weight loss, blood in vomitus, and blood in stools. Major complications include hemorrhage and perforation. Aspirin and similar drugs are typical causes and must be discontinued for a period of time to ensure healing (Landefeld et al., 2004, p. 224).

The goal of treatment is to prevent any complications arising from the initial ulceration, thus allowing it to heal. Medications, including antacids, are prescribed to relieve the condition. Long-term treatment for peptic ulcers remains controversial. The preferred approach appears to be to treat for 12 months; others prefer intermittent courses of treatment (Landefeld et al., 2004, p. 224).

Dyspepsia

Dyspepsia is a chronic or recurrent pain or discomfort in the upper abdomen that is thought to arise in the upper GI tract. Symptoms include nausea, bloating, early satiety, or reflux symptoms. Treatment is difficult (Landefeld et al., 2004, p. 225).

Intestines

Constipation is an irregularity in or lack of elimination of waste materials from the body (Kennie & Warshaw, 1989, p. 24; Landefeld et al., 2004, p. 226). Twenty-four percent of all long-term nursing home residents have reported this to be a problem, and in one study more than 34% of elderly residents used laxatives at least once a week. "Normal" bowel habits studied in 1,500 older residents indicated 99% reported anywhere from 3 bowel movements per day to 3 per week.

Constipation may initially be a decrease in the number of stools passed, progressing to a complete lack of stool or bowel movements. When the person has not been able to pass stool for a long period of time, an impaction (blockage) has probably occurred. The waste in the large intestine has accumulated in one area and become hard because much of the fluid content has been reabsorbed by the body.

Treatment of constipation can include laxative medications, which are commonly prescribed for nursing home residents. Bulk laxatives, osmotic laxatives, suppositories, and enemas are the different forms of medications that may be prescribed. Increased activity is one of the best treatments.

Both over the counter and prescription medications should be reviewed and questions asked about daily fluid and fiber intake as well as exercise (Landefeld et al., 2004, p. 226). A change in the care plan may be indicated.

Hemorrhoids are another painful disturbance that can affect the elimination of waste materials from the body. A hemorrhoid is a vein in either the rectum (internal) or around the anus (external) that becomes enlarged. The external type are usually more painful for the resident. Hemorrhoids may either be the causes or result of chronic constipation (Landefeld et al., 2004, p. 230).

Incontinence is the inability to control the timing of elimination. Some of the causes of this dysfunction may be a neurological disturbance due to disease or trauma to the brain and spinal cord, anal surgery, chronic diarrhea, or mental disturbance. Urinary incontinence is often caused by impaction. Urinary incontinence is a multibillion-dollar health issue that affects almost 60% of nursing home residents. Urinary incontinence is involuntary loss of urine sufficient to be a problem (Landefeld et al., 2004, p. 239). Generally, urinary incontinence is a syndrome, not a single disease, resulting from medical conditions, medications, or lower urinary tract disease. It can herald morbid diseases (e.g., cancer and neurological conditions; Landefeld et al., 2004, p. 239; Malone-Lee, 2006, pp. 1205–1207).

Bacteriuria is also prevalent in this group, and the two conditions are commonly found together (Ouslander et al., 1995, p. 749). A number of researchers feel that urinary incontinence is generally manageable (Palmer, Bennett, Marks, McCormick, & Engel, 1995, p. 19). Incontinence care, however, is a major disruptor of the ability of nursing home residents to "get a good night's sleep" (Engel, 1995, p. 502; Schnelle, Ouslander, Simmons, Alessi, & Gravel, 1993, p. 910). Between 1985 and 1999 the level of incontinence among nursing home residents increased from 55% to 66% (DHHS, 2005, p. 340).

Tube Feedings

Tube feedings are used to provide nutritional substances to residents into the gastrointestinal system. In 1993, 6% were receiving tube feeding compared with a slightly increased rate of 7% in 1999 (Harrington et al., 2000, p. 53).

GERD

Gastroesophageal reflux disease (GERD) is the most common GI disorder affecting the nursing home population (Landefeld et al., 2004, p. 220). This problem occurs when the contents of the stomach move back up into the esophagus due to failure of the valves between the esophagus and stomach. Left untreated GERD can lead to complications of acid reflux disease, peptic strictures, or esophageal ulcers with bleeding (Landefeld et al., 2004, p. 220; Lee, 2006, pp. 430–432).

Treatment

Primary focus is on ensuring adequate nutrition and preventing aspiration. Patients are prescribed diets with food consistency that can be safely swallowed (e.g., soft foods or, at the extreme, pureed foods; Landefeld et al., 2004, p. 223).

5.3.5 NUTRITION

Food

Food provides the body with the nutrients necessary to cell functioning. Adequate nutrition can be of value in the maintenance of fitness and independence as well as prevention of disease (Franz, 1981, p. 40; Maddox & Sussman, 2001, p. 756).

In the earlier section on digestion, the digestive process was described as the time when foods are initially broken down into nutrients so they can be absorbed by the body. The next phase of nutrition is the metabolic process whereby the remainder of the nutrients are absorbed, helping to produce energy and control the various body functions.

The percent of nursing facility residents in the United States who had eating dependency increased from 41% in 1985 to 47% in 1999 (DHHS, 2005, p. 340).

Metabolism is the transformation process in which nutrients undergo various chemical reactions throughout the body, producing energy while also helping cells perform necessary functions. Calories are the units of measurement for determining the amount of energy that is contained in foods or used by the body. Following is a list of some the nutrients considered essential to the body. All of them occur naturally in foods and can be obtained from a well balanced diet.

Protein is a nutrient that can be broken down into components called amino acids. Protein is necessary for growth, repair of damaged tissues, transporting nutrients and chemicals throughout the body, and producing various hormones and enzymes.

Carbohydrates can be broken down quickly into readily available fuel for the body. Two common sources are starches and sugars (Halter, 1995, p. 133). The brain is especially sensitive to any decreased levels of carbohydrates in the body and may be permanently damaged whenever the level is reduced for a period of time.

Fats are considered to be the body's source of energy reserve. Fat forms a protective padding around the major organs, prevents heat loss from the body, and carries vitamins A, D, E and K, helping with their absorption (Evans, 2006, pp. 1215–1217).

Minerals Needed by the Body Include:

Calcium—used to build bones and teeth, giving them their hard structure; also helps to clot blood

Iron—important in building healthy red blood cells that are able to carry oxygen

Sodium—acts as a buffering mechanism, helps dissolve substances in the bloodstream, monitors the amount of fluid in the body

Potassium—contained in fluids and tissues; important in muscle contraction, maintains the body fluid balance, and also acts as a buffering mechanism in the bloodstream.

Vitamins act to control certain body functions and regulate the body's utilization of other foods (Maddox & Sussman, 2001, p. 1046).

Fluids

Internally, the body is bathed in fluids that help to eliminate wastes and assist the cells with chemical reactions. Fluids help maintain the integrity of the body by protecting the skin and distributing nutrients to promote healing.

Some major body fluids include:

- Plasma—carries red blood cells and essential nutrients throughout the body.
- Cerebrospinal fluid—protects the brain and spinal cord.
- Lymphatic fluid—carries white blood cells and fluids from the tissues.

In all phases of life, adequate nutrition sustains the building-up processes of the body and impedes the wearing-out processes (Albanese, 1980, p. 20). However, elderly residents suffering from multiple chronic diseases may need even more nutrients than the healthy adults.

Possible Effects of Aging

The elderly are believed by some researchers to require fewer calories because of reduction in body weight, a decrease in the metabolic rate, and often a decline in physical activity (Landefeld et al., 2004, p. 391; Weindruch, 1995, p. 279). However, at the same time that it may be desirable to reduce the amount of carbohydrates and fats, the elderly person has an increased demand for nutrients to enable them to resist the effects of disease. Thus, the appropriate diet for an older person is complex.

Osteoporosis, a softening of the bones, is a concern among numerous elderly persons. It has been observed frequently in women over 40 (Barzel, 1995, p. 723). A lack of sufficient calcium may contribute to a softening of the bones, making some nursing facility residents especially susceptible to bone breakage in falls or other accidents (Landefeld et al., 2004, p. 41; Maddox & Sussman, 2001, p. 778; Stevens, 2006, p. 592).

Dehydration may occur more easily among older persons if they reduce their fluid intake. Smaller proportions of fat under the skin may permit body fluids to evaporate more readily than previously. Dehydration can occur quickly when an elderly person has a fever (Evans et al., 2000, p. 649) and often has no presenting symptoms or signs (Evans et al., 2000, p. 649). Rapid weight loss (3%) may indicate dehydration.

Aging may affect other structures that aid in digestion. Loss of teeth can result in changes in the types of foods eaten. Loss of weight generally causes problems with fitting of dentures; refitting is often necessary.

A loss in the overall number of cells and muscle mass may decrease body weight. In this situation the body may no longer need as many calories to provide sufficient energy.

As with any person, consumption of more calories than needed while remaining relatively inactive can lead to obesity—more and more fat being stored in the tissues as reserve energy. Obesity has been referred to as a frequent form of malnutrition in the elderly.

One consequence of becoming increasingly unable to eat normally is tube feeding. In 2006, 6.41% of nursing home residents were being fed through insertion of tubes nasogastrically or via gastric (a hole into the stomach) tube feeding (DHHS, 2006, F78, F129–132).

Unplanned weight loss/gain occurred among 7.84% of nursing facility residents in 2006 (DHHS, 2006, F78).

Prescribed Diets *Physician' Order diet*

Although the majority of nursing facility residents will eat normal diets, some residents will have special nutritional needs. Chronic disease and the effects of institutionalization on appetite pose a challenge (Kahana, E., 1995b, p. 512).

Physicians often prescribe special therapeutic diets for this group. The following are among the most common:

- **Soft diet**—for residents who need a diet that is low in fiber, soft in texture, and mild in flavor.
- **Mechanical soft diet**—same as soft diet, except texture is either chopped, pureed, or ground to make foods easier to ingest. (Note: An imaginative dietary staff can use molds that shape the pureed food more nearly back into its regular appearance.)
- **Strict full-liquid diet**—consists of foods and liquids that are liquid at body temperature, but can include cold ice cream and hot soup.
- **High-fiber diet**—to provide bulk; similar to regular diet, but with foods that are difficult to digest; e.g., fruits, vegetables, whole-grain breads and cereals, nuts, and bran.
- **High-calorie–high-protein diet**—may include milk shakes, meats, and similar foods, to provide additional sources of protein.

When residents cannot eat usually, nasogastric, esophagostomy, or gastrostomy tube feeding may be prescribed by the physician (Evans et al., 2000, p. 148).

Nasogastric tubes are inserted through the nose and enter the stomach. Esophagostic tubes pass through the neck into the esophagus. Gastrostomy tubes are surgically inserted directly into the stomach.

Gastrostomy tubes may be preferred for patients/residents needing long-term tube feeding, for example, a cancer resident, because they can be more comfortable, and there is no chance for fluids to flow into the lungs (aspiration, i.e., when the tube is mistakenly inserted into the trachea instead of the stomach cavity). This often leads to aspiration pneumonia. These tubes also will not irritate the lining of the upper gastrointestinal tract as may nasogastric tubes.

Enteral feeding is a recent innovation using such products as Osmolite or Ensure. In this case the feeding tube is inserted nasogastrically, but continues into the duodenum (past the stomach into the opining of the small intestine). A pump feeding tube similar to an IV arrangement delivers the nutrients to enter the duodenum. The obvious advantage is to reduce the possibility of aspiration occurring, because the nutrients are introduced into the small intestine itself. The disadvantage is that a permanently inserted tube between the stomach and duodenum must be reinserted with the use of an X-ray machine, usually in a hospital setting.

In 2006, about one-third (34.74%) of nursing facility residents were receiving mechanically altered diets, 19.2% of residents were on special eating rehabilitation programs and 7.39% of residents used assistive eating devices (DHHS, 2006, F78, F129–F132).

Anemia and Diabetes: Two Metabolic Disease Processes

Two of the most common diseases that disrupt the metabolism of important nutrients are anemia and diabetes (Cohen & Rao, 2006, pp. 139–142; Evans et al., 2000, p. 210; McNamara, 2006, pp. 312–316; Sinclair, 1995, p. 276).

Anemia is a condition in which hemoglobin is deficient, resulting in the body not getting enough oxygen. The red blood cells contain a substance called hemoglobin, which carries the oxygen (Cohen & Rao, 2006, pp. 139–142). Diabetes occurs when the body is unable to metabolize glucose (sugar) because of a problem with a hormone, insulin, which is produced by a ductless gland, the pancreas (Maddox & Sussman, 2001, p. 295).

Total deaths from diabetes mellitus among persons aged 65 and older more than doubled between the years 1980, when 25,000 died of diabetes, and 2003, when 55,000 died of diabetes (DHHS, 2005, Table 32, p. 183). Even so, the length of stay for men hospitalized for diabetes treatment was cut in half between 1990 (11.0 days) and 2003 (5.5 days) (DHHS, 2005, p. 333).

Various types of anemia are found in the nursing facility. It is thought to be due to disease, not old age (Cohen & Rao, 2006; Kane et al., 2004;

Landefeld et al., 2004, p. 314 ff.), and therapy for each type of anemia is varied. About 5% of long-term nursing home residents probably suffer from some form of chronic anemia.

Anemia is the result of a significant decrease in the number of red blood cells produced. Having multiple chronic diseases can lead to anemia. Symptoms of anemia are similar to those for heart disease because they also result in a problem with oxygenation. When anemia is combined with other diseases, such as peripheral vascular disease or coronary artery disease, it may be very serious as well as painful for the resident.

Diabetes

Diabetes affects about 15% of all long-term nursing facility residents. It results from an inability to convert carbohydrates in the body to forms the body can utilize.

Usually, the pancreas produces the hormone insulin, which helps the cells convert sugar (or glucose) into a form of energy for use or storage. Diabetics either produce insufficient amounts of this hormone or have some difficulty in utilizing insulin. The result is large amounts of sugar continually circulating in the bloodstream, causing the condition known as hyperglycemia (high blood sugar).

Chronic hyperglycemia can damage many of the body tissues. Hyperglycemia can cause complications and disabilities in other systems in the body. In its more extreme form diabetes is a factor in the cause of blindness and amputation for elderly patients (Landefeld et al., 2004, p. 339; McNamara, 2006, pp. 312–316).

There are two different classifications of persons with diabetes: insulin dependent and noninsulin dependent. Insulin-dependent diabetes mellitus (IDDM) individuals have generally had the disease since childhood and require daily doses (or the equivalent) for the control of the disease. Almost all of the long-term nursing home population fall into this category. Non-insulin-dependent diabetes mellitus (NIDDM) is usually diagnosed in adults, who are generally able to control the disease by dietary restrictions and the use of oral hypoglycemics (Landefeld et al., 2004, p. 340; McNamara 2006, pp. 312–316).

Much of the treatment provided to nursing home residents involves monitoring the blood sugar level. It is often unclear who is truly a diabetic. Glucose tolerance progressively deteriorates with each decade of life. One researcher, Andres (1989), formulated a percentile system demonstrating decreasing glucose tolerance with age. Thus, the physician practicing in a nursing facility must guard against treating a laboratory value that represents an altered physiologic state as a true case of diabetes.

Glycemic Control

Aggressive glucose control in the resident is important to reduce the risk of vascular complications. Doing glucose checks as ordered in the resident's care plan is important for staff to understand (Landefeld et al., 2004, p. 342).

Risk factors for hypoglycemia

- Therapy with insulin
- Renal insufficiency
- Hepatic dysfunction
- Cognitive impairment
- Poor nutrition
- Alcohol
- Sedative agents
- Complex regimens
- Polypharmacy
- Tight glycemic control
- Recent hospitalization
  (Landefeld et al., 2004, p. 342).

As can be seen, many of these factors are present for a diabetic nursing home resident.

5.3.6 EXTERNAL AND INTERNAL DEFENSE MECHANISMS

The body is equipped with special defense mechanisms to protect it from harmful disruptions in the environment through the use of two different types of defense mechanisms.

The Barrier System of Defense

The first type acts as a barrier preventing harmful substances from entering the body, the largest such organ being the skin (Orentreich, 1995, p. 860). While protecting the body from harmful organisms, the skin also seals in essential body fluids and regulates the body temperature (Franz & Gardner, 1994, p. 17). The respiratory, intestinal, and urinary tracts also have barrier-like components to protect the body from foreign materials that may enter through their systems.

In the respiratory tract, thousands of cilia (small hair like elements) line the passageways and help propel outward any foreign materials that may be inhaled from the air. Coughing expels these particles from the body and back into the environment.

Two additional barrier-like protections are the acid composition of gastric juices and urine, which also act to protect the digestive system and the urinary tract from the entrance of harmful organisms.

The Chemical Defense System

The immune system is often referred to as the second line of defense; it protects the internal structures of the body. Whenever foreign material or an antigen enters the body, the components of the immune system recognize this and mobilize for an attack response. Most often, the foreign material is a small bacterial or viral microorganism.

Different types of antibodies have various means of fighting an infection and use a much more complex interaction than that seen in the cell-mediated response.

Infections   Viral - No Antibiotic

When bacteria or viruses are successful in penetrating the defense mechanisms in large numbers or are allowed to enter the areas of the body where they are not usually found, the resulting disruption is known as an infection (Evans et al., 2000, p. 64). Philip Smith (1989), an infection control epidemiologist who has written extensively in this field, estimates that 1.5 million infections occur each year in U.S. nursing homes. This suggests an average of about one infection per resident per year and that, on average, 5–10% of residents will acquire an infection in any given year. Nursing home residents may be more prone to infections than other population groups because of:

- age-related changes in their bodies
- the presence of multiple chronic diseases (weakening the defenses)
- associated use of multiple medications with side effects that may compromise the body
- increased incidence of immobility and incontinence
- frequent use of invasive devices such as indwelling urinary catheters

These factors all increase nursing home residents' susceptibility to infections and also serve to weaken their body's own natural defense mechanisms.

Three researchers, Beck-Sague, Banerjee, and Jarvis estimate that risk of infection from residing in a nursing home ranges from 3.3% to more than 15% (1993, p. 1739). Kane et al. remain unconvinced, however, that alterations in defense mechanisms predispose the elderly to certain infections. They speculate that environmental factors, specific diseases, and physiological changes other than the immune system may account for increased frequency of certain infections in the elderly (2004, p. 291; see also Goldrick & Larson, 1992, p. 20).

New infectious processes are being identified in nursing homes. More recently documented infections include bacteremia (bacteria in the blood stream occurring with intravascular catheters), conjunctivitis, AIDS (Lashley, 2006b), streptococcal infection, Legionnaires' Disease, and methicillin-resistant staphylococcus aureus (MRSA; Evans et al., 2000, p. 66). More and more nursing facilities are being asked to care for and are accepting MRSA residents who have special requirements for care in enforcing the universal precautions when receiving care. Of particular concern is whether the MRSA is colonized or noncolonized upon admission. A colonized MRSA means the infectious agents are encapsulated and much less likely to spread infection. Noncolonized MRSA can spread infection via airborne particles and touching objects in the patient's physical vicinity. MRSA was isolated from 320 of 422 emergency room admissions suggesting that MRSA is present on the skin of more than half of ER patients (Moran et al., 2006).

Additional infection risk factors are emerging as nursing facilities accept transfer from hospitals of patients who are quite ill, some of whom have tracheostomies, central IV catheters, hyperalimentation, or AIDS (Smith, 1989, p. 8). The emergence of vancomycin-resistance in *Staph. aureus* is of increasing concern for the nursing facility that receives such patients from the hospital (Evans et al., 2000, p. 66).

Nosocomial Infections   Home Grown

Infections that are associated with institutionalization or acquired while in a health care facility are called nosocomial infections. Nursing home residents are considered to be at a particular risk of developing these infections because of the levels of group interaction and activities among residents.

Half of all infections in the chronic-care facility studied may be due to nosocomially acquired pneumonia or urinary tract infections and that these two infections are commonly responsible for morbidity (illness) in the elderly population. Pneumonia immunization is recommended for persons over 65 (Evans et al., 2000, p. 85; McNeil, 2006, pp. 569–572). Some of the other types of nosocomial infections often seen in the nursing home include infections of the skin, soft tissues, and gastrointestinal tract. Because of more frequent and longer hospitalizations nursing facility residents are at increased risk for Staphylococcus and gram negative infections (Kane et al., 2004). Infection control has generally improved in recent years according to research by Raymond Otero who focused on methicillin-resistant *Staphylococcus aureus* (MRSA; Otero, 1993, pp. 48–49). A study of central line catheter infection rates in hospitals reduced the median rate of 2.7 catheter-related blood infections per 1,000 patient days to nearly zero infections by using proper hygiene, disinfecting the catheter site, and removing catheters more quickly.

The Inflammation Response *itis* *inflammation*

Inflammation occurs in the physical responses by the other body systems when fighting off infection of some external threat. The blood vessels dilate (expand) bringing more cells to combat the unwanted component. This is often the cause of redness surrounding areas of skin that may become infected. The debris from the antigen often become pus, which may drain from the infection as well.

Special Difficulties in Identifying Infections

Infections in the elderly may be more difficult to diagnose because it is possible to confuse the symptoms with those of other chronic diseases. Also, even when symptoms are present, the elderly resident may be reluctant to complain about these disruptions, so they are less likely to be reported.

Most infections are not considered to be chronic diseases because they respond to treatment, and their damage to the body can often be reversed. Some of the possible effects of aging on the immune system are discussed in the next section.

Possible Effects of Aging

The skin contains fibers that change as persons age. These changes may make the skin and other connective tissue drier and less resilient (Balen & Lin, 1995, p. 222; Kenney, 1982, p. 34; Tonna, 1995c, p. 196).

Skin, nail, and hair cells, which are among the fastest to grow during younger years, often do not replace themselves as quickly when persons age. Together, these changes help explain why many elderly people have some degree of tough, dry, wrinkled skin. Kligman also suggests that these types of changes work to diminish the barrier function of the skin as a person ages (1979, p. 40).

A study by Tindall and Smith of 163 persons 64 years of age and older showed that 94% of them had "lax" skin, secondary to changes in connective tissue, which contributed to wrinkling and other related manifestations (1963, p. 1039).

The greatest alteration in the internal immune system is the involution (decrease in size) of the thymus gland. This change is suspected to influence the function of the immune system, but it is still too early to determine the full range of implications this may have on the health of elderly individuals. Some impairment of the immune response makes elderly individuals more susceptible to infection.

Disease Processes

Some of the more prevalent diseases or disruptions that affect either of the body's defense mechanisms are discussed in the following sections. Tuberculosis and pneumonia have already been dealt with in greater detail.

Facility Responses to the Presence of Infections: The Infection Control Program

The federal requirements in the Medicare program require nursing facilities to establish infection control programs to monitor facility performance in this area. The federal Department of Labor has issued the Universal Precautions required of all facilities.

Depending on the nature of the infection, various isolation precautions need to be taken to protect other residents, staff, and visitors from acquiring the infection as well. The administrator must also make sure that residents with certain communicable diseases are reported to the state health department. Each state, in cooperation with the U.S. Public Health Service, specifies diseases that must be reported to the state health department.

Infections complicate the elderly residents' disease status and may even increase their chance of death (mortality). Besides this risk, infections may increase the likelihood that a resident will need to be transferred to a hospital for more intensive care.

Risk Control—Infection Control—the Infection Control Practitioner (ICP)

The risk of an epidemic is always present in the nursing facility. An epidemic is a cluster of infections involving multiple individuals. Nursing home epidemics include influenza, Staphylococcal skin infections, antibiotic-resistant

586   PATIENT / RESIDENT CARE

bacteria, infectious diarrhea, scabies, and tuberculosis. A survey of Nebraska nursing homes found more than 50% of the facilities experienced an epidemic in the previous year involving an average of 35 residents and 14 employees. Influenza was the most common cause. A careful following of the Department of Labor's Universal Precautions (Bloodborne Pathogens) rules will do much to reduce epidemics. Along with federal and state requirements each facility is expected to individualize and enforce its own infection control policies coordinated by a trained part-time or full-time infection control practitioner (ICP).

+ Hand Washing   One Way to Stop Spreading Handwashing *effective Way*

Lack of hand washing remains a major source of the spread of infections in the health care setting. Studies indicate that compliance with hand washing guidelines remains under 50% in the health care setting.

The reader is urged to download Guideline for Hand Hygiene in Health-Care Settings Recommendations of the Healthcare Infection Control Practices Advisory Committee and the HICPAC/SHEA/APIC/IDSA Hand Hygiene Task Force issued October 25, 2002/ *Morbidity and Mortality Weekly Report,* Volume 51, No. RR-16 from the CDC Web site www.cdc.gov. In their search box type in hand hygiene 2002.

Skin Disease

Herpes Zoster (Shingles)

One of the diseases that primarily affects elderly individuals is herpes zoster, more commonly called shingles (Evans et al., 2000, p. 60). This infection is caused by the herpes varicella virus (not to be confused with herpes simplex), which travels along nerve pathways to infect skin cells. Skin covering the chest region and areas surrounding the eye are among the areas more commonly infected by this disease. Residents who suffer from a debilitating disease, such as cancer, are also at greater risk of developing this infection.

Signs and symptoms include itching, usually preceding a rash, reddened areas of the skin (usually along a nerve pathway), vesicles (fluid-filled pimples) often erupting over reddened areas, and burning accompanied by stabbing pain.

At present there is no cure for this form of herpes infection, so treatment consists of attempts to alleviate the associated symptoms rather than effect a cure. Steroids are often used to reduce inflammation, which may shorten the length of the infection and provide comfort. Antibiotics are sometimes prescribed to prevent secondary infections and analgesics to relieve pain.

Decubitus Ulcers   *pressure ulcer*

Pressure sores is the federal government's preferred term for these infections known also as bed sores, decubitus ulcers, and stasis ulcers (ulcers resulting from tissue death due to reduced blood flow), all terms for the same process—tissue breakdown. Stasis ulcers are the sores that result from extremely poor peripheral circulation or peripheral vascular disease (Evans et al., 2000, p. 103; Garagusi, 1989, p. 204; Landefeld et al., 2004, p. 191).

Tissue breakdown often occurs over a bony prominence (buttocks, elbow, heel, hip, shoulder). These ulcers do not develop from an infection, but rather from some form of constant unrelieved pressure on one area of the body.

With all of these ulcers the end result is the same: Tissues do not receive an adequate amount of oxygen, so they break down and begin to die. This process is similar to what happens to the heart muscle in coronary artery disease.

Residents at most risk for developing these ulcers are those chronically immobile (paralyzed) because of a stroke or some other incapacitating illness and those experiencing poor nutritional status, constant pain, incontinence, or dementia (Gubitz, 2006, p. 206–208; Landefeld et al., 2004, p. 281 ff.). These ulcers often enlarge to form cavities of dead tissue prone to the development of infection and once enlarged, are more difficult to heal.

Decubitus Ulcer Formation   *pressure ulcer*

The formation of an ulcer usually occurs with the weight of the body exerts pressure on internal soft tissues by compressing them between skeletal bone and another hard surface; (Evans et al., 2000, p. 59). Residents who are immobilized or unable to move by themselves are particularly at risk for developing bedsores. Because these patients cannot, on their own, change position frequently, there is the danger of continuous pressure on one area of their body.

Many of these residents spend much of their time lying on their back, also knows as the decubitus position ("decubitus" means lying down). When this occurs, the areas most likely to develop sores are the buttocks, hips, heels, shoulders, ears, and elbows. Similarly, residents who spend long periods sitting up in a chair without moving are also at risk of developing these sores.

Signs and symptoms of decubitus ulcers include:

- tingling, pale skin color, or other signs that there is a loss of circulation to an area
- reddened area of skin over a bony prominence
- a sore that will not heal
- edema (swelling) of the lower legs and shiny skin

However, these signs are often difficult to recognize before tissue has already died and the ulcer itself has already developed (Evans et al., 2000, p. 105; Rowe & Besdine, 1982, p. 51).

Pressure sores are typically classed as Grade I, I, III, and IV.

Grade I: acute inflammatory response, often over a bony prominence; skin red, but unbroken

Grade II: extension of the acute inflammatory response through the dermis to subcutaneous fat

Grade III: extension through fat to deep fascia, base of ulcer infected

Grade IV: deep ulceration reaching the bone (Kane et al., 2004, p. 236).

Following are some of the main treatments the facility may use:

- providing special equipment, such as a water mattress
- keeping the resident clean and dry
- eliminating the source of pressure
- working to improve the resident's circulation
- assuring frequent position change (at least every 2 hours) for those who are unable or unlikely to do so themselves
- padding feet, elbows, and other areas at high risk of tissue breakdown (e.g., using "bunny boots" on the feet)
- frequently assessing the integrity of a resident's skin
- changing diet to include foods higher in protein, Vitamin C, and calorie content to promote healing
- preventing infection by applying dressings and dispensing antibiotic medications as prescribed
- using elastic stockings or Ace wrap bandages, which are often prescribed for the person with peripheral vascular insufficiency (poor blood circulation in their arms and legs).
- other: A number of experimental treatments are constantly being offered to nursing facilities. Use of a hypobaric chamber, which facilitates the flow of oxygen to injured areas is one such approach. (Landefeld et al., 2004, p. 284).

Maintaining a moist wound environment increases the rate of healing. Dressings that maintain a moist wound environment are occlusive.

Topical Dressings

- Polymer films—impermeable to liquid but permeable to both gas and moisture vapor. Polymer films do not eliminate dead space and do not absorb exudates.
- Hydrogels—are three layer hydrophilic polymers that are insoluble in water but absorb aqueous solutions. These are poor bacterial barriers and do not adhere to the wound.
- Hydrocolloid dressings—are complex dressings similar to ostomy barrier products. They are impermeable to moisture vapor and gases (hence oxygen needed to heal the wound),
- Alginates—complex polysaccharide dressings that are highly absorbent in exudative wounds. If the wound is allowed to dry, damage to the epithelial tissue may occur with removal.
- Biomembranes—offer bacterial resistance but are expensive and not readily available.
- Saline-soaked gauze—if not allowed to dry can be effective. Moist saline gauze and occlusive type dressings have similar ulcer healing abilities. Thus, the use of occlusive type dressings has been shown to be more cost effective due to decreased nursing time in wound dressing changes.
- Phenytoin—has been associated with a shorter time to complete healing and formation of granulation tissue.
  (Landefeld et al., 2004, p. 284 ff.)

Debridement

Necrotic debris increases the possibility of bacterial infection and delays wound healing. The preferred method of debriding pressure ulcers remains controversial (Landefeld et al., 2004, p. 286). Some facilities use mechanical debridement with dry gauze dressings and the like, others use surgical sharp instruments or suction devices (Landefeld et al., 2004, p. 286).

Both pressure sores and stasis ulcers are significant disruptions of the skin's protective barrier defense. A study by Garibaldi, Brodine, and Matsumiya (1981) concluded that 32% of infections originated from this source. One of the most severe types of infections that may result is called sepsis, a condition in which the circulating bloodstream carries infectious organisms throughout the body.

Residents Especially at Risk: The Bedfast and Chairbound

Residents who are bedfast or chairbound for long periods of time are at high risk of developing pressure sores. Figure 5.9 reveals that over the years 1993 to 1999 nearly half of all residents were chairbound. This includes residents who were in a bed or recliner for 22 or more hours per day in the week before the federal survey. The percent of bedfast residents increased from 5% of residents in 1993 to 7% of residents in 1999. The average percent of bedfast residents ranged from 2% in North Dakota to 16% in Hawaii in 1999. Even a slight increase in the number of such residents increases nursing load carried by a facility.

A number of residents depend on a chair for mobility or are unable to walk without extensive or constant support from others. Figure 5.10, illustrating skin integrity, indicates that this is an extensive problem in the typical nursing facility

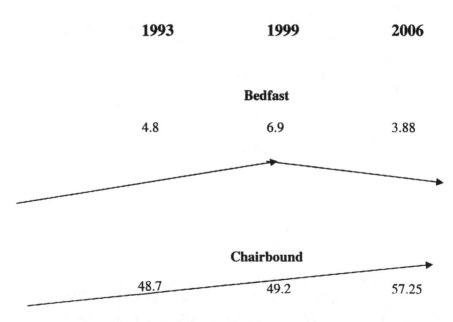

FIGURE 5.9 Percentage and trend lines of residents in U.S. nursing homes who are bedfast or chairbound, 1993, 1999, and 2006.
Source: DHS, 2006, F78, F100–106.

Nonroutine Skin Care

Figure 5.10 reveals some headway in reducing the percent of residents with pressure sores, dropping from 7.5% of residents in 1991 to 7.1% of residents in 1999. This reduction in pressure sores may be due to the consistent increase in percent of residents receiving special skin care from 30% in 1993

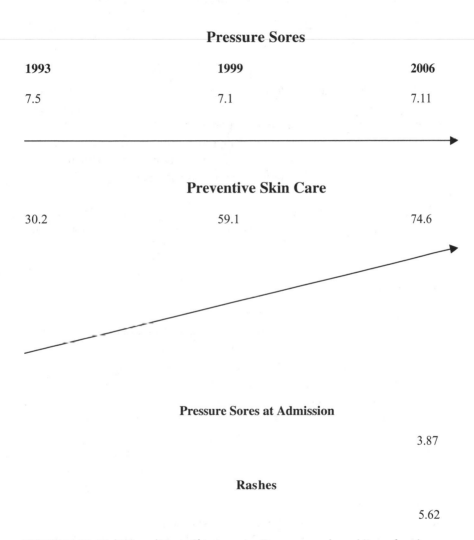

Pressure Sores

1993	1999	2006
7.5	7.1	7.11

Preventive Skin Care

| 30.2 | 59.1 | 74.6 |

Pressure Sores at Admission

3.87

Rashes

5.62

FIGURE 5.10 Medical condition—Skin integrity. Percentage and trend lines of residents with pressure sores and receiving special skin care in U.S. nursing facilities , 1993, 1999, and 2006. Pressure sores at admission and rashes, 2006.
Source: DHHS, 2006, F78, F115–118.

to 60% in 1999. Special skin care is nonroutine care according to a resident care plan or physician's order, usually designed to prevent or reduce pressure ulcers of the skin.

Facilities must ensure that residents without pressure sores do not develop them if avoidable. In both 1993 and 1999, about 18% of facilities received deficiencies for failing to meet this nursing care challenge. The deficiency rate dropped during 1994 to 1996, but began rising in 1997 (Harrington et al., 2000, p. 97).

Attention of the Administrator

The *in-house acquired preventable decubitus ulcer rate* is one of the three or four yardsticks by which the quality of the care given in the facility is judged. Good nursing care is the best form of overall treatment. Lehman identifies the administrator's roles as assuring that evaluation and screening for residents at high risk for developing these ulcers is routinely done. Approximately two-thirds of these ulcers develop within the first weeks that a patient is institutionalized.

The DHHS Agency for Health Care Policy and Research (AHCPR) has developed clinical practice guidelines for the management of pressure sores (1995, p. 15).

Hypothermia

Hypothermia (low body temperature) is an issue of special concern to nursing home staff. Usually, the body temperature is maintained between 97 and 99 degrees Fahrenheit. Patients in a nursing home facility may be endangered by subtle changes in temperature. The elderly resident often may have less insulation from body fat, increasing the risk of hypothermia.

Hypothermia is the sudden appearance of a low body temperature (less than 95 degrees). Often it is difficult to diagnose hypothermia because symptoms may be similar to those of a minor stroke.

When the body temperature drops below 95 degrees, residents are no longer able to feel cold and may be suffering from confusion, so they are often unable to complain of other symptoms, such as skin that is pale, dry, and cool with low pulse or blood pressure.

Many complications may result from hypothermia, including dehydration, renal failure (Evans et al., 2000, p. 658; White & Sullivan, 2006, pp. 163–168), pneumonia, and cardiac arrhythmias (Evans et al., 2000, p. 373). Treatment is aimed at slowly rewarding the patient back to a normal body temperature, usually with blankets. Residents with multiple chronic diseases may not survive an episode of hypothermia.

Because of the threat of hypothermia, loss of heat in the nursing facility can be a life-threatening situation for the patients.

Cancer

Cancer is actually a group of chronic diseases that affect different areas of the body. Approximately 5% of nursing home residents suffer from some form of cancer. In 2003, deaths from malignant neoplasms (cancer) were dramatically high among older Americans.

Death rate per 100,000 population for malignant neoplasms selected ages

Age	
25–34	9.4
55–64	343
65–74	770
75–84	1,302
85 and older	1,698

(DHHS, 2005, Table 38, p. 199).

Cancer is the second leading cause of death among persons aged 65 and over and has increased in numbers in recent decades. In 1980, 258,000 older persons died of cancer compared to 388,000 in 2003 (DHHS, 2005, Table 32, p. 183).

Cancer is discussed here as a disorder of the immune system because cancer cells act as antigens and are known to attack many organs or cells throughout the body.

The growth of cancer cells is markedly different from that of normal cells. They grow much more rapidly and are often released or break out from their initial area of growth (tumor) and travel into the bloodstream or lymphatic channels and then throughout the body. Damage may result either from this rapid cell growth, depleting normal cell food supply, or from actual expansion and crushing of the organ affected.

Another mode for cancer growth occurs when cancerous cells travel from the initial growth to new sites, forming metastases or other cancer sites throughout the body. Metastasis is the transfer of disease from one organ or part of the body to another not directly connected with it, due either to transfer of pathogenic microorganisms or transfer of cells.

The cause of cancer is still unknown, but among the different factors believed to play possible roles in this disease are environmental exposure to harmful substances, chronic chemical or biologic irritation (drugs, alcohol, smoking, viral infections, radiation), inherited genetic predisposition to the disease, dietary and even behavioral.

It has been suggested that some combination of these factors probably best explains the cause of cancer. Often these factors may expose the body to a substance known as a carcinogen, which alters the body's immune response capabilities and allows these substances to enter the body and promote the growth of cancerous cells.

According to Birchenall and Streight (1982), the leading types of cancer seen in nursing facility residents, listed in order of prevalence by sex, are as follows:

Males—lung, colon, rectum, and prostate

Females—breast, colon, rectum, and lung

Variations in Cancer Treatments

Physicians may choose to manage cancer patients with different forms of treatments, depending on the specifics of the disease. Surgery, radiation, and use of chemical therapy are the three most common forms of cancer treatment. There are more than 250 different kinds of cancer; forms of treatment will vary for individual patients according to the severity of their illness.

Problems Associated With Cancer Treatments

There are many problems associated with cancer treatment. The patient with colon cancer may have undergone surgery to remove the diseased portion of the bowel. If a large enough area has been removed, then the patient will usually also have a colostomy, which is an opening on the abdomen where the end of the bowel is brought to the surface and digestive waste materials are collected in a bag attached to an appliance surrounding the site. Depending on the level of independence, residents with colostomies may require additional assistance with this special type of elimination process.

The two other types of cancer treatment (radiation and chemotherapy) may be quite painful for residents because of their associated side effects. One of these is anorexia (continual lack of appetite). When this persists, physicians may prescribe special high-calorie food supplements to maintain the patient's strength and energy, as well as treatments for pain and nausea.

In 2006, under 1% (0.22%) of nursing home residents were receiving radiation therapy and under 1% (0.36%) were receiving chemotherapy (DHHS, 2006, F78–F119).

5.3.7 MUSCULOSKELETAL SYSTEM

The muscles and skeleton working together provide two important functions: (a) a supporting framework for all of the other body structures, and (b) mobility, which is closely related to the nursing facility resident's degree of independence and autonomy (Hofland, 1995, p. 100; Maddox & Sussman, 2001, p. 111).

The Skeleton and Muscles

One of the basic elements of the supporting framework of the body is the skeleton, which is composed of the many bones that meet to form joints. The muscles are attached to the skeleton. The skeleton also protects soft tissues and organs inside the body. This framework dictates an individual's posture, directly affecting personal appearance.

Joints

In the body there are 68 joints, which are the points where the ends of two bones meet. These joint bones are covered by cartilage and surrounded by a capsule containing fluid that lubricates the area to enhance movement. The joint is held in place by ligaments.

Movement

In order for movement to occur, the muscles must first receive a nerve impulse from the brain directing them to contract, then relax. Because the muscles are attached to the bones, when they move, the bone moves also. The joints respond like mechanical levers to assist in completing this movement. Thus, mobility requires coordination between both the nervous and musculoskeletal systems.

Possible Effects of Aging

The individual bones contain an inner component—bone marrow—that produces the red blood cells. The remainder of bone consists of a network of fibrous tissue containing salts, which are primarily minerals, such as calcium, that serve to harden and strengthen the bone (Hayflick, p. 118).

There is some consensus that during the aging process the total amount of bone in the body is decreased. However, to determine the loss, one needs to have measured the amount of bone the individual had at age 35.

Higher Risk for Women

Women are at a high risk of experiencing some degree of bone loss following menopause (Evans et al., 2000, p. 618; Giangregorio, Papaioannou, & Adachi, 2006, pp. 883–885). It has been established that this loss results from a withdrawal of estrogen, which apparently helps promote the body's use of dietary calcium for the purpose of bone growth (Evans et al., 2000, p. 189 ff.).

When bone loss occurs, some of the observable changes are shortened stature and a slumped posture due to a compression of the vertebrae (bones in the spine) and the cartilage discs between them.

Often, because of these changes, elderly individuals become stooped and appear to have a hump back. They are also more likely to fracture one of their bones.

While a certain amount of bone loss is associated with aging, much of it in the elderly is a result of osteoporosis (Evans et al., 2000, p. 193; Giangregorio et al., 2006, pp. 883–885). There is considerable controversy over the extent to which these changes in the bone can be attributed to normal aging rather than to osteoporosis, which will be described later.

Both muscles and bones are made up of connective tissue and collagen (Balen & Vilenchik, 2006, pp. 259–262; Maddox & Sussman, 2001, p. 217). Similar to the collagen-related changes associated with age, muscles, also become less elastic as a result of this same process. The most significant age-related muscle change for the elderly is a decrease in the amount throughout the body. In addition, degenerative changes in the nervous system may disturb impulses, decreasing muscle skills. However, it is unclear to what extent, if any, these changes in bone and muscle size and strength are related to age, rather than to the possible effects of decreased activity.

Disease Processes

The discussion of age-related changes in the musculoskeletal system reflects the considerable uncertainty as to whether the changes in bones are a manifestation of the aging process or a distinct disease process.

The term rheumatism has often been used by the elderly to describe any painful disorder of the muscles, joints, and their surrounding areas. Following is a discussion of some of the common disruptions of musculoskeletal functioning as experienced in the nursing home population.

Osteoporosis

Osteoporosis has already been described as a condition of decreased skeletal mass without alteration of any chemical components of bone (Giangregorio et al., 2006, pp. 883–885, Rossman, 1979, p. 285). Thus, while there may be less total amount of bone, the components of bone are still present in necessary proportions.

The cause of osteoporosis remains unclear, but the mechanism of bone loss apparently is through increased reabsorption of bone tissue by the body. Osteoporosis may result from prolonged use of medication, immobility, or some other underlying disease.

Symptoms of osteoporosis include bone pain, often in the lower back, recurrent bone fractures, and frequent falls (Giangregorio et al., 2006, pp. 883–885; Landefeld et al., 2004, p. 75) and related injuries.

Treatment can include managing the symptoms of pain, treating complications such as fractures, rehabilitation to correct physical inactivity, and increasing protein and vitamin intake. Medications often used are calcium supplements and hormones, usually estrogen, to improve the body's ability to absorb calcium.

Simply taking extra calcium without estrogen replacement appears to be dramatically less effective, according to Glowacki, who also believes reports that estrogen replacement therapy causes endometrial (inner lining of the uterine wall) cancer are exaggerated. There is no evidence, he asserts, that estrogen replacement therapy causes breast cancer (Glowacki, 1989, p. 294).

Arthritis

Arthritis is an inflammation of a joint (Evans, 2006, p. 80; Evans et al., 2000, p. 545; Kerr, 2006, pp. 80–81; Landefeld et al., 2004, p. 264; Maddox & Sussman, 2001, p. 91). Nearly 25% of nursing home residents suffer from some form of this disease. However, there are many different types of arthritis; two that commonly afflict nursing home residents are osteoarthritis and rheumatoid arthritis.

Osteoarthritis   DJD   Pain Control

This is the most prevalent form, also called degenerative joint disease. As the disease progresses, the cartilage and other components of the joint begin to wear away or degenerate (Evans et al., 2000, p. 566). The joints that bear most of the weight on a continual basis are most commonly affected, including the knee, hips, and ankles.

Symptoms include aching pain in the affected joint, most often a backache, and decreased mobility because the pain becomes worse following exercise.

Treatment consists of relieving symptoms. Use of an anti-inflammatory agent such as enteric-coated aspirin is usually recommended (Kane et al.,

1989, p. 224; Kane et al., 2004). Continual degeneration of the hip joint may require a surgical replacement if the patient still has good walking skills.

Rheumatoid Arthritis

This is a much more serious form of arthritis. It can affect any age group. This is considered an autoimmune (Heidrick, 1995, p. 100; Kerr, 2006; Landefeld et al., 2004, p. 264) disease because it is thought the body begins to attack its own cells in the joint, causing an inflammatory reaction.

Signs and symptoms include

- symmetric inflammation of joints on both sides of the body
- frequent flare-ups and remissions of pain
- stiffness and joint swelling, usually in the hands
- pain, often occurring in the morning hours and decreasing with exercise

Treatments include

- a balance of rest and exercise
- physical therapy
- heat and cold applications
- whirlpool baths

Medications include

- aspirin, to decrease the inflammation
- analgesics, to relieve the pain
- Prednisone, 15–20 mg daily

See Arthritis Foundation, www.arthritis.org

Falls

More than 70% of deaths that result from all falls occur among persons over 65 years of age. Falling is a major cause of disability and death in the elderly and may be due to factors such as chronic illness or orthostatic hypotension (decreased blood pressure upon standing; Evans et al., 2000, pp. 93, 111; The Johns Hopkins Medical Letter, 1994, p. 5; Kippenbrock & Soja, 1993, p. 205; Landefeld et al., 2004, p. 75; Stevens, 2006, p. 592, Tideiksaar, 1995, p. 361). This phenomenon is sometimes associated with reduced blood pressure among residents after eating, known as postprandial hypotension (Evans et al., 2000, p. 119).

Patients in the facility dining room who have just finished a large meal are especially vulnerable. It appears that the blood (Cohen, 1995c) supply is being routed to the digestive system, causing even lower blood pressure when the resident stands up from the meal.

Osteoporosis, gait disorders (Evans et al., 2000, p. 825), and decreased blood supply to the brain may also be found in the typical nursing home resident, leaving them more prone to falls than the noninstitutionalized elderly population (Evans et al., 2000, p. 93).

It is estimated that due to privacy in rooms, only 25% of falls in institutions are witnessed and that 25%–50% of residents fall each year. Eighty percent of all individuals falling are age 75 or older.

Facility environments can often be unsafe. An emphasized and smoothly running risk management program focusing on incident reports can identify changes needed in the facility environment to reduce falls.

Review Medications

- Falls are often associated with prescriptions, which may lead to increased falling as a side effect.
- Psychotropic medications. Substantial evidence links neuroleptics, benzodiazepines, and antidepressants with falls and fractures.
- Neuroleptics. Risk of sedating.
- Benzodiazepines. Both long and short acting can increase risk of falling due to drowsiness or sedation.
- Antidepressants. The lowest dose possible may reduce the likeliness of falls.
- Cardiovascular medications. Digoxin and antihypertensive medications may cause dizziness upon standing or finishing a meal (postprandial hypotension).
  (Blazer, 2006; Landefeld et al., 2004, pp. 81–82).

A resource tool for the nursing facility "A Took Kit to Prevent Senior Falls: Falls in Nursing Homes" can be downloaded from the CDC's (Centers for Disease Control) National Center for Injury Prevention and Control from www.cdc.gov/ncipe/factsheets/nursing.htm.

Fractures

Frequently, when facility residents fall, they fracture one of the bones in their body. Often this is in either the spine or the hip (Landefeld et al.,

2004, p. 272 ff.). When a nursing home resident fractures the hip, two treatment approaches are used.

One is to place the resident on bed rest. Lyon and Nevins suggest that this conservative form of treatment is safer and less likely to lead to further mental decline or other complications (1984, p. 391). The other approach is for the resident to have surgery to repair the hip. Often the patient is provided with an artificial prosthesis. Gordon (1989) argues for definitive treatment within the first 24 to 72 hours, early ambulation with physical therapy.

The danger of hip fracture increases dramatically with age: In women ages 75–79 the incidence of hip fracture is 6 of 1,000 falls, for those 85–89 the incidence of hip fracture rises to 48.6 per 1,000 falls (Landefeld et al., 2004, p. 273; Maddox & Sussman, 2001, pp. 377, 489).

It is important for the nursing facility to record in the patient's records and on incident reports whether the fracture was due to a fall or force (e.g., being lifted out of bed by a nursing assistant) or was a pathological fracture due to bone giving way under normal use (e.g., standing up).

Amputees

Amputees are another group of nursing facility residents who need special assistance when walking.

Three-fourths of all amputations are performed on patients 65 years of age and older. The most common type of amputation is the removal of the leg either above or below the knee (abbreviated as AKA or BKA). An amputation is the treatment of last resort for residents with a severe infection, peripheral vascular disease, or injury that is often related to diabetes. Many devices are available to restore lost function. In the absence of suitable prosthetic devices, the environment can be changed to accommodate to the resident's skills.

Contractures

Often patients with chronic rheumatoid arthritis develop contractures in their hands. Contractures are a deformity that result when the muscle has shortened and pulls the adjacent joint into a flexed position. After a period of time the joint becomes fixed in this position and results in a permanent deformity in which the joint cannot be straightened. Contractures are another disruption likely to occur in the immobilized resident.

Other joints that are likely to develop contractures, besides those in the hand and wrist, include the foot, hips, and legs.

The best form of treatment for contractures is to help prevent them by exercising the joints of those who are unable to do so for themselves. These are called passive range-of-motion exercises and can be taught to the resident's family. Proper positioning in bed helps prevent the development of these contractures. Special devices and splints are available for that purpose. Contractures are major health problems that must be identified and addressed as early as possible. All health care staff including nurses aides must be made responsible for early identification of the onset of a contracture.

In 2006, more than one out of every four (28.92%) of nursing facility residents suffered from some form of contractures (DHHS, 2006, F78, F100–F106).

Rehabilitation Services

Rehabilitation services are provided under the direction of a rehabilitation professional (usually a physical therapist, occupational therapist, or speech therapist) to improve functioning. The rate at which residents received these services declined slightly from 19% in 1993 to 16% in 1999. These services varied from 7% of residents in South Dakota facilities to 38% in Alaska (Harrington et al., 2000, p. 49).

Over recent decades the availability of both occupational and speech therapists has been increasing. The number of active occupational therapists increased from 25,000 in 1980 to 72,000 in 2000 and for speech therapists the number practicing increased from 50,000 to 121,000 during that same time period (DHHS, 2005, Table 108, p. 346).

Limited Range of Motion Services

Residents with limited range of motion must receive appropriate treatment and services to increase their range and to prevent declines in range of motion. During the years 1993–1999 between 8% and 9% of facilities received deficiencies for failure to provide sufficient range of motion therapies.

5.3.8 GENITOURINARY (RENAL) SYSTEM

The renal system consists of the two kidneys, which filter wastes from the blood, and two ureters, which transmit the filtered materials (urine) from the kidneys to the bladder, where the urine is stored until discharged through the urethra (Lindeman, 2006, pp. 630–632; Malone-Lee, 1995, p. 402).

In addition to removing waste materials from the bloodstream, the kidneys also help regulate the amount of fluids in the body. At the same time, the kidneys also monitor the level of important electrolytes including sodium (Na), potassium (K+), and calcium (Ca+++).

Channels within the kidney filter the blood and collect a concentration of waste products and excess fluids. The newly filtered blood supply is returned to the general circulation by the renal vein and the concentration of waste materials or urine travels from within the kidney to the bladder by connecting tubes (ureters).

The bladder is a balloon-like muscular structure that serves as a holding tank for the continuous stream of urine produced by the kidneys. When a sufficient amount of urine has collected in the bladder, signals are sent to the brain identifying the need to urinate.

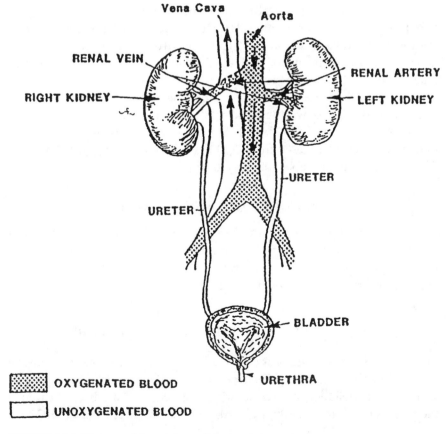

FIGURE 5.11 Diagram of the urinary and renal system.

Individuals have voluntary control over the bladder in responding to this need to urinate. A nerve impulse sent back to the bladder signals it to contract and expel urine through the urethra, at which point it leaves the body. See Figure 5.11 for an illustration of the location of the renal system for both men and women.

Effects of Aging on the Renal System

The average 80-year-old adult, according to some studies, has approximately one-half of the renal function of a normal 30-year-old (Evans et al., 2000, pp. 56, 648; Landefeld et al., 2004, p. 247).

Because the kidneys are so closely associated with the circulatory system, age-associated atherosclerotic (hardening) changes in blood vessels can also affect the kidney. Because of the location of the renal organs, age-related changes in the reproductive organs also influence their ability to function. A diagram of the urinary system is presented in Figure 5.11.

Studies have shown that the ability of the kidneys to concentrate urine probably decreases with age. A progressive loss of renal mass (size) is also believed to occur (Lindeman, 2006, pp. 630–632; Rowe, 1982, p. 223). However, these changes have not been associated with an overall decline of kidney function. Because the bladder is a muscle, its capacity to hold large amounts of urine also seems to decrease with age.

Alterations in Renal Function

Disruptions in renal function may be caused by problems in an associated system or systems, such as arteriosclerotic changes in blood vessels and changes in body nutrients, as in diabetes, leading to renal failure.

A disruption may also be due to a malfunction of the kidney itself or to some type of internal blockage within the kidney and ureters, as with kidney stones or tumors. Approximately 10% of nursing home residents are estimated to have kidney problems.

Chronic Renal Failure

Renal failure is the inability of the kidney to filter out body waste products. This can be either an acute (short-term) or more likely, a chronic (long-term) process.

Chronic renal failure may be caused by cardiovascular changes leading to a decreasing amount of blood being filtered through the kidneys. This decrease in blood flow can result in permanent damage to some of the kidney's internal filtering mechanisms (nephrons) that require continual use for optimal functioning. The most obvious physical sign of renal failure is uremia, or a decrease in urine output, which may progressively lead to oliguria, or no urine output.

The symptoms of chronic renal failure, much like the disease itself, develop gradually. Some of the initial symptoms include dehydration, electrolyte imbalance, osteoporosis, nocturia (producing much urine at night), and anemia (Landefeld et al., 2004, p. 251; Malone-Lee, 2006, pp. 1205–1210). Most patients experience symptoms of fatigue and weakness. With worsening or renal failure, buildup of nitrogenous wastes leads to gastrointestinal symptoms (nausea, anorexia, hiccups) and later to neurological symptoms (sleepiness, confusion, irritability). Urinary frequency and nocturia are common because of a loss of concentrating function (Landefeld et al., 2004, p. 252).

When little or no urine is produced by the body, toxic waste materials may build up, which could damage other organs and cause painful symptoms, including itching and dry skin, mental confusion, weakness, muscle cramps, nausea, vomiting, and diarrhea. The elderly are particularly prone to developing end state renal disease and are the largest group entering kidney dialysis programs (Faubert, Shapiro, Porush, & Kahn, 1989, pp. 245–246; Lindeman, 2006, pp. 630–632).

In 2003, 35,000 U.S. residents aged 65 and over died of nephritis (DHHS, 2005, Table 32, p. 183).

End Stage Renal Disease

Chronic renal failure that has progressed to the stage where little or no urine is being produced is called end stage renal disease (ESRD). The two most common forms of treatment are kidney transplantation and dialysis (Lindeman, 2006, pp. 630–632; Maddox & Sussman, 2001, p. 423).

Kidney dialysis (hemodialysis, i.e., filtering the blood) requires special equipment that performs much like the kidney in filtering unwanted waste materials and fluids from the blood. The process is usually performed in special clinics and takes several hours. The patient's blood is circulated externally through a small machine that filters the blood in much the same fashion as the kidney itself. Feinstein and Friedman (1979) report that from its inception hemodialysis has been successful when used for older patients.

Peritoneal dialysis may be performed for the bedridden patient; it involves filtering out excess fluids from the peritoneum, which lines the abdominal organs (i.e., the serious membrane lining the walls of the abdominal and pelvic cavities, containing the viscera). This procedure is similar to kidney dialysis. The waste products are filtered out through dialyzing the peritoneal cavity instead of the kidneys themselves.

In 2006, under 2% of nursing home residents (1.47%) were receiving kidney dialysis (DHHS, 2006, F78–F93).

Renal Calculi

Kidney stones, or renal calculi, are formed in the kidney as a result of an imbalance in body chemistry. These stones are hard crystalline stone-like substances that become a problem when they block urine flow out of the kidney or block any other area of the renal system.

The group of residents most at risk for developing kidney stones are those unable to move or who are on chronic bed rest. In the previous section we discussed how these residents are likely to suffer from increased osteoporosis. The extra calcium that the body absorbs may also form kidney stones when enough of this mineral is filtered.

Symptoms are blood in urine, decrease in urine outflow, and pain in the back or side. Treatment consists of relief of pain symptoms and medications to relax ureters, allowing the stones to pass. If retrieved, the stones are analyzed to determine their composition and the necessity for any further treatment. In recent years, the need for surgical removal of kidney stones has been greatly reduced by the use of a machine called a lithotripter, which bombards and breaks the kidney stones into small fragments by directing electrical shock waves that pass harmlessly through body tissue to break up the kidney stones.

Urinary Incontinence

Urinary incontinence is the inability to control the timing of urination. Bladder or urinary incontinence more often than one time a week is a common problem in nursing facility residents (Harrington et al., 2000, p. 55; Lindeman, 2006, pp. 631–632). There are many reasons why a resident may become incontinent, including neurologic damage, chronic constipation, and impactions. A defect in the nervous system (stroke patients who lose nervous control of the bladder), urinary tract infections, and constant pressure on the bladder from other disorders such as constipation all may cause incontinence (Evans et al., 2000, p. 672; Kane et al., 2004, p. 152; Malone-Lee, 2006, pp. 1205–1207).

Figure 5.12 indicates that a persistent half of all residents have bladder incontinence. The percentage of residents in a bladder incontinence training program nearly doubled from 5.0% in 1993 to 9.92% in 2006.

Problems in mobility that prevent the resident from reaching the toilet in time may also lead to incontinence. The nursing staff must be prompt in

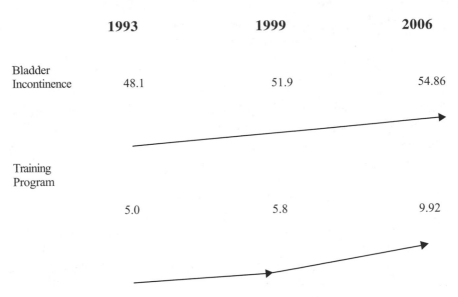

1993	1999	2006

Bladder
Incontinence   48.1   51.9   54.86

Training
Program

5.0   5.8   9.92

FIGURE 5.12 Trends and percent of U.S. nursing home residents with bladder incontinence
and percent in a bladder incontinence training program, 1993, 1999, and 2006.
Source: DHHS, 2006, F78–F99.

assisting the resident to the bathroom on a regular schedule. The resident is
more able to empty the bladder if placed on the commode.

Bladder retraining is used to assist the resident in using the bathroom at appropriate times. There are several types of bladder retraining programs (Kane
et al., 2004). Once assurance has been obtained that there is no impaction,
the nurses monitor the amount of fluid consumed by the resident and assist
the patient to use the toilet about 2 hours afterwards. A persistent 5% to 6% of
all residents were in a bladder training program during the years 1993–1999
(Harrington et al., 2000, p. 55).

Residents who are unable to use a bathroom are catheterized. Urine is released intermittently about every 2 hours following fluid intake. Special devices are also used to assist the resident in voiding (urinating). These include
bed pans, urinals for men, and bedside commodes for the resident who can
get up out of bed.

If none of these treatments are successful, some type of drainage system
can be ordered for the resident. Men may use either a condom-like or an
indwelling type of catheter. Women may use only the indwelling catheter,
which is inserted into the urethra and threaded up into the bladder. Urine
flows out of the bladder and through the catheter. It is then collected in a
clear plastic drainage bag. This is a closed system to attempt to control the
introduction of bacteria or other harmful microorganisms into the urinary

tract, but it is a last choice because urinary tract infections are associated with this approach (Kane et al., 2004; Lindeman, 2006, pp. 630–632; Maddox & Sussman, 2001, p. 423).

See National Association for Continence—www.nafc.org.

Urinary Tract Infections

Increased risk for urinary tract infections (UTI) includes prostatic hypertrophy and loss of estrogen effect, neurogenic bladder from stroke or diabetes, incontinence, and use of indwelling and condom cathethers (Gubitz, 2006, pp. 206–208; Landefeld et al., 2004, p. 349; Malone-Lee, 2006, pp. 1205–1207).

Asymptomatic Bacteriuria

Asymptomatic bacteriuria (>100,000 colonies/mL on 2 consecutive specimens in an asymptomatic patient) is common in the nursing home population (Landefeld et al., 2004, p. 349). In the nursing home asymptomatic bacteriuria is more likely to be antibiotic resistant than in the general population. Distinguishing asymptomatic from symptomatic infection is difficult. Pyuria is almost always present, frequently there is no fever and the resident is often unable to describe symptoms. Thus, in the absence of some objective evidence of infection, such as fever, pain, or change in cognitive or functional status, treatment for a positive culture should be withheld and the resident carefully observed (Landefeld et al., 2004, p. 349; Malone-Lee, 2006, pp. 1205–1207). The most commonly isolated organisms are Escherichia coli, Klebsilla pneumoniae, Proteus mirabilis, and staphlococci (Landefeld et al., 2004, p. 349). Residents with suspected sepsis from UTI should be sent to the hospital. Recommended medications include Ciprofloxacin®, Levofloxacin®, Amoxacillin®/clavulanic acid, or Ceftriaxone®.

According to Kurtz, of all age groups, the elderly most frequently have UTI and associated illnesses (1982, p. 54). Together, UTI and pneumonia were found to be responsible for more than half of all infections in a chronic-care facility studied (Evans et al., 2000, p. 56; Farber, Brennen, Punteri, & Brody, 1982, p. 518). Sterile catheter insertions tend to become infected within 3 weeks regardless of preventive efforts (Evans et al., 2000, p. 700 ff.).

Infection from urinary catheters is, therefore, usually impossible to prevent. The bladder is usually sterile. Urinary tract infections are the most common form of catheter-related infections and account for 30% of all nosocomial infections. The female rate of urinary tract infections is higher than the male rate because pathogenic organisms traveling up the outside of the catheter have a shorter distance to travel in women (2") compared to men (6" to 8"). When urinary catheters are used for extended periods of time the risk for acute UTI complicated by pyelonephritis (inflammation of the kidney) occurs. Sepsis from pyelonephritis is a major cause of death in patients with long indwelling catheters.

The most commonly associated causes of UTI, as identified by Bjork and Tight, include lack of hand washing between patient contacts (an example of poor infection control practices by staff), close proximity of residents with catheters, and the prevalence of residents who have indwelling urinary catheters (1983, p. 1675). Other causes, such as poor insertion techniques and poor positioning of drainage bags, have been identified as causes of infection.

Indwelling Catheter Rates

Indwelling catheters are tubes used to drain the bladder. In 1993, about 8% of facility residents were catherized declining to 7% in 1999 (Harrington et al., 2000, p. 59). There has been a constant push to reduce the number of residents with indwelling catheters.

Residents with urinary catheters often show no symptoms associated with the initial stages of this infection. Residents who do not have indwelling catheters may complain of **symptoms,** including burning and painful urination, cloudy and foul smelling urine, fever, and chills. The indwelling catheter should be cleaned daily with soap and water where it enters the urethra and the catheter itself changed aseptically every month.

An initial form of **treatment** is to obtain a sample of urine, which may be studied to determine the organisms present. Antibiotic therapy is usually held off for as long as possible. There is only a limited number of antibiotics available to treat UTI, and residents with chronic indwelling catheters are likely to become resistant to these antibiotics quickly, at which point there is little alternative treatment available. As many as 50% of urinary tract infections are recurrent.

A frequently encountered nursing facility problem is that many elderly women have asymptomatic bacteriuria (Evans et al., 2000, p. 703). Treatment protocols may indicate a constant need for treatment in these cases. However, chronic suppressive antibiotic administration to these residents can be counterproductive because it can lead to development of antibiotic-resistant organisms leading to a super infection.

In an effort to avoid overuse of antibiotics, a new trend among geriatric physicians is to treat UTI only if it is symptomatic, that is, burning discomfort or pain; not treating when the culture is positive but the patient is asympotomatic.

UTI is an ongoing treatment challenge in the nursing facility. New approaches are constantly being sought. Practical experience suggests that no matter how careful or sterile the procedures, infection often spreads, not on the inside but up the outside of the inserted tube. Despite every staff effort an incontinent female patient may be at risk of infection within minutes after incontinence occurs.

Facilities have been cited at about the rate of 11% of facilities over the years 1993 to 1999 for improper bladder care (Harrington et al., 2000, p. 99).

Bowel Incontinence Rates

Bowel incontinence more often than one time a week is also a common problem among nursing facility residents. Over the years 1993 through 1999 a persistent 42% of all residents were afflicted with bowel incontinence (Harrington et al., 2000, p. 57). About 4% of residents were in a bowel training program.

Ostomy Care Rate

Ostomy care includes special care for a skin opening to the intestine or urinary tract such as a colostomy (opening to the colon). Ostomy care was provided to between 2% and 3% of residents during the years 1993 to 1999 (Harrington et al., 2000, p. 49).

5.3.9 REPRODUCTIVE SYSTEM

The reproductive system in the younger adult has the capacity to promote the creation of new life and facilitate the expression of intimacy through human contact. Some of the most notable changes in the elderly include the woman's loss of reproductive capabilities following menopause (change of life), whereas a man retains reproductive capabilities. However, both sexes have continued needs to express their sexuality throughout the life span (Wallace, 1992, p. 309).

The first part of this section is a description of the reproductive organs and age-associated changes for each sex; the second is a discussion of sexuality and the nursing home resident.

Women

The reproductive organs in women include the ovaries, which produce eggs that travel down the fallopian tubes to the uterus about once every month. Hormones act to control these reproductive cycles. Estrogen is the female sex hormone that directs most of these processes.

The organs of the lower reproductive tract are the cervix, the uterus, and the vagina. The cervix is the opening of the uterus leading into the vagina. The vagina is a barrel-shaped organ that leads to the external genitals in the female reproductive tract, such as the labia and the clitoris. During mid-life most women go through menopause (cessation of egg production and therefore of menstruation) and are no longer fertile.

Diseases of the uterus tend to decrease with age. Changes in the reproductive system are closely related to decreases in secretions of the hormone estrogen.

Some of the physical changes that may be experienced by elderly women include a loss of tone and elasticity in the breast, uterus, cervix, and vagina; a thinning and drying of the vaginal walls, which may cause uncomfortable irritations; infections and bleeding; decrease in size of the uterus, fallopian tubes, and vagina; loss of pubic hair; and decrease in the number of ducts or milk glands of the breasts.

Elderly women do not tend to suffer from diseases of the uterus or reproductive tract per se. However, the incidence of breast cancer does continue to rise with age, and it remains the most common type of cancer affecting elderly women (Balducci, 2006, pp. 155–158). The signs and symptoms of breast cancer are a hardened lump or thickening in the breast and change in size of the breast and the nipples. Treatment depends of the extent of the disease and may include surgery, radiation, or chemotherapy, as well as the relief of associated symptoms.

Another age-related change is genital prolapse. This occurs when the tone of the genital organs becomes so weakened that they begin to drop and may seem to fall out of the vagina. Women with weak muscles are at risk. Some of the signs and symptoms associated with genital prolapse include constant pressure on the bladder, incontinence of urine and a sense of weight in the pelvis. Usually this disorder can be repaired surgically.

Decrease in the production of the female sex hormone estrogen may also lead to osteoporosis (discussed under the previous section on the musculoskeletal system). With the exception of arthritis, the rate of chronic disease among women is about equal to the rates of men (Evans et al., 2000, p. 22; Giangregorio et al., 2006, pp. 883–885).

Men

The primary organs of the male reproductive tract are the testes, scrotum, prostate, and penis.

The testes are encased within the scrotum and produce the male hormone testosterone and sperm cells. These cells mature as they travel through the surrounding epididymis until released into the vas deferens. The sperm travel through the vas deferens until they are released from the ejaculatory ducts into the urethra. Nearby ducts secrete seminal fluid from the prostate gland, which provides food for the sperm as well as enhancing their motility. When the male ejaculates, the sperm travel down the urethra through the penis and are emitted from the body (Balducci, 2006, pp. 155–158; Maddox & Sussman, 2001, p. 641).

Some of the age-related changes in the male reproductive tract are an enlargement of the prostate gland, decreased production of testosterone, which may result in slight decreases in sexual desire, and a reduction in muscle bulk and strength. Sperm production continues into advanced old age, so males continue with the ability to impregnate into old age.

Problems with the prostate gland are a major concern for many elderly men. Enlargement of the prostate is a common age-related change in men. For some men, this enlargement may interfere with the ability to urinate or may cause incontinence (Balducci, 2006, pp. 155–158; Maddox & Sussman, 2001, p. 385). Prostatitis is an inflammation of this gland that often develops following the initial enlargement of the prostate gland and can be very painful. Other symptoms include painful urination and blood in the urine.

This enlargement may develop into cancer of the prostate, which is the second most common form of cancer in elderly men. Cancer of the prostate is considered a "geriatric disease," with 95% of all cases seen in elderly men. The initial symptoms for this disease are the same as those experienced with prostatitis, including a decrease in urination and discomfort. Surgery is usually performed to remove the cancerous or extremely large prostate. Chemotherapy or hormone treatments may also be used.

Coping With Sexuality

Sexual needs persist into old age, with continued activity considered healthy and health preserving. The elderly nursing home resident, like those in the community, continues to have needs for a positive self-image and self-esteem (Maddox & Sussman, 2001, p. 903), which are closely associated with the needs for intimacy and sexuality. Too often, society and individuals discourage sexual activity in the nursing home because of existing stereotypes and misunderstandings about sex and old age (Verrillo, 2006, pp. 1191–1192).

Sexuality is not achieved exclusively by sexual intercourse, but may also incorporate a variety of activities related to touch and displays of affection. Older people may be more likely to express their sexuality in these more diffuse and varied terms.

The sexual partners of those who have confirmed HIV antibody tests are themselves at risk for developing AIDS. Education to prevent disease transmission in the facility may become important.

Impotence, or the inability to perform sexually, is more often attributed to the male. The extent of this disorder in old age is not known, but an early American Medical Association (1967) report revealed that, rather than organic problems, anxiety and internalization of societal pressures account for most of the problems related to impotence (Kay & Neeley, 1982; Evans et al., 2000, p. 1000). Nursing homes are often perceived as disapproving and as actively discouraging displays of love or affection among residents. A frequent suggestion in the literature is that nursing home staff be educated concerning sexuality in old age and that more efforts be made to deal with problems of morality that may arise.

Stillwell and O'Conner (1989) attempt to dispel some of the myths concerning sexuality with the observation that

- older people do remain interested in sex
- older people find each other physically attractive
- sexuality contributes to overall well-being

Contrary to public perceptions, the incidence of a heart attack or stroke during sexual intercourse is actually very low, and sexual activity is sometimes recommended for patients with diseases such as arthritis because of the therapeutic effects of exercise and intimacy.

One research study suggests allowing for privacy of some residents to develop closer relationships. Another encourages the development of programs to deal with quality-of-life issues such as loneliness and isolation that are important to residents. Sexual expression would be only one component of this effort (Kahana, B., 1995, p. 526).

5.3.10 EMOTIONAL AND MENTAL WELL-BEING

A number of the physical system disruptions discussed previously can have profound effects on the mental well-being of the nursing home resident.

Effects of Aging

Differences of opinion exist as to whether intelligence declines with age. One difficulty is the use of tests that may not be appropriate measures for the elderly.

Aging is associated with special problems that may not be as disruptive for younger individuals. Burnside identifies two of these as behavioral problems and mental illness (1981, p. 63). The range of behaviors residents employ to cope with these problems will vary, but studies often show that many of the recurrent problems in a nursing home are related to behavioral problems.

When residents are admitted to the facility, they may display initial symptoms of anxiety and apprehension regarding their new surroundings (Trella, 1994, p. 313). Chronic illness and the process of dying are anxiety-provoking and necessarily are an aspect of life with which nursing home residents must constantly cope.

Anxiety may be experienced by most individuals, and each deals with it in a particular way. Some manifestations of anxiety include fantasizing, hostile or dependent behavior, avoidance of eye contact, fidgeting, insomnia, and isolation from other.

Insomnia

Insomnia, or sleep disorder, is common among the elderly. Studies of human sleep patterns have shown that the elderly spend more time in bed, have more difficulty getting to sleep, or tend to awaken during sleep periods.

Sleep problems may result from the use of multiple medications as well as from anxiety. To assist the residents to cope, sleeping medications may be prescribed, along with increases in daily activities and attempts to alleviate the source of anxiety.

Loneliness

Behaviors associated with loneliness are similar to those of a mild depressive mood and include isolation, constipation, weight loss, insomnia, fatigue, and loss of appetite. Depression is often associated with losses, some of which are depicted in Figure 5.13. Identifying and addressing mild depression is a major issue in nursing facility care. A significant proportion of nursing home residents experience mild depression, which often remains unidentified and unaddressed by the facility staff.

Treatment for these residents is to discern the cause of depression and try to help them cope effectively with those feelings (Aller & Van Ess Coeling,

FIGURE 5.13 Losses, adjustments, and gains of persons admitted to long-term care.

1995, p. 21; Moore & Gilbert, 1995, p. 7). If these behaviors persist and worsen, the resident may be progressing toward mental illness. Antidepressive medications may also be prescribed in these cases (see Ade-Ridder & Kaplan, 1993, p. 13; Blazer, 2006, pp. 303–305; and Engel & Graney, 1993, p. S18)

The deaths per 100,000 resident population aged 65 years and over has been falling: 7% in 1990, down to 4% in 2003 (DHHS, 2005, Table 46, p. 223).

Mental Illness

Some studies have revealed that about 10% of elderly citizens have severe mental illness, and the incidence of mental illness tends to increase as people age. It is estimated that the rate of mental illness in nursing homes is somewhere between one-fourth and one-half of all residents. This high prevalence of mental illness may be a result of preexisting problems.

Often the term senile is used to describe a variety of behaviors in mental illness, ranging from slight forgetfulness to a generalized decline in mental functioning of the elderly.

Those with a history of mental illness often have been transferred to the nursing home from a psychiatric facility, a phenomenon brought about by the development of psychotropic drugs in the 1950s and 1960s. This population may also be suffering from mental retardation.

Psychotrophic drugs are those that exert an effect on the mind. They are usually used to calm and control patient behavior. Equipped with these new medications and a belief that mentally ill persons are better cared for in the community setting, most states dramatically reduced the number of persons held in the state mental hospitals. It is believed that a significant portion of persons who were deinstitutionalized during this movement have entered the nursing home as a substitute for the mental hospital. As time passes, and the states continue to keep lower the number of hospital beds available for the mentally ill, this phenomenon is likely to continue (Mosher-Ashley & Henrikson, 1993, p. 34).

Psychoactive Drug Rates

The percentage of residents receiving psychoactive drugs is rising (see Figure 5.14). By 1999, half of all residents were on psychoactive medications. This progressively increased over the years 1999 to 2006. By 2006, two-thirds of residents were receiving psychoactive drugs. Such drugs include antidepressants, antianxiety drugs, sedatives and hypnotics, and antipsychotics. There has been pressure from the federal government for facilities to prescribe fewer psychoactive drugs while at the same time encouraging facilities to diagnose patients and prescribe more antidepressant drugs.

The second group of mentally ill patients often become emotionally disturbed because they are no longer able to cope with the physical and social changes associated with the aging process (Miller, 1994, p. 35).

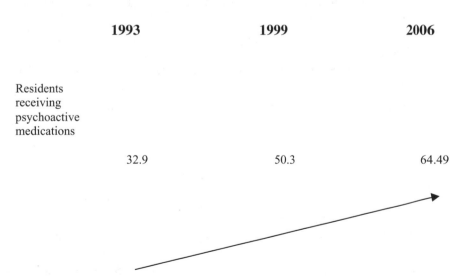

1993   **1999**   **2006**

Residents
receiving
psychoactive
medications

32.9   50.3   64.49

FIGURE 5.14 Trend among residents in U.S. nursing facilities receiving psychoactive medications, 1993, 1999, and 2006.
Source: DHHS, 2006, F78.

Who is mentally ill? What is mental illness? These are difficult questions in the setting of the nursing facility (Haight, 1995, p. 105; Scott, Bramble, & Goodyear, 1991, p. 21). The changes brought about by chronic physical illnesses and by the "normal" social changes faced by older persons are sometimes powerful enough to overwhelm even a well-adjusted person. The line between disabling mental illnesses and the day-to-day effects of attempting to cope with aging, especially in the institutionalized setting of the nursing facility, is often blurred.

Organic Brain Syndrome

Organic brain syndrome, brain failure, and senility are all different words describing the same disorder (Golden & Cohen, 1995, p. 717; Gwyther, 1995, p. 62). Dementia and Alzheimer's disease have already been discussed as problems of the nervous system.

The two most common causes of organic brain syndrome are (a) Alzheimer's disease, and (b) cerebrovascular insufficiency, or reduced blood flow to the brain. The brain tissue responds to any impairments resulting from these disorders with a variety of symptoms that initially can involve memory loss, leading to levels of disorientation and confusion and to difficulty following even simple directions. These symptoms of confusion progress until the resident is no longer aware of reality (Blustein, 1993, p. 6; Emanuel & Emanuel, 1992, p. 2067).

Affected residents may engage in such problematic behaviors as suicidal threats or attempts, destructiveness, hostility, nosiness, and wandering off (Busse & Pfeiffer, 1973, p. 173; Rantz & McShane, 1995, p. 23). These behaviors can become especially troublesome in the group setting of a nursing home. Psychiatric consultation is usually desirable in these instances.

Diagnostic Tests

- brain scans: not always indicated if there are no focal neurological findings, gait is normal.
- MRI (magnetic resonance imaging): shows more detail and white matter changes.
- CT (cat scan): adequate to rule out treatable problems such as clots, stroke, hydrocephalus.
  (Jones, 2004)

Treatment can include

- reality orientation (continually reminding residents of the date, time and place to keep the oriented to their environment; Maddox & Sussman, 2001, p. 859). (Note: Some observers, however, feel reality orientation increases anxiety whereas behavioral disturbances may decrease if staff enter the resident's reality.)
- choosing compatible roommates and company for these residents
- avoiding sudden changes or surprises
- increasing the amount of assistance available to these residents to perform the activities of daily living (Fillenbaum, 1995, p. 9)
- providing a supportive environment

The most disoriented patients are typically those with advanced dementia (Baldwin, 1995, p. 286). Results of a study of Rhode Island facilities showed that about 26% of nursing home residents studied were disruptive at least once in 2 weeks, for example, physical abuse, screaming, wandering (Maddox & Sussman, 2001, p. 305; National Center for Health Services, 1989, p. 8).

Restraints

The restraint issue is one of the most debated in the nursing home industry (Landefeld et al., 2004, p. 41; Strumpf & Evans, 1995, p. 819). Restraints are variously defined. In essence, a restraint is anything that restricts a resident beyond their will (Maddox & Sussman, 2001, p. 883). Restraints may be physical, for example, a vest or a gerichair that keeps the resident from getting out of the chair, or mental, for example, the use of psychotropic drugs to control anxiety or agitation. Some nursing chains have achieved a restraint free environment in groups of facilities after mounting a conscious program (Technical Assistance Services, March/April, 1995).

The use of restraints, particularly physical restraints, is one of the thorniest issues in long-term care. Cogent arguments for and against them can be marshaled (Aller & Van Ess Coeling, 1995, p. 21; Bourbonniere, Evans, & Strumpf, 2006, pp. 1027–1029; Brooke, 1991–1992, p. 9; Burger, 1994, p. 3; Janelli, Kanski, & Neary, p. 18; Johnson, 1995, p. 75; Magee et al., 1993, p. 31; Menscer, 1993, p. 145; Moss & La Puma, 1991, p. 22; Scherer, Janelli, Kanski, Neary, & Morth, 1991, p. 14; Watzke & Wister, 1993, p. 24; Werner, Cohen-Mansfield, Koroknay, & Braun, 1994, p. 19). Reducing chemical restraints has also been of concern and is a source of contention.

Restraint use is now closely regulated with monthly reviews and justifications mandated under nursing home reform requirements. Many facilities have moved toward a restraint free environment, because, in the their view, restraints kill the human spirit.

Figure 5.15 reveals an increase in the number of contractures identified among residents during the years 1993 to 2006. Restraint use, however, has decreased 50% over these same years, from 20% in 1993 to 10% in 1999, continuing downward to 6.58% in 2006.

By 2006, after a strong effort by the federal and state governments and private organizations, percent of nursing home residents being restrained had gone down to 6.91%. Only 1.4% of residents had physician orders for restraints (DHHS, 2006, F78, F100–F106).

Increasingly, facilities are moving toward a "no restraint" policy.

Depression

Depression is probably the most common mental illness in the elderly (Blazer, 1995, p. 266; Blazer, 2006, pp. 303–305; Landefeld et al., 2004, p. 464;

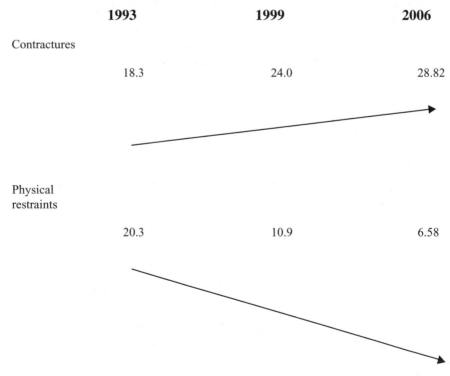

	1993	**1999**	**2006**
Contractures	18.3	24.0	28.82

	1993	**1999**	**2006**
Physical restraints	20.3	10.9	6.58

FIGURE 5.15 Percent of residents in U.S. nursing homes with contractures and percent with physical restraints.
Source: DHHS, 2006, F100–F106.

Teuth, 1995, p. 43). Residents must be assessed to determine whether they are merely in a depressed mood or if the disease has progressed to a mental illness (Kane et al., 2004). Often depression may be associated with another underlying chronic disease (e.g., arthritis or Parkinson's disease) or may be a result of a reaction to medications. Depression can be a symptom or precursor of other chronic diseases. Depression often looks just like dementia in residents. Symptoms begin or worsen over weeks or months and should be treated.

Importance of Treating Depression

- depression worsens patients' functioning of activities of daily living
- increases the likelihood of illnesses
- increases the possibility of death in less than a few years
- affects sleep, energy level, and quality of life.
  (Jones, 2004)

How to Identify a Depression on Top of a Dementia

- less interested in usual activities
- increase or decrease in usual appetite
- insomnia or sleeping too much
- more nervous, agitated, or pacing more than usual
- more forgetful of daily routine suddenly
- like medical delirium, pays less attention to you and others
- not able to sit as well for looking at magazines, watching TV
- talks about being dead or wanting to kill him/herself
- may become more withdrawn, emotions may seem "frozen"

Additional signs of depression include loss of appetite resulting in weight loss, feelings of sadness, loss of interest in people, and a sense of great effort needed to perform daily activities. The elderly may also complain of symptoms that are actually attributable to depression. Often the real problem is loss of control over their daily lives and lack of decision-making opportunities (Everard, Rowles, & High, 1994, p. 520).

Treatment of depression can include the use of antidepressant medications, usually tricyclic antidepressant drugs or newer ones such as Prozac and Paxil (The Johns Hopkins Medical Letter, January, 1995, p. 5; Landefeld et al., 2004, p. 103). These drugs themselves, however, also have strong side effects (Kane et al., 2004; Landefeld et al., 2004, p. 102).

Electrocortical shock treatment is a powerful form of treatment used to stimulate a specified area of the brain. The use of electro shock treatments for depression and other mental disorders has been a subject of intense controversy for decades (Kane et al., 2004).

Counseling, group activities, and social functions appear to be productive therapeutic techniques available to the nursing home staff.

In essence, efforts by the staff to restore a sense of worth and importance to the resident may be among the most powerful tools available. Some of these include daily exercise, such as aerobics geared to the resident's level of physical capacity, dance therapy, recreation therapy, work therapy, and bibliotherapy (reading books; Maddox & Sussman, 2001, p. 369; Osgood, 1995, p. 548; Waldo, Ide, & Thomas, 1995, p. 12).

5.4 Final Observations on a Career in Nursing Home Administration

Fix It (the Facility) All the Time

Nobel laureate Albert Szent-Gyorgyi observed that there is a tendency for all living things to keep growing, changing, and evolving. Everything around us is constantly changing: the health system, the economic system, the aging population itself, and its relationship to everything else. The relationships among hospitals, nursing homes, assisted-living facilities, life care communities, home health agencies, third-party payers, health maintenance organizations, managed care processes, and government regulations are always in flux. If the nursing facility does not change and grow, improve and evolve, it will face extinction. The nursing facility is a living organism. Treat it as alive and you and it will survive.

Fix It (Your Own Career) All the Time

In the unlikely event that at some point in your career in nursing home administration you feel yourself on a plateau, having achieved all you had hoped in your facility, consider the following.

An aboriginal tribe made it a practice to move on whenever the food was plentiful from lush harvests. When life was this easy they knew they were in danger of becoming fat, lazy, and unprepared for the inevitable seasons of scarcity when their survival skills would be necessary.

Finished Never Is

The Japanese concept of *kaizen* means continuous improvement, a commitment to the idea that "finished never is."

David Harrington, a violinist with the avant-guard Kronos Quartet, finds being an artist a source of perpetual renewal because it is a task that has no ending point.

Pablo Casals, the cellist, was asked why, at the age of 94, he continued to practice as hard each day as he had decades earlier, because he remained clearly the preeminent cellist in the world. He replied that he practiced because he hoped to improve.

REFERENCES

Ade-Ridder, L., & Kaplan, L. (1993). Marriage, spousal care giving, and a husband's move to a nursing home. *Journal of Gerontological Nursing, 19*(10), 13–23.

Agency for Health Care Policy and Research. (1995, March-April). Guidelines on pressure sores released. *Research Activities* (Agency for Health Care Policy and Research, No. 183, AHCPR Pub. No. 95–0051), p. 15.

Albanese, A. A. (1980). *Nutrition for the elderly.* New York: Liss.

Albert, M. (1995). Alzheimer's disease: Clinical. In G. L. Maddox (Ed.), *The encyclopedia of aging* (2nd ed., pp. 56–57). New York: Springer Publishing Company.

Aller, L. J., & Van Ess Coeling, H. (1995). Quality of life: Its meaning to the long term care resident. *Journal of Gerontological Nursing, 21*(2), 20–25.

American Medical Association. (1967). *The extended care facility: A handbook for the medical society.* Chicago: Author.

Anderson, W. F. (1976). *Practical management of the elderly* (3rd ed.). Oxford, England: Blackwell.

Andres, R. (1989). Relation of physiologic changing in aging to medical changes of disease in the aged. In W. Reichel (Ed.), *Clinical aspects of aging* (3rd ed.). Baltimore: Williams & Wilkins.

Aronow, W. S. (2006). Homocysteine. In Richard Schulz (Ed.), *The encyclopedia of aging* (4th ed., pp. 533–536). New York: Springer Publishing Company.

Baldwin, B. A. (1995). Disruptive behaviors. In G. L. Maddox (Ed.), *The encyclopedia of aging* (2nd ed., pp. 284–286). New York: Springer Publishing Company.

Balducci, L. (2006). Cancer control. In Richard Schulz (Ed.), *The encyclopedia of aging* (4th ed., pp. 155–158). New York: Springer Publishing Company.

Balen, A. K., & Lin, A. N. (1995). Connective tissues. In G. L. Maddox (Ed.), *The encyclopedia of aging* (2nd ed., pp. 220–222). New York: Springer Publishing Company.

Balen, A. K. & Vilenchik, M. M. (2006). Connective tissue. In Richard Schulz (Ed.), *The encyclopedia of aging* (4th ed., pp. 259–262). New York: Springer Publishing Company

Barzel, U.S. (1995). Osteoporosis. In G. L. Maddox (Ed.), *The encyclopedia of aging* (2nd ed., pp. 722–723). New York: Springer Publishing Company.

Basen, M. (1977). The elderly and drugs: Problem overview and program strategy. *Public Health Reports, 92*(1), 43–48.

Beck-Sague, C., Banerjee, S., & Jarvis, W. R. (1993). Infectious diseases and mortality among U.S. nursing home residents. *American Journal of Public Health, 83*(12), 1739–1742.

Bennett, D. A., & Knopman, D. S. (1994). Alzheimer's disease: A comprehensive approach to patient management. *Geriatrics, 49*(8), 20–26.

Birchenall, J. M., & Streight, M. E. (1982). *Care of the older adults* (2nd ed.). Philadelphia: Lippincott.

Bjork, D., & Tight, R. (1983). Nursing home hazard of chronic indwelling urinary catheters. *Archives of Internal Medicine, 143*(9), 1675–1676.

Blazer, D. G. (1995). Depression. In G. L. Maddox (Ed.), *The encyclopedia of aging* (2nd ed., pp. 265–266). New York: Springer Publishing Company.

Blazer, D. (2006). Depression. In Richard Schulz (Ed.), *The encyclopedia of aging* (4th ed., pp. 303–305). New York: Springer Publishing Company.

Blustein, J. (1993). The family in medical decision making. *Hastings Center Report, 23*(3), 6–13.

Bourbonniere, M., Evans, L. K., & Strumpf, N. E. (2006). Restraints: physical/chemical. In Richard Schulz (Ed.), *The encyclopedia of aging* (4th ed., pp. 1027–1029). New York: Springer Publishing Company.

Brody, H. (1995a). Central nervous system (brain and spinal cord). In G. L. Maddox (Ed.), *The encyclopedia of aging* (2nd ed., pp. 166–171). New York: Springer Publishing Company.

Brody, H. (1995b). Nerves. In G. L. Maddox (Ed.), *The encyclopedia of aging* (2nd ed., pp. 674–675). New York: Springer Publishing Company.

Brooke, V. (1991–1992, Winter). Meeting the challenge: Involuntary restraints in the nursing home. *The Journal of Long Term Care Administration, 19*, pp. 9–14.

Brown, W.T. (2006). Genetic programming theories. In Richard Schulz (Ed.), *The encyclopedia of aging* (4th ed., pp. 445–447). New York: Springer Publishing Company.

Bruns, H. J. (1995). Gastrointestinal system. In G. L. Maddox (Ed.), *The encyclopedia of aging* (2nd ed., pp. 390–392). New York: Springer Publishing Company.

Burger, S. G. (1994). Avoiding physical restraint use: New standards in care. *Long Term Care Advances* (Duke University Center for the Study of Aging and Human Development), *5*(2), 1–9.

Burnside, I. (Ed.). (1981). *Nursing and the aged.* New York: McGraw Hill.

Busse, E., & Pfeiffer, E. (1973). *Mental illness in later life.* Washington, DC: American Psychological Association.

Carter, D., & Balin, A. (1983). Dermatological aspects of aging. *Medical Clinics of North America, 67*(2), 531–534.

Chui, H. (1995b). Vascular dementia. In G. L. Maddox (Ed.), *The encyclopedia of aging* (2nd ed., pp. 173–174). New York: Springer Publishing Company.

Cohen, F. L. (1995a). Survival. In G. L. Maddox (Ed.), *The encyclopedia of aging* (2nd ed., p. 50). New York: Springer Publishing Company.

Cohen, F. L. (1995b). Tuberculosis. In G. L. Maddox (Ed.), *The encyclopedia of aging* (2nd ed., pp. 945–947). New York: Springer Publishing Company.

Cohen, H.J. & Rao, A.V. (2006). Blood. In R. Schulz (Ed.), *The encyclopedia of aging* (4th ed., pp. 139–142). New York: Springer Publishing Company.

Cooper, J. (1978). Drug therapy in the elderly: Is it all it could be? *American Pharmacist, 18*(7), 25–33.

Corso, J. (1981). *Aging: Sensory systems and perception.* New York: Praeger.

Department of Health and Human Services. (2005). Centers for Disease Control and Prevention, National Center for Health Statistics. Hyattsville, MD: Author.

Department of Health and Human Services. (2006). Centers for Medicare and Medicaid Services, Oscar Form 672: F24–F145.

DePorter, C. (2006, July). Personal communication. Division of Facilities Services, NC.

Emanuel, E. J., & Emanuel, L. L. (1992). Proxy decision making for incompetent patients. *Journal of the American Medical Association, 267,* 2067–2071.

Engel, B. T. (1995). Incontinence. In G. L. Maddox (Ed.), *The encyclopedia of aging* (2nd ed., pp. 501–502). New York: Springer Publishing Company.

Engel, V. F., & Graney, M. J. (1993). Stability and improvement of health after nursing home admission. *Journal of Gerontology, 48*(1), pp. S17–S23.

Everad, K., Rowles, G. D., & High, D. (1994). Nursing home room changes: Toward a decision-making model. *The Gerontologist, 34,* 520–527.

Evans, J. G., Williams, T. F., Beattie, B. L., Michel, J-P, & Wilcock, G. K. (2000). *Oxford textbook of geriatric medicine* (2nd ed.). New York: Oxford University Press.

Evans, J. G. (2006). Vitamins. In Richard Schulz (Ed.), *The encyclopedia of aging* (4th ed., pp. 1215–1217). New York: Springer Publishing Company.

Farber, B., Brennen, C., Punteri, A., & Brody, J. (1982). Nosocomial infections in a chronic care facility. *Journal of the American Geriatric Society, 32,* 513–519.

Faubert, P. F., Shapiro, W. B., Porush, J. G., & Kahn, A. I. (1989). Medical renal disease in aged. In W. Reichel (Ed.), *Clinical aspects of aging* (3rd ed., pp. 228–247). Baltimore: Williams & Wilkins.

Feinstein, E., & Friedman, E. (1979). Renal disease in the elderly. In I. Rossman (Ed.), *Clinical geriatrics* (2nd ed.). Philadelphia: Lippincott.

Fillenbaum, G. G. (1995). Activities of daily living. In G. L. Maddox (Ed.), *Theencyclopedia of aging* (2nd ed., pp. 7–9). New York: Springer Publishing Company.

Franz, M. (1981, Summer). Nutritional requirements of the elderly. *Journal of Nutrition for the Elderly,* 1.

Franz, R. A., & Gardner, S. (1994, September). Clinical concerns: Management of dry skin. *Journal of Gerontological Nursing,* pp. 15–18.

Garagusi, V. F. (1989). Infectious disease problems in the elderly. In W. Reichel (Ed.), *Clinical aspects of aging* (3rd ed., p. 204). Baltimore: Williams & Wilkins.

Garibaldi, R., Brodine, S., & Matsumiya, S. (1981). Infections among patients in nursing homes. *New England Journal of Medicine, 305,* 731–735.

Giangregorio, L. A, Papaioannou, A., & Adachi, J.D. (2006) Osteoporosis. In R. Schulz (Ed.), *The encyclopedia of aging* (4th ed., pp. 883–885). New York: Springer Publishing Company.

Gibbons, J. C., & Levy, S. M. (1989). Gastrointestinal diseases in the aged. In W. Reichel (Ed.), *Clinical aspects of aging* (3rd ed., p. 197). Baltimore: Williams & Wilkins.

Glowacki, G. A. (1989). Geriatric gynecology. In W. Reichel (Ed.), *Clinical aspects of aging* (3rd ed.). Baltimore: Williams & Wilkins.

Golden, C. J., & Cohen, D. I. (1995). Organic brain syndrome. In G. L. Maddox (Ed.), *The encyclopedia of aging* (2nd ed., pp. 686–687). New York: Springer.

Goldrick, B. A., & Larson, E. (1992). Assessing the need for infection control programs: A diagnostic approach. *Journal of Long Term Care Administration, 20*(1), 20–23.

Gordon, J. C. (1989). Musculoskeletal injuries in the elderly. In W. Reichel (Ed.), *Clinical aspects of aging* (3rd ed.). Baltimore: Williams & Wilkins.

Gubitz, G. (2006). Cerebrovascular disease: stroke and transient ischemic attack. In R. Schulz (Ed.), *The encyclopedia of aging* (4th ed., pp. 206–208). New York: Springer Publishing Company.

Guideline for Hand Hygiene in Health-Care Settings Recommendations of the Healthcare Infection Control Practices Advisory Committee and the HICPAC/SHEA/APIC/IDSA Hand Hygiene Task Force issued October 25, 2002/ Morbidity and Mortality Weekly Report, Volume 51, No. RR-16.

Gwyther, L. (1983). Alzheimer's disease. *North Carolina Medical Journal, 44*(7), 435–436.

Gwyther, L. P. (1995). Alzheimer's disease: Special care units. In G. L. Maddox (Ed.), *The encyclopedia of aging* (2nd ed., pp. 60–62). New York: Springer Publishing Company.

Haight, B. K. (1995). Suicide risk in frail elderly people relocated to nursing homes. *Geriatric Nursing, 16*(3), 104–107.

Halter, J. B. (1995). Carbohydrates. In G. L. Maddox (Ed.), *The encyclopedia of aging* (2nd ed., pp. 131–133). New York: Springer Publishing Company.

Harrington, C. H., Carrillo, M. S., Thollaug, S. C., Summers, P. R., & Wellin, V. (2000). *Nursing facilities, staffing, residents, and facility deficiencies, 1993 through 1999.* San Francisco: University of California at San Francisco, Department of Social & Behavioral Sciences.

Harris, R. (1989). Exercise and physical fitness for the elderly. In W. Reichel (Ed.), *Clinical aspects of aging* (3rd ed., pp. 90–91). Baltimore: Williams & Wilkins.

Hayflick, L. (1965). The limited in vitro lifetime of human diploid cell strains. *Experimental Cell Research, 37*(3), 614–636.

Hayflick, L. (1995). Biological aging theories. In G. L. Maddox (Ed.), *The encyclopedia of aging* (2nd ed., pp. 113–118). New York: Springer Publishing Company.

Hefti, F. (1995). Neurotrophic factors and aging. In G. L. Maddox (Ed.), *The encyclopedia of aging* (2nd ed., pp. 686–687). New York: Springer Publishing Company.

Heidrick, M. L. (1995). Autoimmunity. In G. L. Maddox (Ed.), *The encyclopedia of aging* (2nd ed., pp. 99–100). New York: Springer Publishing Company.

Heidrick, M. L. (2006). Autoimmunity. In R. Schulz (Ed.), *The encyclopedia of aging* (4th ed., pp. 95–96). New York: Springer Publishing Company.

Herdman, R. C. (1992). *Special care units for people with Alzheimer's and other dementias: Consumer education, research, regulatory and reimbursement issues* (Office of Technology Assessment 0–328–415 Q1 3, p. 7). Washington, DC: U.S. Government Printing Office.

Hing, E. (1977). *Characteristics of nursing home residents' health status and care received* (NCHS Series 13, No. 51). Washington, DC: Public Health Service.

Hofland, B. F. (1995). Autonomy and aging. In G. L. Maddox (Ed.), *The encyclopedia of aging* (2nd ed., pp. 100–101). New York: Springer Publishing Company.

Howlett, S. E. (2006). Cardiovascular system: Vasculature. In R. Schulz (Ed.), *The encyclopedia of aging* (4th ed., pp. 168–170). New York: Springer Publishing Company.

Janelli, L. M., Kanski, G. W., & Neary, M. A. (1998, June). Physical restraints: Has OBRA made a difference? *Journal of Gerontological Nursing, 49,* pp. 17–21.

Johnson, S. H. (1995, Fall). Law and quality in long term care. *Journal of Long Term Care Administration,* pp. 75–77.

Johnson, S. (2006). Nutrition. In R. Schulz (Ed.), *The encyclopedia of aging* (4th ed., pp. 854–859). New York: Springer Publishing Company.

Jones, B. N. (2004). *Psychosis and agitation in the elderly,* NCHCFA presentation, Winston-Salem, NC.

Jones, J. K. (1989). Drugs and the elderly. In W. Reichel (Ed.), *Clinical aspects of aging* (3rd ed., pp. 50–60). Baltimore: Williams & Wilkins.

Kahana, B. (1995). Isolation. In G. L. Maddox (Ed.), *The encyclopedia of aging* (2nd ed., pp. 526–527). New York: Springer Publishing Company.

Kahana, E. (1995a). Deinstitutionalization. In G. L. Maddox (Ed.), *The encyclopedia of aging* (2nd ed., pp. 254–256). New York: Springer Publishing Company.

Kane, R. L., Ouslander, J. G., & Abrass, I. B. (1989). *Essentials of clinical geriatrics* (2nd ed.). New York: McGraw Hill.

Kane, R. L., Ouslander, J. G., & Abrass, I. B. (2004). *Essentials of clinical geriatrics* (5th ed.). New York: McGraw Hill.

Karcher, K. A. (1993, March). Is your risk management program designed to deal with Alzheimer's disease? *Nursing Homes,* pp. 34–36.

Kart, C., Metress, E., & Metress, J. (1978). *Aging and health: Biological and social perspectives.* Menlo Park, CA: Addison Wesley.

Kaszniak, A. W. (1995). Parkinson's disease. In G. L. Maddox (Ed.), *The encyclopedia of aging* (2nd ed., pp. 727–729). New York: Springer Publishing Company.

Kay, B., & Neeley, J. (1982). Sexuality and aging: A review of current literature. *Sexuality and Disability, 5*(1), 38–46.

Kenney, R. (1982). *Physiology of aging: A synopsis.* Chicago: Year Book Medical.

Kennie, D. S., & Warshaw, G. (1989). Health maintenance and health screening in the elderly. In W. Reichel (Ed.), *Clinical aspects of aging* (3rd ed., p. 24). Baltimore: Williams & Wilkins.

Kerr, L. D. (2006). Arthritis. In R. Schulz (Ed.), *The encyclopedia of aging* (4th ed., pp. 80–81). New York: Springer Publishing Company.

Kippenbrock, T., & Soja, M. E. (1993). Preventing falls in the elderly: Interviewing patients who have fallen. *Geriatric Nursing, 14*(4), 205–209.

Kligman, A. (1979). Perspectives and problems in cutaneous gerontology. *Journal of Investigative Dermatology, 73*(1), 39–46.

Kline, D. (2006). Vision: system, function and loss. In R. Schulz (Ed.), *The encyclopedia of aging* (4th ed., pp. 1212–1214). New York: Springer Publishing Company.

Kurtz, S. (1982). Urinary tract infection in older persons. *Comprehensive Therapy, 8*(2), 54–58.

Landefeld, C. S., Palmer R. M., Johnson M. A., Johnston C. B., & Lyons W. L. (2004). *Current geriatric diagnosis & treatment.* New York. Lange Medical Books/McGraw-Hill.

Landfield, P. W. (1995). Stress theory of aging. In G. L. Maddox (Ed.), *The encyclopedia of aging* (2nd ed., pp. 903–905). New York: Springer Publishing Company.

Lashley, F.R. (2006a). AIDS/HIV. In R. Schulz (Ed.), *The encyclopedia of aging* (4th ed., pp. 48–51). New York: Springer Publishing Company.

Lashley, F.R. (2006b). Tuberculosis. In R. Schulz (Ed.), *The encyclopedia of aging* (4th ed., pp. 1196–1198). New York: Springer Publishing Company.

Leaf, A. (1973). Getting old. *Scientific American, 229*(3), 44–52.

Lee, M. (2006) Gastrointestinal functions and disorders. In R. Schulz (Ed.), *The encyclopedia of aging* (4th ed., pp. 430–432). New York: Springer Publishing Company.

Lehman, K. Administrator's role in prevention and care of decubitus ulcers. *Journal of Long Term Care Administration, 11*(2), 22.

Libow, L. (1981). *The core of geriatric medicine: A guide for students and practitioners.* St. Louis: Mosby.

Lindeman, R. D. (1989). Application of fluid and electrolyte balance principles to the older patient. In W. Reichel (Ed.), *Clinical aspects of aging* (3rd ed., p. 286). Baltimore: Williams & Wilkins.

Lindeman, R. D. (2006). Kidney and urinary system. In R. Schulz (Ed.), *The encyclopedia of aging* (4th ed., pp. 630–632). New York: Springer Publishing Company.

Lyon, L., & Nevins, M. (1984). Management of hip fracture in nursing home patients: To treat or not to treat? *Journal of the American Geriatrics Society, 32*(5), 391–395.

MacHudis, M. (1983). In W. Reichel (Ed.), *Clinical aspects of aging: A comprehensive text* (2nd ed.). Baltimore: Williams & Wilkins.

Maddox, G. L., & Sussman, S. W. (2001). *The encyclopedia of aging* (3rd ed.). New York: Springer Publishing Company.

Magee, R. (1993, April). Institutional policy use of restraints in extended care and nursing homes. *Journal of Gerontological Nursing,* pp. 31–39.

Malone-Lee, J. (1995). Genitourinary system. In G. L. Maddox (Ed.), *The encyclopedia of aging* (2nd ed., pp. 400–402). New York: Springer Publishing Company.

Malone-Lee, J. (2006). Urinary tract symptoms, assessment, and management. In R. Schulz (Ed.), *The encyclopedia of aging* (4th ed., pp. 1205–1207). New York: Springer Publishing Company.

McCaddon, A., & Kelly, C. L. (1994). Familial Alzheimer's disease and vitamin B12 deficiency. *Age and Aging, 23,* 334–337.

McNeil, S. A. (2006). Immunizations. In R. Schulz (Ed.), *The encyclopedia of aging* (4th ed., pp. 569–572). New York: Springer Publishing Company.

Massoud, E. (2006) Hearing. In R. Schulz (Ed.), *The encyclopedia of aging* (4th ed., pp. 508–512). New York: Springer Publishing Company.

Medvedev, Z. A. (1995). Wear-and-tear theories. In G. L. Maddox (Ed.), *The encyclopedia of aging* (2nd ed., pp. 964–965). New York: Springer Publishing Company.

Medvedev, Z. A. (2006). Wear-and-tear theories. Article title. In R. Schulz (Ed.), *The encyclopedia of aging* (4th ed., pp. 1224–1225). New York: Springer Publishing Company.

McNamara, C. (2006). Diabetes. In R. Schulz (Ed.), *The encyclopedia of aging* (4th ed., pp. 312–316). New York: Springer Publishing Company.

Meites, J., & Quadri, S. K. (1995). Neuroendocrine theory of aging. In G. L. Maddox (Ed.), *The encyclopedia of aging* (2nd ed., pp. 677–681). New York: Springer Publishing Company.

Menscer, D. (1993). Let the people go: Caring for the demented elderly without using restraints. *North Carolina Medical Journal, 54*(4), 145–150.

Miller, R. I. (1994). Managing disruptive responses to bathing by elderly residents. *Journal of Gerontological Nursing, 20*(11), 35–39.

Moore, J. R., & Gilbert, D. A. (1995). Elderly residents: Perceptions of nurses' comforting touch. *Journal of Gerontological Nursing, 21*(1), 6–13.

Moran, G. J., Krishnadasan, A., Gorwitz, R. J., Fosheim, G. E., McDougal, L. K., Carey, R. B., et al. (2006, August 17). *New England Journal of Medicine, 355,* 666–674.

Mosher-Ashley, P. E., & Henrikson, N. M. (1993, July-August). Long-term care alternatives for the mentally ill. *Nursing Homes,* pp. 34–36.

Moss, A. J. (1989). Diagnosis and management of heart disease in the elderly. In W. Reichel (Ed.), *Clinical aspects of aging* (3rd ed., p. 65). Baltimore: Williams & Wilkins.

Moss, R. J., & La Puma, J. (1991, January-February). The ethics of mechanical restraints. *Hastings Center Report,* pp. 22–24.

National Center for Health Services. (March, 1989). National Center for Health Services research and health care technology assessment. *Research activities.* Rockville, MD: Author, no. 115.

National Center for Health Services. (September, 1989). National Center for Health Services research and health care technology assessment. *Research activities.* Rockville, MD: Author, no. 121.

O'Brien, A.A.J., & Bulpitt, C. J. (1995). Hypertension in the elderly. In G. L. Maddox (Ed.), *The encyclopedia of aging* (2nd ed., pp. 489–491). New York: Springer Publishing Company.

Orentreich, D. S. (1995). Skin. In G. L. Maddox (Ed.), *The encyclopedia of aging* (2nd ed., pp. 860–861). New York: Springer Publishing Company.

Osgood, N. J. (1995). Leisure programs. In G. L. Maddox (Ed.), *The encyclopedia of aging* (2nd ed., pp. 546–548). New York: Springer Publishing Company.

Otero, R. B. (1993, May). Current approaches to infection control. *Nursing Homes,* pp. 48–49.

Ouslander, J. G., Schapira, Schnelle, Uman, Fingold, Tuico, & Nigam. (1995). Does eradicating bacteriuria affect the severity of chronic urinary incontinence in nursing home residents? *Annals of Internal Medicine, 122*(10), 749–754.

Paffenbarger, R. S., Wing, A. L., & Hsieh, C. (1986). Physical activity, all-cause mortality and longevity of college alumni. *New England Journal of Medicine, 314,* 605.

Pierce, R. I. (1995). Pulmonary system. In G. L. Maddox (Ed.), *The encyclopedia of aging* (2nd ed., pp. 783–786). New York: Springer Publishing Company.

Poe, W., & Holloway, D. (1980). *Drugs and the aged.* New York: McGraw Hill.

Rafuse, P. E., & Kelly, M.E.M. (2006). Eye: clinical issues. In R. Schulz (Ed.), *The encyclopedia of aging* (4th ed., pp. 405–410). New York: Springer Publishing Company.

Rantz, M. J., & McShane, R. E. (1995). Nursing interventions for chronically confused nursing home residents. *Geriatric Nursing, 16*(1), 22–27.

Ray, W. A. (1993). Reducing antipsychotic drug use in nursing homes. *Archives of Internal Medicine, 153,* 713–720.

Redford, J. B. (1989). Rehabilitation and the aged. In W. Reichel (Ed.), *Clinical aspects of aging* (3rd ed., pp. 177–186). Baltimore: Williams & Wilkins.

Reichel, W. (Ed.). (1983). *Clinical aspects of aging: A comprehensive text* (2nd ed.). Baltimore: Williams & Wilkins.

Reichel, W., & Rabins, E. V. (1989). Evaluation and management of the confused, disoriented or demented elderly patient. In W. Reichel (Ed.), *Clinical aspects of aging* (3rd ed., pp. 137–153). Baltimore: Williams & Wilkins.

Reisberg, B. (1995). Senile dementia. In G. L. Maddox (Ed.), *The encyclopedia of aging* (2nd ed., pp. 837–847). New York: Springer Publishing Company.

Rimer, B. K. (1995). Cancer control and aging. In G. L. Maddox (Ed.), *The encyclopedia of aging* (2nd ed., pp. 130–131). New York: Springer Publishing Company.

Ripich, D. N., Wykle, M., & Niles, S. (1995). Alzheimer's disease caregivers: The focused program. *Geriatric Nursing, 16*(1), 15–19.

Roberts, J., & Snyder, D. L. (1995). Drug interactions. In G. L. Maddox (Ed.), *The encyclopedia of aging* (2nd ed., pp. 289–291). New York: Springer Publishing Company.

Rogaeva, E. Y., & George-Hyslop, P. (2006). Alzheimer's disease: Genetic factors. In R. Schulz (Ed.), *The encyclopedia of aging* (4th ed., pp. 54–57). New York: Springer Publishing Company.

Rossman, I. (Ed.). (1979). *Clinical geriatrics* (2nd ed.). Philadelphia: Lippincott.

Rowe, J. (1982). Renal function and aging. In Reff and Schneider (Eds.), *Biological markers of aging* (pp. 661–664). Washington, DC: USDHHS, NIH, Public Health Service.

Rowe, J., & Besdine, R. (1982). *Health and disease in old age.* Boston: Little, Brown.

Scherer, Y. K. (1991). The nursing dilemma of restraints. *Journal of Gerontological Nursing, 17*(2), 14–17.

Schiffman, S. S. (2006). Taste and smell. In R. Schulz (Ed.), *The encyclopedia of aging* (4th ed., pp. 1168–1170). New York: Springer Publishing Company.

Schnelle, J. F., Ouslander, J. G., Simmons, A. (1993). The nighttime environment, incontinence care and sleep disruption in nursing homes. *Journal of the American Geriatrics Society, 41*(9), 910–914.

Scott, R. R., Bramble, K. J., & Goodyear, N. (1991). How knowledge and labeling of dementia affect nurses' expectations. *Journal of Gerontological Nursing, 17*(1), 21–24.

Selma, T. P., Palla, K., Padding, B., & Brauner, D. J. (1994). Effect of OBRA 1987 on antipsychotic prescribing in nursing home residents. *Journal of the American Geriatrics Society, 42,* 648–652.

Sengstaken, E. A., & King, S. A. (1993). The problems of pain and its detection among geriatric nursing home residents. *Journal of the American Geriatrics Society, 41,* 541–544.

Shashaty, G. G. (1989). Thromboembolism in the elderly. In W. Reichel (Ed.), *Clinical aspects of aging* (3rd ed., p. 101). Baltimore: Williams & Wilkins.

Sinclair, A. J. (1995). Diabetes mellitus. In G. L. Maddox (Ed.), *The encyclopedia of aging* (2nd ed., pp. 274–276). New York: Springer Publishing Company.

Sinex, F. M. (1977). The molecular genetics of aging. In C. Finch & L. Hayflick (Eds.), *Handbook of the biology of aging.* New York: Van Nostrand Reinhold.

Smith, P. W. (1989). Making infection control an art. *Provider, 15*(12), 7–9.

Starr, I. (1964). An essay on the strength of the heart. *American Journal of Cardiology, 14*(6), 771–783.

Sterritt, P. F., & Pokorny, M. E. (1994). Art activities for patients with Alzheimer's and related disorders. *Geriatric Nursing, 15*(3), 155–159.

Stillwell, E., & O'Conner, C. (1989). Sexuality, intimacy, and touch. In W. Reichel (Ed.), *Clinical aspects of aging* (2nd ed., p. 542). Baltimore: Williams & Wilkins.

Stevens, J. A. (2006). Injury. In R. Schulz (Ed.), *The encyclopedia of aging* (4th ed., p. 590). New York: Springer Publishing Company.

Strumpf, N. E., & Evans, L. K. (1995). Restraints: Physical–chemical. In G. L. Maddox (Ed.), *The encyclopedia of aging* (2nd ed., pp. 817–819). New York: Springer.

Sullivan, R. J. (1995). Cardiovascular system. In G. L. Maddox (Ed.), *The encyclopedia of aging* (2nd ed., pp. 133–138). New York: Springer Publishing Company.

Swanson, E. A., Maas, M. S., & Buckwalter, K. C. (1993). Catastrophic reactions and other behaviors of Alzheimer's residents: Special unit compared with traditional units. *Archives of Psychiatric Nursing, 7*(5), 292–299.

Technical Assistance Services. (1995, March, April). Washington, DC: National Citizens Coalition for Nursing Home Reform.

Teuth, M. J. (1995). How to manage depression and psychosis in Alzheimer's disease. *Geriatrics, 50*(1), 43–49.

Thompkins, C. A., & Scharp, V. L. (2006). Aphasia. In R. Schulz (Ed.), *The encyclopedia of aging* (4th ed., pp. 71–74). New York: Springer Publishing Company.

Thompkins, C. A., Scharp, V. L., & Meigh, K. M. (2006). Communication disorders. In R. Schulz (Ed.), *The encyclopedia of aging* (4th ed., pp. 234–239). New York: Springer Publishing Company.

Tideiksaar, R. (1995). Falls. In G. L. Maddox (Ed.), *The encyclopedia of aging* (2nd ed., pp. 359–361). New York: Springer Publishing Company.

Tindall, J., & Smith, J. (1963). Skin lesions of the aged. *Journal of the American Medical Association, 186,* 1037–1040.

Tonna, E. A. (1995a). Cartilage. In G. L. Maddox (Ed.), *The encyclopedia of aging* (2nd ed., pp. 146–147). New York: Springer Publishing Company.

Tonna, E. A. (1995b). Collagen. In G. L. Maddox (Ed.), *The encyclopedia of aging* (2nd ed., pp. 146–147). New York: Springer Publishing Company.

Tonna, E. A., updated by Evans, J. G. (1995c). Arthritis. In G. L. Maddox (Ed.), *The encyclopedia of aging* (2nd ed., pp. 79–80). New York: Springer Publishing Company.

Trella, R. (1994). From hospital to nursing home: Bridging the gaps in care. *Geriatric Nursing, 15*(6), 313–316.

USDHEW (1976), p. 13, Washington, D.C.

Vallarino & Sherman. (1981). Stroke, hip fractures, amputations, pressure sores, and incontinence. In L. Libow (Ed.), *The core of geriatric medicine: A guide for students and practitioners.* St. Louis: Mosby.

Van Vliet, L. (1995a). Aphasia. In G. L. Maddox (Ed.), *The encyclopedia of aging* (2nd ed., pp. 75–76). New York: Springer Publishing Company.

Van Vliet, L. (1995b). Communication disorders. In G. L. Maddox (Ed.), *The encyclopedia of aging* (2nd ed., pp. 198–200). New York: Springer Publishing Company.

Verrillo, R. T. (2006) Touch. In R. Schulz (Ed.), *The encyclopedia of aging* (4th ed., pp. 1191–1192). New York: Springer Publishing Company.

Waldo, M. J., Ide, B. A., & Thomas, D. P. (1995, February). Postcardiac-event elderly: Effect of exercise on cardiopulmonary function. *Journal of Gerontological Nursing,* pp. 12–19.

Wallace, M. (1992). Management of sexual relationships among elderly residents of long term care facilities. *Geriatric Nursing,* 308–322.

Watzke, J. R., & Wister, A. V. (1993). Staff attitudes: Monitoring technology in long term care. *Journal of Gerontological Nursing,* November, pp. 23–29.

Weindruch, R. (1995). Diet restriction. In G. L. Maddox (Ed.), *The encyclopedia of aging* (2nd ed., pp. 276–279). New York: Springer Publishing Company.

Weiner, D. K. (2006). Pain and pain management. In R. Schulz (Ed.), *The encyclopedia of aging* (4th ed., pp. 890–895). New York: Springer Publishing Company.

Werner, P., Cohen-Mansfield, Koroknay, & Braun. (1994). Reducing restraints: Impact on staff. *Journal of Gerontological Nursing,* 19–24.

White, H. K., & Sullivan, R. K., Jr. (2006). Cardiovascular system: Overview. In R. Schulz (Ed.), *The encyclopedia of aging* (4th ed., pp. 163–168). New York: Springer Publishing Company.

Zinn, J. S., & Mor, V. (1994). Nursing home special care units: Distribution by type, state, and facility characteristics. *Geriatrics,* 34(3), 371–376.

Index

ownership, 342–346
risk, 316–318, 322–323
stocks, 338–340
therapeutic actions of drugs, 519–520
Term insurance, 346
Theory X, 190, 191
Theory Y, 190–191
Theory Z, 191
Thioridazine (Mellaril), 514–515
Third-party payers, 267
Thomas, William, 136–137
3M (Minnesota Mining and
    Manufacturing), 97
Time period concept, 231
Toileting, 138
Toilet rooms, 474
Toilet stalls, 471, 480
Top-down budgeting, 297–298
Topical dressings, 589
Tort-feasor, 315
Torts, 314–315
Total quality management (TQM),
    83–84, 119
Total variable costs, 288–289
Tours, personal, 111
Toyota Motor Company, 334
TQM (total quality management),
    83–84, 119
Trade unions. See Unions
Training employees, 79, 148,
    180–186, 196
Tranquilizers, 514–515
Transactions, recording, 236–243
Transferring employees, 211–212
Transferring residents, 138
Transient ischemic attacks, 539
Transportation, influence on recruitment,
    158
Treasury stock, 340
Trend analysis, 12
Trial balance, 243
Triple net leases, 336
Tripping, 502
Tube feeding, 575, 578–579
Tuberculosis, 552–553
Turnover, employee, 181, 205
Turnover rate in percent ratio, 259
Tylenol, 515

Type A personalities, 195
Type B personalities, 195

Ulcers, 572–573
Unemployment compensation, 435
Unequal treatment, 419
*Uniform Guidelines on Employee Selection
    Procedures,* 164
Unions
    bargaining unit, 416
    dispute-settling rules, 415–416
    history, 410–412
    nurses in, 417–418
    in nursing homes, 416–418
    prohibited behavior, 412
    proportion of workers in, 411–412, 418
    rights of members, 414
    Taft-Hartley Act, 412–413
United States
    baby boomers, 361–362
    demographic trends, 360–366
    early management-labor relations,
        409–411
    early nursing home administration,
        356–357
    life expectancy, 360
    men/women ratio, 361
    population 65 years of age and older,
        360–361, 362
Unity of command, 66
Unqualified opinion, 326
Upholstered furniture, 447
Upper-level managers, 8, 50
Upward communication, 58
Urinals, 472
Urinary incontinence, 574, 605–607
Urinary tract infections, 607–609
Urologists, 511
Useful life, asset, 283
Users, in consumer decision making, 111

Validity of information, 166–167, 177
Value Line Investment Survey, 340
Values, 62
Variable costs, 287
Variance analysis, 303
VA (Veterans Administration), 264, 490
Veins, 535

SPRINGER / PUBLISHING COMPANY

Nursing Home Federal Requirements

Guidelines to Surveyors and Survey Protocols

James E. Allen, PhD, MSPH, CNHA

Larger Format! Accessible and user-friendly, this updated edition of **Nursing Home Federal Requirements** contains information that is essential for nursing home administrators as well as educators and professionals preparing for licensure. It presents the latest federal guidelines and the procedures used by federal surveyors in certifying facilities for participation in Medicare and Medicaid. It is the only text that provides a comprehensive index to nursing home federal requirements.

New to this edition:

- Updated Definitions of Medicare and Medicaid
- Compliance Requirements with Title VI of the Civil Rights Act of 1964
- Skilled Nursing Facility (SNF)/Hospice Requirements when SNF serves Hospice Patients
- SNF-Based Home Health Agencies
- Life Safety Code Requirements Effective March 10, 2006
- Definitions of Certified Beds, Dually-Participating and Distinct Parts
- Changes in SNF Provider Status
- Surveyor Qualifications Standards
- Management of Complaints and Incidents

October 2006 · 592 pp · 978-0-8261-0267-6 · softcover

11 West 42nd Street, New York, NY 10036-8002 • Fax: 212-941-7842
Order Toll-Free: 877-687-7476 • Order Online: www.springerpub.com

The Licensing Exam Review Guide in Nursing Home Administration

Fourth Edition

James E. Allen, PhD, MSPH, CNHA

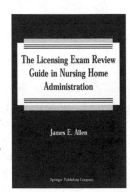

Praise for the previous edition:

"Serves as an excellent study guide for students or as a source of course examination questions for the instructor...The author has skillfully taken the format of the National Association of the Boards of Examiners of Nursing Home Administrators and utilized them as a basis for this text."
—**Journal of Health Administration Education**

This revised and updated study guide is based on the same format as the actual exam and provides an easy-to-use, effective way to review essential concepts and practice test-taking skills.

Serving as the key companion to **Nursing Home Administration, 5th Edition,** this updated guide reflects the latest changes in the domains of practice for nursing home administrators.

The Guide features:

• Over 800 test questions

Core Information on:

• Management, governance, leadership

• Finance

• Environment/federal requirements

• Over 1,000 key terms and concepts

• Nursing: resident/patient care

• Answer key

2002 · 192pp · 978-0-8261-5923-6 · softcover

11 West 42nd Street, New York, NY 10036-8002 • Fax: 212-941-7842
Order Toll-Free: 877-687-7476 • Order Online: www.springerpub.com